The Twenty-ninth Hahnemann Symposium

Drugs and Hematologic Reactions

The Twenty-ninth Hahnemann Symposium

Drugs and Hematologic Reactions

Editors

Nikolay V. Dimitrov, M.D.

Associate Professor, Department of Medicine, Division of Hematology and Medical Oncology, and Research Associate Professor, Department of Biological Chemistry, Hahnemann Medical College and Hospital, Philadelphia, Pennsylvania

John H. Nodine, M.D.

Associate Professor, Department of Medicine, Division of Clinical Pharmacology, Hahnemann Medical College and Hospital, Philadelphia, Pennsylvania

GRUNE & STRATTON
A Subsidiary of Harcourt Brace Jovanovich, Publishers
New York and London

Library of Congress Cataloging in Publication Data
Main entry under title:

Drugs and hematologic reactions.

Includes bibliographical references.

1. Hematopoietic agents—Congresses. 2. Drug interactions—Congresses. I. Dimitrov, Nikolay V., ed. II. Nodine, John H., ed. III. Hahnemann Medical College and Hospital of Philadelphia. [DNLM: 1. Hematologic diseases—Etiology—Congresses. 2. Hematopoietic system—Drug effects—Congresses. 3. Latrogenic disease—Congresses. WH140 D704 1973]
RM335.D78 615'.718 73-10366
ISBN 0-8089-0812-X

Grune & Stratton, Inc.
111 Fifth Avenue
New York, New York 10003

Library of Congress Catalog Card Number 73-10366
International Standard Book Number 0-8089-0812-X
Printed in the United States of America

Contents

Preface

Recent developments in the study of drug effects on the various elements of the hematopoietic system have produced many new concepts that have often been isolated in specialized publications or have not even been published. The authors of the various chapters of this book have been involved extensively in this new scientific frontier. Their chapters not only aim at organizing this new material into a unified scientific presentation, but they also attempt to evaluate the practical significance and to place the whole topic in proper scientific perspective.

While one cannot doubt that outstanding benefits have been accrued from the rapid development of new and highly effective drugs during the last two decades, even more benefits can be expected with more knowledge of often occult effects that may interfere with therapy and may even be life threatening. Dissemination of these new facts to medical students, practicing physicians, and research scientists allows for more judicious use of drugs and enables those in the profession to become more alert to potential problems so that these problems can be prevented or caught in an earlier stage and ultimately managed more effectively. In addition, dissemination provides a basis for further research in providing safer drugs, evaluating potential new hazards, and giving new approaches to management through soundly based research.

The hematopoietic system as well as the cellular elements are included separately with additional emphasis on coagulation mechanisms and basic biochemical changes. Wherever possible, the mechanisms are amplified to provide a comprehensive understanding of the whole process.

Finally, the particular therapeutic approaches are discussed and evaluated to give perspective to the overall management of these conditions. While the ultimate aim is practical application, the presentation is aimed at providing an understandable basis for the rational handling of patients. The material provides a comprehensive picture and is organized and indexed to also permit the use of the book as a reference in the detailed follow-up of special problems when they are encountered.

Nikolay V. Dimitrov, M.D.
John H. Nodine, M.D.

Contributors

NABIH I. ABDOU, M.D., PH.D., Assistant Professor of Medicine, Division of Allergy and Immunology, School of Medicine, University of Pennsylvania and Veterans Administration Hospital, Philadelphia, Pennsylvania.

YEON S. AHN, M.D., Assistant Professor of Medicine, University of Miami School of Medicine, Miami, Florida.

WILLIAM S. BECK, M.D., Associate Professor of Medicine, Harvard Medical School; Director of the Hematology Research Laboratory, Massachusetts General Hospital, Boston, Massachusetts.

BENJAMIN CALESNICK, M.D., Professor of Pharmacology and Clinical Professor of Medicine; Director, Division of Human Pharmacology, Hahnemann Medical College and Hospital, Philadelphia, Pennsylvania.

DALE H. COWAN, M.D., Department of Medicine, Case Western Reserve University School of Medicine at Cleveland Metropolitan General Hospital, Cleveland, Ohio.

NIKOLAY V. DIMITROV, M.D., Associate Professor of Medicine, Research Associate Professor of Biochemistry, Hahnemann Medical College and Hospital; Head, Section of Hematology and Medical Oncology, Hahnemann Medical Division, Philadelphia General Hospital, Philadelphia, Pennsylvania.

JØRGEN ELLEGAARD, M.D., PH.D., Research Fellow, Marselisborg Hospital, Aarhus, Denmark.

ALLAN J. ERSLEV, M.D., Cardeza Research Professor of Medicine; Director, Cardeza Foundation for Hematologic Research, Department of Medicine, Jefferson Medical College of Thomas Jefferson University, Philadelphia, Pennsylvania.

VIGGO ESMANN, M.D., Professor of Medicine, University of Aarhus, Aarhus, Denmark.

JAMES D. FAIX, B.S., Research Associate, Hahnemann Medical College and Hospital, Philadelphia, Pennsylvania.

THOMAS G. GABUZDA, M.D., Associate Professor of Medicine, Jefferson Medical College of Thomas Jefferson University; Chief, Department of Hematology, The Lankenau Hospital, Philadelphia, Pennsylvania.

FRANK H. GARDNER, M.D., Professor of Medicine; Director, Hematology Research Laboratory, Presbyterian-University of Pennsylvania Medical Center, Philadelphia, Pennsylvania.

R. L. GORDON, D.O., Fellow in Hematology and Medical Oncology, Hahnemann Medical College and Hospital, Philadelphia, Pennsylvania.

ROBERT G. GRAW, Jr., M.D., Senior Investigator, Hematology and Supportive Care Branch, National Cancer Institute, Bethesda, Maryland.

EDWARD S. HENDERSON, M.D., Chief, Medicine A, Roswell Park Memorial Institute, Buffalo, New York.

JOHN D. HINES, M.D., Associate Professor of Medicine, Department of Medicine, Case Western Reserve University School of Medicine at Cleveland Metropolitan General Hospital, Cleveland, Ohio.

PAUL HOLLISTER, M.D., Assistant Professor, Department of Medicine, Michigan State University, East Lansing, Michigan.

S. B. KAHN, M.D., Associate Professor of Medicine; Co-Director, Clinical Cancer Training Program, Hahnemann Medical College and Hospital, Philadelphia, Pennsylvania.

ROBERT W. KELLERMEYER, M.D., Associate Professor of Medicine and Pharmacology, University Hospitals of Cleveland, Case Western Reserve University, Cleveland, Ohio.

GERALD W. KING, M.D., Postdoctoral Fellow, Division of Hematology and Oncology, Ohio State University Hospital, Columbus, Ohio.

JAN KOCH-WESER, M.D., Associate Professor of Pharmacology, Harvard Medical School; Associate Physician and Chief of Clinical Pharmacology Unit, Massachusetts General Hospital, Boston, Massachusetts.

JACK LEVIN, M.D., Associate Professor of Medicine, The Johns Hopkins University School of Medicine and Hospital, Baltimore, Maryland. (Dr. Levin is a John and Mary R. Markle Scholar in Academic Medicine and recipient of a Research Career Development Award from the National Heart and Lung Institute, National Institutes of Health, Bethesda, Maryland.)

JAMES W. LINMAN, M.D., Professor of Medicine; Director, Osgood Leukemia Center, University of Oregon Medical School, Portland, Oregon.

ALBERT F. LoBUGLIO, M.D., Associate Professor of Medicine, Division of Hematology and Oncology, Ohio State University Hospital, Columbus, Ohio.

SCOTT MURPHY, M.D., Assistant Professor of Medicine, University of Pennsylvania Medical School; Associate Director, Hematology Research Laboratory, Presbyterian-University of Pennsylvania Medical Center, Philadelphia, Pennsylvania.

ANTHONY V. PISCIOTTA, M.D., Professor of Medicine, The Medical College of Wisconsin; The Milwaukee County General Hospital, Milwaukee, Wisconsin.

PETER QUESENBERRY, M.D., Department of Medicine, St. Elizabeth's Hospital and Tufts Medical School, Boston, Massachusetts. (Dr. Quesenberry is a Scholar of the Leukemia Society of America.)

PERRY A. SCHEINOK, PH.D., Professor; Director, Division of Biometrics and Computing, Department of Physiology and Biophysics, Hahnemann Medical College and Hospital, Philadelphia, Pennsylvania.

SANDOR S. SHAPIRO, M.D., Professor of Medicine, Department of Medicine, Cardeza Foundation for Hematologic Research, Jefferson Medical College of Thomas Jefferson University, Philadelphia, Pennsylvania.

WILLIAM C. SHERWOOD, M.D., Associate Professor of Medicine, Jefferson Medical College of Thomas Jefferson University; Medical Director, Penn Jersey Regional Red Cross Blood Program, Philadelphia, Pennsylvania.

FREDERICK STOHLMAN, JR., M.D., Department of Medicine, St. Elizabeth's Hospital and Tufts Medical School, Boston, Massachusetts.

LEIF G. SUHRLAND, M.D., Professor, Department of Medicine, Michigan State University, East Lansing, Michigan.

SCOTT N. SWISHER, M.D., Chairman, Department of Medicine, Michigan State University, East Lansing, Michigan.

ARTHUR A. TROWBRIDGE, M.D., Fellow in Hematology, University of Oregon Medical School, Portland, Oregon.

HARVEY J. WEISS, M.D., Associate Professor of Medicine, Columbia University College of Physicians and Surgeons; Director, Division of Hematology, The Roosevelt Hospital, New York, New York.

HAROLD A. WURZAL, M.D., Associate Professor of Pathology and Medicine, University of Pennsylvania; Director of Blood Bank, Hospital of the University of Pennsylvania, Philadelphia, Pennsylvania.

ADEL A. YUNIS, M.D. Professor of Medicine and Biochemistry; Director, Division of Hematology and The Howard Hughes Laboratories for Hematological Research, University of Miami School of Medicine and The Howard Hughes Medical Institute, Miami, Florida.

PART I

Mechanisms Involved in Drug Effects on the Hematopoietic System

Benjamin Calesnick
and Perry A. Scheinok

1
Adverse Drug Reactions and Drug Interactions

There are two sensitive areas in drug therapy which have become increasingly important to practicing physicians.[1] First, with few exceptions, drugs do not have a single effect on a single target cell, tissue, or organ. Hence, when a patient receives a drug one must anticipate that its total potential pharmacodynamics may be expressed.[2] This means that in addition to its therapeutic response, its toxic effects must be considered because, under appropriate circumstances, all known drugs are toxic. As a matter of fact, one might postulate that a nontoxic chemical is highly unlikely to be of interest as a drug. Hence, dosages have to be tailored carefully so that most patients may obtain the maximum therapeutic response and minimum toxic effects. This has become the principal function of the clinical or human pharmacologist.

Second, multiple drug ingestions or administrations have become a major factor for adverse drug reactions. This is the result, in some instances, when physicians and the general public use drugs indiscriminately and unwisely. The resulting drug interactions occur when the effects of one drug are modified by prior or concurrent administration of another drug or drugs. During the past several years there has been an awareness of this problem, especially when one drug alters the expected therapeutic response of another.

For convenience, we have classified drug-induced toxic effects as adverse effects due to primary pharmocologic attributes, untoward or side effects produced by secondary attributes, and iatrogenic or chemically induced diseases.

ADVERSE EFFECTS DUE TO PRIMARY PHARMACOLOGIC ATTRIBUTES

These are the most predictable toxic reactions, and therefore a thorough preclinical pharmacologic study should elicit such possible toxic effects and carefully assess the chance that they will be important clinically. Various types follow.

Misdosage (Dose-related)

DELIBERATE MISUSES

Deliberate misuses—criminal, suicidal, or other illicit uses—result in a variety of reactions:

Acute intoxication. This is caused by overdoses of: (a) CNS depressants, the symptoms of which include depressed respiration, coma, hyperpyrexia and miosis (opiates); (b) CNS stimulants, producing agitation, auditory and visual hallucinations, tachycardia, convulsion, and mydriasis; and (c) anticholinergics, producing agitation, auditory and visual hallucinations, tachycardia, convulsions, mydriasis, hyperpyrexia, and beet-red skin.

Withdrawal symptoms (acute abstinence syndrome). These occur with the CNS depressants—alcohol, sedatives, tranquilizers, and opiates. They are classified in the table.

Stage	Alcohol, Sedatives and Tranquilizers	Opiates
First	Agitation, tachycardia, elevated BP, sweating, anorexia, and insomnia	Yawning, lacrimation, rhinorrhea, and sweating
Second	Hallucinations and amnesia	Gooseflesh, mydriasis, anorexia, tremors, and low back pain
Third	Delusions, disorientations, delirium, and amnesia	Insomnia, restlessness, air-hunger, elevated BP, hyperglycemia and hyperpyrexia
Fourth	Convulsions	Emesis, diarrhea, and weight loss

Withdrawal symptoms are also observed with the CNS stimulants, i.e., amphetamines, (excessive doses of which cause severe depression and suicidal tendencies).

Flashbacking. LSD is the usual cause.

MEDICATION ERROR

Medication errors are generally due to accidental misdoses.

TITRATION

An undesirable effect may develop while the proper dosage of the medication is being established in an individual patient, i.e., diarrhea during the treatment of acute gouty arthritis with colchicine.

Pharmacologic (Dose-related)

UNDESIRED EXPECTED EFFECTS

These are true side effects, i.e., sinus tachycardia observed when epinephrine is administered as a bronchodilator or the sedative effects of antihistamines in the treatment of allergies.

DESIRED EXCESSIVE EFFECTS

Desired excessive effects are the exaggerated desired pharmacologic effects of a drug when it is administered in doses within the approximate therapeutic range, i.e., hypolycemic reaction to insulin.

UNDESIRED UNEXPECTED EFFECTS

These effects are an expression of the basic pharmacologic action of a drug when it is administered in doses within the approximate therapeutic range, i.e., dehydration and electrolyte imbalance with diuretics.

Nonpharmacologic (Not Dose-related)

DRUG ALLERGY

This is a reaction that has an immunologic basis. Prior sensitization is required with the same or closely related chemical structure and an antigen-antibody interaction results. This effect is independent of the normal action of the drug and may result in dermatitis, urticaria, conjunctivitis, gastrointestinal disturbances, or fatal anaphylactic shock. This reaction is not dose-related and is characterized by the presence of circulating humoral or tissue antibodies. An example is the high incidence of penicillin allergy.

IDIOSYNCRACY

An abnormal reaction to a drug, qualitatively different from the effect usually obtained in a majority of the population. Prior sensitization is not required, as in drug allergy, and may be explained by a biochemical abnormality in an individual with a genetic defect. One example is the nonthrombocytopenic purpura which develops in a small percentage of individuals receiving quinine. Another is the photosensitivity induced by the phenothiazines, sulfonamides, griseofulvin, and tetracyclines.

PHARMACOGENETICS

Pharmacogenetics is the term applied to reactions due to hereditary factors which influence biotransformation and drug response and may help explain hypersensitivity, drug allergy, or idiosyncrasy.[3,4]

MUTAGENESIS

Mutagenesis is a cellular process in which there is a molecular alteration of chromosomes. The efficacy of the mutagen is obviously dependent on its gaining entrance into the cells, whether they be somatic or germ cells. The problem of somatic mutagens is clinically important in the production of defects in the developing embryo or fetus and is called teratogenesis. It is not always possible to establish a clearcut relationship between embryotoxic and embryopathic mutagenesis. Everyone now knows that thalidomide caused some of the pregnant women who received it to give birth to grossly deformed infants. The effect produced by teratogenic agents is determined by dosage and the developmental stage of the embryo at the time of treatment. (a) The amount of drug must be appropriate. All agents can be administered in such small quantities as to cause no effect. On the other hand, excessive amounts of the drug may overwhelm the embryo and produce death (embryotoxic). The so-called "teratogenic zone" is somewhere between the ineffective and lethal level. (b) The embryo becomes quite susceptible to teratogenesis as soon as cellular differentiation appears; this is called the critical period. (c) Developmental deviation decreases when embryonic processes are nearly complete, with the result that larger doses are needed to produce the effect. If dosage is increased, the severity precludes survival. Germ cell mutagens, which includes x-ray and halogenated pyrimidines, produce changes in sex chromosomes and may create problems in hereditary disease.

CARCINOGENICITY

Many chemical substances are capable of producing malignant tumors in man. Some of these carcinogenic substances are particularly dangerous, if they are taken even in small doses over a long period of time. Modern pharmacology is producing more and more compounds (e.g., hormonal preparations and psychotropic drugs) taken in just this way. Special care has to be exercised if the drug has a chemical structure related to that of a known carcinogen.

DRUG DEPENDENCY

Drugs that affect the central nervous system may cause dependence. Thus, a stimulant of the central nervous system may produce euphoria, a condition that predisposes to abuse of the drug. A drug that causes hallucination or any other disorders of perception are also potentially dangerous. Another example is the wide use of cathartics by individuals who depend on them for daily bowel movements.

UNTOWARD EFFECTS OR SIDE EFFECTS PRODUCED BY SECONDARY ATTRIBUTES

Drug-induced toxic effects can also be produced by the secondary attributes of a drug, as for example the yellow discoloration associated with the administration of quinacrine (Atabrine).

IATROGENIC OR CHEMICALLY INDUCED DISEASES

These diseases may develop during the acute or chronic administration of a drug. The effect may be species-specific in that it was not discernible in preclinical studies and appeared only after man received the agent. It may affect any cell, tissue, or organ of the body.

Chemically Induced Diseases

The chemically induced diseases are hepatic disease,[5–7] renal diseases,[8,9] blood dyscrasias,[10–14] and porphyria.[15]

HEPATIC

The chemically induced hepatic diseases are (a) the hepatocullular diseases induced by carbon tetrachloride and by ethanol; (b) acute cholangiolitis associated with the sex steroids; (c) allergic cholangiolitis, caused by the phenothiazines; and (d) steatosis, associated with the tetracyclines.

RENAL

Chemically induced renal diseases may be a direct, indirect, allergic, chronic, or predisposing effect of the toxic agent. A direct effect is the acute toxic necrosis associated with heavy metals, carbon tetrachloride, trimethadione (Tridione) and paramethadione (Paradione), the aminoglycoside antimicrobial agents (streptomycin, neomycin, kanamycin, and gentamycin).

Acute renal ischemia is caused by the antihypertensive drugs that reduce circulatory perfusion pressure, such as large doses of the pressor agents used in the treatment of shock.

A nephrotic syndrome or angiitis is one manifestation of an allergic response to the sulfonamides, bee venom, or poison ivy.

Toxic manifestations classified as chronic are those observed after prolonged exposure, such as lead nephropathy.

Predisposing effects are the aggravation of a preexisting renal lesion, for example: potassium deficiency is a predisposing effect in pyelonephritis.

BLOOD DYSCRASIAS

These are manifest as anemia, agranulocytosis, or thrombocytopenia.

Anemia may be due to (a) impaired red cell production, i.e.—aplastic anemia—such as that produced by chloramphenicol, chloroquine (Aralen), gold, sulfonamides, and phenylbutazone; (b) deficiencies of iron (acetyl salicylic acid and adrenal steroids), folate (diphenylhydantoin, oral contraceptives, pyrimethamine (Daraprim), or pyridoxine (isoniazid); or (c) accelerated red blood cell destruction—hemolytic anemia—i.e., enzyme deficiencies such as G–6–PD (primaquine, Neo-quipenyl), nitrofurantoin, (Furadantin), acetanilid; unstable hemoglobin—Hb Zurich—(sulfonamides ?); or immune mechanisms of the penicillin type, Stibophen type (Fuadin), or α-methyldopa (Aldomet) type.

Agranulocytosis is the most common blood dyscrasia, induced either through immunologic (aminopyrine, sulfonamides) or nonimmunologic mechanisms (phenothiazines).

Thrombocytopenia may be induced through immunologic mechanisms (quinidine, chlorothiazide, acetazolamide, phenylbutazone), or platelet toxicity (ristocetin Spontin).

PORPHYRIA

Drugs inducing porphyria are griseofulvin (Fulvicin, Grifulvin) and benzene hexachloride (Kwell).[15]

DRUG INTERACTIONS

Thus far we have been discussing the toxicity of single drugs. Recently, interest has been renewed in adverse reactions that may occur when patients take two or more drugs during a given period of time.[16] Actually, one of the earliest reports of this type appeared in 1951,[17] clearly demonstrating that the concurrent administration of quinidine, meperidine, and procaine resulted in synergistic cardiotoxicity.

Drug interactions present a complex problem and may result in changes of absorption, distribution, biotransformation, and/or excretion of drug(s) by other drug(s), due to the following possible mechanisms:

1. Antagonism, chemical and physical
2. Protein binding during transport of drugs
3. Drug metabolism
4. Antagonism at receptors
5. Changes in renal clearance of drugs

We would like to review briefly some important factors that might be altered in the aforementioned mechanisms.

Antagonism

In general, there is a firm relationship between the degree of absorption, lipoid solubility, and ionization constant (pKa) of a drug in that the drug must be un-ionized and lipoid soluble.[18] Most weekly acidic drugs, such as aspirin, are well absorbed from the stomach, whereas weakly basic drugs, such as dextromethorphan, are absorbed from the small intestine. Anything that slows the emptying rate of the stomach, such as anxiety, fatty meal, drugs such as codeine, or increased peristalsis (cathartics) can delay the onset of weak basic drugs. If the drug is acid-unstable, then it might decompose extensively, if it remains in the stomach too long. Tetracyclines form insoluble complexes with aluminum and calcium salts, which is the reason these antibiotics must not be taken with aluminum antacids or milk. Mucin in the gastrointestinal tract has been shown to bind and prevent the absorption of streptomycin. Many oral antibiotics, especially the aminoglycosides and tetracyclines, will suppress vitamin K_1 production and decrease the intestinal absorption of glucose, iron, vitamin B_{12}, and penicillin G.

Protein Binding

A drug which has a greater affinity for protein binding sites will displace another drug from plasma or tissue binding.[19] For example, the displacement of warfarin from serum protein by chloral hydrate, ethacrynic acid (Edecrin), nalidixic acid (NegGram), indomethacin (Indocin), phenylbutazone (Butazolidin), and bishydroxycoumarin by clofibrate (Atromid-S) makes increased amounts of anticoagulant available and bleeding may result. Probenecid (Benemid), phenylbutazone, and acetylsalicylic acid displace penicillins and sulfonamides from serum carrier sites and thus increased antibiotic activity is produced. Finally, methotrexate (Amethopterin) is displaced by sulfadimethoxine (Madribon) and sulfamethoxypyridazine (Kynex, Midicel), thereby enhancing the toxicity of methotrexate.

Drug Metabolism

Many drugs can stimulate certain mechanisms involved in the metabolism of drugs.[20–23] For example: coumarins are metabolized more rapidly in the presence of barbiturates, glutethimide (Doriden), ethchlorovynol (Placidyl), griseofulvin, and DDT and therefore inhibit the action of coumarin. Drugs like methylphenidate (Ritalin), disulfiram (Antabuse), chloramphenical, and phenyramidol (Analexin) inhibit the metabolism of these anticoagulants, so increasing response and bleeding may result.[24] Vitamin K or estrogens can stimulate the syntheses of clotting factor. Continuous administration of certain other drugs may stimulate their own metabolism, for example: phenylbutazone, tolbutamide (Orinase), probenecid, diphenhydramine (Benadryl), and chlorcyclizine (Di-Paralene).

Drug Interaction at the Receptor Sites

A basic concept of drug action is that the pharmacologic action of a compound is ultimately due to the drug exerting its effect on a specific site in the cell or organism which we call the receptor site. Drug interactions can occur when two or more drugs occupy the same receptor, and the net result depends on the characteristics of each drug; if each produces the same effect, then their combined effect will usually be equal to or greater than the sum of their individual effects. This is called summation or an additive effect. On the other hand, if only one drug produces an effect, then the combined effect can either be less than the effect of the active drug or no effect may be produced. This is called antagonism.

Examples of *summation* or *additive* effects are given in Table 1.

Table 1
Types of Drug Interaction

Drug +	Drug =	Interaction
Tubocurarine (Succinylcholine)	Aminoglycosides (neomycin, kanamycin, streptomycin, gentamicin) Polymyxins (polymyxin B, colistin) Bacitracin	Myasthenia, apnea
Methoxyflurane (Penthrane)	Tetracyclines	Nephrotoxicity
Aminoglycosides	Ethacrynic acid (Edecrin)	Ototoxicity
Cephaloridine	Ethacrynic acid (Edecrin) furosemide (Lasix)	Nephrotoxicity

Examples of *antagonism* are illustrated in Table 2.

Table 2
Examples of Drug Antagonism

Agonist	Antagonist
Acetylcholine	Atropine
Succinylcholine	Gallamine (Flaxedil)
Guanethidine (Ismelin)	Amphetamine or tricyclic antidepressant(s)
Isoproterenol	Propranolol (Inderal)

Patients who are taking monamine oxidase inhibitors, such as Parnate, Niamid, Nardil, or Eutonyl may develop a severe hypertensive crisis when they also take sympathomimetic amines such as ephedrine, phenylephrine, phenylpropanolamine (found in various "cold" preparations), or amphetamines; if they ingest certain foods having a high tyramine content, like aged cheese, beer, wine, bananas, broad beans, or pickled herring.

Renal Clearance

Most drugs are excreted by the kidney either as free drug or as water-soluble metabolites. If the drug is an ionizable substance, then tubular reabsorption can be influenced by the pH of tubular fluids, as is the situation in the mechanism of absorption found in the gastrointestinal tract. Therefore, urinary pH can influence the rate of renal clearance. If a drug is in its un-ionized form, it will be more readily reabsorbed into the blood. As a matter of fact, it has been observed that the effects of a single dose of amphetamine can last for several days if urinary pH is made sufficiently alkaline by the concurrent administration of sodium bicarbonate or by placing the patient on a vegetable diet. Acid drugs, such as salicylic acid, sulfonamides, and phenobarbital are excreted much faster when urinary pH is alkaline. Therefore, the concurrent administration of drugs that increase pH, such as sodium bicarbonate and carbonic anhydrase inhibitors (Diamox, Cardrase), with the above drugs cause a rapid clearance of acid drugs. On the other hand, basic drugs, such as the antihistamines, meperidine (Demerol), and imipramine (Tofranil), are excreted faster when urinary pH is made acidic by the administration of ammonium chloride or glutamic acid.

Other drugs, such as penicillin, probenecid (Benemid), the salicylates, ethacrynic acid (Edecrin), the thiazide diuretics (Diuril, Hydrodiuril, Esidrix), and indomethacin (Indocin) are excreted by a special biochemical system in the kidney. When these drugs are taken concurrently they can interfere with the excretion of the other. For example: probenecid and the salicylates can inhibit the excretion of indomethacin. Probenecid can delay the excretion of penicillin and enhance blood levels of the antibiotics. Phenylbutazone, by interfering with excretion of hydrohexamide, the active metabolite of acetohexamide (Dymelor), can produce exaggerated hypoglycemic effects.

Certain antibiotics are more active in an alkaline urine (Nitrofurantoin, Nalidixic, Erythromycin, and aminoglycosides); whereas, others are active in an acid urine (Methenamine mandelate and Trimethoprin or Syraprim).[25]

FREQUENCY OF DRUG INTERACTIONS

We are sure at this point in our discussion that many of you might be asking yourselves: "How frequently can I anticipate such problems in treating patients with drugs?" It has been predicated, in one study, that drug interactions could have developed in over 8% of the patients treated.[26] It has also been projected that polypharmacy today may result in a geometric progression of drug interactions which can be expressed mathematically as 2^n, where n is the number of drugs administered concomitantly.[27] Thus, if a patient is taking six different drugs then 2^6 or 64 different drug interactions are possible.

In an extensive and sophisticated exercise in statistics involving the principle of "combinations and permutations," we have come up with a most interesting conclusion (see appendix to this chapter for details of calculations).[28] If we assume that every drug administered to a patient is active and the order in which each drug is given is important, then the maximum total number of possible drug interactions and drug toxicities are those summarized in Table 3. As can be seen from this table, if we assume that the average hospitalized patient receives eight different chemical entities during a 24-hour period, then there is a theoretic possibility that over 100,000 different drug-induced toxicities or drug interactions are possible. Furthermore, speaking as a mathematician rather than a pharmacologist, the maximum number of individuals required to demonstrate each type of drug interaction is summarized in Table 4. Again, in the average hospitalized patient, it would require almost 400,000 different individuals to demonstrate all of the different drug-induced toxicities or drug interactions that are possible. You may say that this is a far cry from the realities observed in clinical practice. Yet, these figures do tend to illustrate the extreme importance of bearing in mind the theoretic possibilities of the incidences of these problems.

Table 3
Total Number of Possible Drug Interactions and Drug Toxicities

Number of Drugs	Number of Drug Interactions	Number of Drug Induced Toxicities
2	2	4
3	12	15
4	60	64
5	320	325
6	1,950	1,956
7	13,692	13,699
8	109,592	109,600
9	986,400	986,409
10	9,864,090	9,864,100

Table 4
Number of Possible Patient Complexes Due to Different Interactions

Number of Drugs	Number of Patient Complexes
1	0
2	2
3	12
4	72
5	500
6	4,050
7	37,632
8	394,352
9	4,596,552
10	60,755,472

Since many of the drug-induced toxicities and drug interactions discussed have been produced under experimental conditions, you may question the clinical significance of these findings. You may well be justified in asking: "Are these facts or fantasy?" Let us point out that prescribing drugs is a serious matter. Only when the physician knows which toxicities may result from the prescription of certain drugs and the incidence of such toxicities can he properly estimate the risks involved in prescribing a given drug for a particular patient. In establishing a diagnosis, certain eventualities have to be considered. This includes the natural history of the disease and the pharmacology of the drug to be used.

SUMMARY

Two important problems are associated with the clinical use of drugs: (a) their toxic effects and (b) interactions. Since all drugs are toxic under appropriate conditions, a working knowledge of possible toxic effects that may occur is necessary. These effects may be due to overdosage, acute abstinence syndrome, flashbacking, undesired and unexpected effects. On the other hand, non-dose-related phenomena may develop, such as allergy, idiosyncrasy, mutagenesis, carcinogenesis, or drug dependency.

A new area of discussion involves iatrogenic or chemically induced diseases which may be produced by the acute or chronic administration of drugs on blood forming elements, kidneys, or liver.

With the resurgence of polypharmacy, there is a tremendous interest in drug interactions. The interaction between two or more drugs may effect changes in the chemical or physical properties of one or more drugs, interfere with protein binding, drug metabolism, receptor reactivity, or changes in renal clearances.

In a detailed statistical study of the theoretic possibilities of drug-induced toxicities and drug interactions, it is postulated that if the average hospitalized patient receives eight different chemical entities during a 24-hour period, then there is a theoretic possibility that over 100,000 different drug-induced toxicities or drug interactions may occur. Furthermore, the maximum number of individuals required to demonstrate each possible type of drug interaction amounts to over 400,000.

APPENDIX

Possible Number of Interactions

Let us suppose that the patient receives n number of drugs, each one being a single compound. The question we wish to answer is what is the possible number of interactions? It is assumed that: (a) *no* drug is inactive, and (b) drug A interacting with drug B is different from drug B interacting with drug A.

For example: nalorphine (Nalline) behaves as a narcotic antagonist only if a strong narcotic has been previously administered; otherwise, it acts in many respects as a narcotic itself. If administered intravenously in full therapeutic doses without prior administration of a narcotic, nalorphine or levallorphan (Lorfan) produce marked respiratory depression in man. In mild respiratory depression produced by small doses of narcotics, nalorphine or levallorphan may not only have negligible antagonist effects but may also increase the narcotic-induced depression. Similarly, these drugs may augment respiratory depression due to non-narcotic drugs or causes.

Another example is the interaction between phenobarbital and the anticoagulants bishydroxycoumarin (Dicumarol) or warfarin (Coumadin, Panwarfin). If the patient is initially stabilized on a fixed daily dose of one of these anticoagulants, then the addition of phenobarbital may increase the metabolism of the anticoagulant and thereby reduce anticoagulant effectiveness with a risk of possible thrombus formation. On the other hand, if the patient has been stabilized with one of these anticoagulants in the presence of phenobarbital, the discontinuation of phenobarbital will result in a decrease in enzyme-stimulating effect. The anticoagulant will not be metabolized as fast and hemorrhage may result.

Actually, we note that there are two concepts involved. First, there is the actual overall number of separate interactions and secondly, there is the way they can be combined within a particular patient, which we shall call a patient-complex. Thus, if every patient had a unique combination of interactions when he is given n drugs, how many different patients do we need to exhaust all possibilities.

To answer the first question, we note that there are $n(n-1)(n-2)\ldots(n-k+1)=(n)_k$ different ways we can form ordered sets of sizes k from a set of size n. Here $(n)_n=(n)_{n-1}=n!$ (n factorial). Thus, under the assumption that order makes a difference (assumption 2), we have:

$$n!+n!+(n)_{n-2}+(n)_{n-3}+\ldots+(n)_2=\sum_{k=2}^{n}(n)_k=P_n$$

Unfortunately, there is no mathematical expression in closed form for this relationship. We can do the following, however. If one denotes by P'_n the sum of the total number of possible permutations

$$P'_n = \sum_{k=0}^{n} (n)_k = P_n + n + 1$$

it is easily seen that $P'_n = nP'_{n-1} + 1$, $(P'_0 = 1)$. In addition, since

$$P'_n = P_n + n + 1$$

one gets the recurrence relationship

$$P_n = nP_{n-1} + n(n-1), \ (P_0 = P_1 = 0).$$

If one defines the generating function for the terms P'_n to be

$$P'(s) = \sum_{k=0}^{\infty} P'_k \, s^k/k!$$

so that

$$P'_k = \sum_{j=0}^{k} (n)_j$$

is the coefficient of $s^k/k!$, then it is well known that $P'(s) = e^s/(1-s)$ (where e is the base of natural logs)[1]. The coefficients P_n of interest are $P_n = P'_n - n - 1$, and thus the generating function for

$$P(s) = \sum_{k=2}^{\infty} \frac{P_k s^k}{k!} = \frac{s^2 e^s}{1-s}$$

In Table 3, we see the values for P_n, $n = 1, \ldots, 10$.

For the second concept, we define the following notation:

By:

$$(n_1, n_2, n - n_1, n - n_2), \qquad n_1, n_2, n - n_1, n - n_2 > 0$$

we denote a partition of n drugs within a patient such that n_1 drugs interact separately, n_2 drugs interact separately, and $n - n_1 - n_2$ drugs interact separately.

Thus, suppose we give a patient four drugs. Then one can have the following combinations of interactions: (4), (3, 1), (2, 2), (2, 1, 1), (1, 1, 1, 1). In other words, if one denotes the drugs by A, B, C, and D, then the partition (3, 1) represents all of the interactions one can get from three drugs interacting separately and one drug acting alone. Some of these permutations would be (ABC)(D), (ACB)(D), (BAC)(D), (BCA)(D), (CAB)(D), and (CBA)(D). It is clear that there are 24 such possibilities, where the remaining 18 have A, B, and C acting separately in turn. Overall, since we take the attitude that we need at least two drugs for an interaction, we will ignore the situation (1, 1, 1, 1). In order to simplify matters we shall use the following notation. By [ABC][DE] (square brackets), we denote all permutations of the partition (3, 2) of five drugs, or equivalently *all* permutations of three drugs interacting separately and two drugs interacting separately. On the other hand, by (ACB)(DE) (round brackets) we denote a specific permutation within the partition. Since we always write partitions with the greater numbers preceding the smaller, (3, 2) is the same partition as (2, 3). When partition sizes are unequal, we have no difficulty in counting the number of different permutations. We use the fact that if one starts with a set of n elements, and wishes to make up m subsets of sizes $k_1, k_2, \ldots k_m$, such that $k_1 + k_2 + \ldots + k_m = n$, then this can be done in

$$\frac{m!}{k_1!\, k_2! \ldots k_m!}$$

ways. In addition, since we know that each subset of size k_j, $j = 1, \ldots, m$ can be permuted in $k_j!$ ways, we note that by the product rule we obtain

$$\frac{n!}{k_1!\, k_2! \ldots k_m!}\, k_1!\, k_2! \ldots k_m! = n!$$

different permutations.

However, when some of the partitions are of the same size, we need to modify $n!$ by a numerical factor. We see this as easiest for the case of four drugs. Note that for our purpose the permutation (AB)(CD) is identical to (CD)(AB). For, if it were different, we would be arguing that somehow giving drugs (AB) and (CD) leads to a different set of interactions than giving (CD) and then (AB). But this would really imply that we were dealing with a permutation of [ABCD], and not [AB][CD], and thus we are concerned with only half the expected total (4!), so that the partition (2, 2) has (½)4! different permutations. In this case, they can be written as:

(AB)(CD); (BA)(CD); (AB)(DC); (BA)(DC)
(AC)(BD); (CA)(BD); (AC)(DB); (CA)(DB)
(AD)(BC); (DA)(BC); (AD)(CB); (DA)(CB)

for a total of 12 = (¼)4!

In Table 5 are listed all possible partitions for $n = 1, 2, \ldots, 10$, and Table 4 lists the number of different patient complexes due to different drug interactions for $n = 1, \ldots, 10$, the latter being the total number of effectively different permutations we can have within a partition. How totals were computed for $n = 6$ is illustrated in Table 6.

If one were interested in just the total number of partitions x_n for each number n (and not the permutations), there is again no closed formula for this quantity. As before, however, there is a way of getting x_n by using generating functions.

The result in this area is as follows.[1] Let x'_n be the number of unrestricted partitions of n, ($x'_0 = 1$), and define

$$X'(t) = \sum_{\nu=0}^{\infty} x'_\nu\, t^\nu$$

to be its generating function. Note that $x'_\nu = xX_\nu + 1$, since the partition (1, 1, . . . , 1) is always disregarded when considering $x_\nu X'(t) = (1 + t + t^2 + t^3 + \ldots)(1 + t^2 + t^4 + \ldots) \ldots (1 + t^k + t^{2k} + t^{3k} + \ldots) \ldots = 1/(1 - t)(1 - t^2) \ldots (1 = t^k) \ldots .$

Table 5
The Different Partitions for $n = 1$ to $n = 10$

$n = 1$	(1)
$n = 2$	(2), (1, 1)
$n = 3$	(3), (2, 1), (1, 1, 1)
$n = 4$	(4), (3, 1), (2, 2), (2, 1, 1), (1, 1, 1, 1)
$n = 5$	(5), (4, 1), (3, 2), (3, 1, 1), (2, 2, 1), (2, 1, 1, 1), (1, 1, 1, 1, 1)
$n = 6$	(6), (5, 1), (4, 2), (3, 3), (4, 1, 1), (3, 2, 1), (2, 2, 2), (3, 1, 1, 1), (2, 2, 1, 1), (2, 1, 1, 1, 1), (1, 1, 1, 1, 1, 1)
$n = 7$	(7), (6, 1), (5, 2), (4, 3), (5, 1, 1), (4, 2, 1), (3, 3, 1), (3, 2, 2), (4, 1, 1, 1), (3, 2, 1, 1), (2, 2, 2, 1), (3, 1, 1, 1, 1), (2, 2, 1, 1, 1), (2, 1, 1, 1, 1, 1), (1, 1, 1, 1, 1, 1, 1)
$n = 8$	(8), (7, 1), (6, 2), (5, 3), (4, 4), (6, 1, 1), (5, 2, 1), (4, 3, 1), (4, 2, 2), (3, 3, 2), (5, 1, 1, 1), (4, 2, 1, 1), (3, 2, 2, 1), (3, 3, 1, 1), (2, 2, 2, 2), (4, 1, 1, 1, 1), (3, 2, 1, 1, 1), (2, 2, 2, 1, 1), (3, 1, 1, 1, 1, 1), (2, 2, 1, 1, 1, 1), (2, 1, 1, 1, 1, 1, 1), (1, 1, 1, 1, 1, 1, 1, 1)
$n = 9$	(9), (8, 1), (7, 2), (6, 3), (5, 4), (7, 1, 1), (6, 2, 1), (5, 3, 1), (4, 4, 1), (5, 2, 2), (4, 3, 2), (3, 3, 3), (6, 1, 1, 1), (5, 2, 1, 1), (4, 2, 2, 1), (4, 3, 1, 1), (3, 3, 2, 1), (3, 2, 2, 2), (5, 1, 1, 1, 1), (4, 2, 1, 1, 1), (3, 3, 1, 1, 1), (3, 2, 2, 1, 1), (2, 2, 2, 2, 1), (4, 1, 1, 1, 1, 1), (3, 2, 1, 1, 1, 1), (2, 2, 2, 1, 1, 1) (3, 1, 1, 1, 1, 1, 1), (2, 2, 1, 1, 1, 1, 1), (2, 1, 1, 1, 1, 1, 1, 1), (1, 1, 1, 1, 1, 1, 1, 1, 1)
$n = 10$	(10), (9, 1), (8, 2), (7, 3), (6, 4), (5, 5), (8, 1, 1), (7, 2, 1), (6, 3, 1), (5, 4, 1), (6, 2, 2), (5, 3, 2), (4, 4, 2), (4, 3, 3), (7, 1, 1, 1), (6, 2, 1, 1), (5, 3, 1, 1), (4, 4, 1, 1), (5, 2, 2, 1), (4, 3, 2, 1), (3, 3, 3, 1), (4, 2, 2, 2), (3, 3, 2, 2), (6, 1, 1, 1, 1), (5, 2, 1, 1, 1), (4, 3, 1, 1, 1), (4, 2, 2, 1, 1), (3, 3, 2, 1, 1), (3, 2, 2, 2, 1), (2, 2, 2, 2, 2), (5, 1, 1, 1, 1, 1), (4, 2, 1, 1, 1, 1), (3, 3, 1, 1, 1, 1), (3, 2, 2, 1, 1, 1), (2, 2, 2, 2, 1, 1), (4, 1, 1, 1, 1, 1, 1), (3, 2, 1, 1, 1, 1, 1), (2, 2, 2, 1, 1, 1, 1), (3, 1, 1, 1, 1, 1, 1, 1), (2, 2, 1, 1, 1, 1, 1, 1), (2, 1, 1, 1, 1, 1, 1, 1, 1), (1, 1, 1, 1, 1, 1, 1, 1, 1, 1)

If one performs the multiplication, then as needed, the coefficient of t^n will be $x'_n = x_n + 1$.

Possible Number of Adverse Effects

Under the same conditions as above, what is the possible number of adverse effects that may be produced?

Note that the problem here is again expressible on two levels. First, how many different reactions were there, and, second, how many different complexes of reactions can a patient present. Again, we have the two assumptions above.

Examination of the first part clearly indicates that for n drugs, the number of adverse reactions equals:

Table 6
The Total Number of Possible Patient Complexes Due to Different Interactions for $n = 6$

Partition	Form	Number
(6)	[ABCDEF]	6!
(5, 1)	[ABCDE][F]	6!
(4, 2)	[ABCD][EF]	6!
(3, 3)	[ABC][DEF]	6!/2
(4, 1, 1)	[ABCD][E][F]	6!/2
(3, 2, 1)	[ABC][DE][F]	6!
(2, 2, 2)	[AB][CD][EF]	6!/6
(3, 1, 1, 1)	[ABC][D][E][F]	6!/6
(2, 2, 1, 1)	[AB][CD][E][F]	6!/4
(2, 1, 1, 1, 1)	[AB][C][D][E][F]	6!/24

Total Equals 5.6! + 6![5/8] = 4050

$n! + n! + (n)_{n-2} + (n)_{n-3} + \ldots + (n)_2 + (n)_1 = P_n + n = P_n' + 1 = P_n''$ (with $P_0'' = 0$) since each individual drug can give an adverse reaction. Using the material above, we get a recurrence relationship $P_n'' = nP''_{n-1} + n$. In addition, the generating function

$$P_n''(s) = \sum_{k=1}^{\infty} P_k''s^k = se^s/1 - s$$

For the second concept the element (1, 1, . . . , 1) is included for the case of n drugs, and thus there is one more partition than before. We are now dealing with restricted partitions of n elements, which were denoted above by x_n', and the generating function is

$$X'(t) = \sum_{j=1}^{\infty} (1 - t^j)^{-1}$$

as elucidated above. In addition, each number in Table 4 must be augmented by 1 to cover the total number of different permutations or patient complexes.

REFERENCES

1. Martin EW: Hazards of Medication. Philadelphia, Lippincott, 1971
2. Food and Drug Administration: Appraisal of the Safety of Chemicals in Foods, Drugs and Cosmetics. Topeka, Kansas, The Association of Food and Drug Officials of the United States, 1959
3. Kalow W: Pharmacogenetics; Heredity and the Response to Drugs. Philadelphia, Saunders, 1962
4. McKusick VA: Medical Genetics, 1958-1960. An Annotated Review. St Louis, Mosby, 1961
5. Remmer HMD: The role of the liver in drug metabolism. Am J Med 49:617, 1970

6. Rubin E, Beattie DS, Toth A et al: Structural and Function effects of ethanol on hepatic mitochondria. Fed Proc 31:131, 1972
7. Tumen HS, Cain JC, Haubrich WS et al: Hepatic reactions to drugs. JAMA 191:405, 1965
8. Heymann W: Nephrotic syndrome after use of trimethadione and Paramethadione in petit mal. JAMA 202:893, 1967
9. Kunin CM: Nephrotoxicity of antibiotics, JAMA 202:204, 1967
10. Beutler E: Drug-induced anemia. Fed Proc 31:141, 1972
11. Beutler E: Drug-induced blood dyscrasias, JAMA 189:143, 1964
12. Crosby WH, Kaufman RM: Drug-induced blood dyscrasias. JAMA 189:417, 1964
13. Erslev AJ: Drug-induced blood dyscrasias. JAMA 188:531, 1964
14. Huguley CM: Drug-induced blood dyscrasias. JAMA 188:817, 1964
15. Tschudy DP, Bonkowsky HL: Experimental porphyria. Fed Proc 31:147, 1972
16. Yesair DW, Bullock FJ, Coffey JJ: The pharmacodynamics of drug interactions, Drug Metab Rev 1:35, 1972
17. Calesnick B, Smith MH, Beutner R: Combined action of cardiotoxic drugs. J Pharmacol Exp Ther 102:138, 1951
18. Milne MD: Influences of acid-base balance on efficacy and toxicity of drugs. Proc R Soc Med 58:946, 1965
19. Brodie BB: Displacement of one drug by another from carrier or receptor sites. Proc Soc R Med 58:946, 1965
20. Burns JJ, Conney AH: Enzyme stimulation and inhibition in metabolism of drugs. Proc R Soc Med 58:955, 1965
21. Conney AH: Drug metabolism and therapeutics. N Engl J Med 280:653, 1969
22. Prescott LF: Drug metabolism and therapeutics. Scot Med J 16:121, 1971
23. Schoene B, Fleischmann RA: Determination of drug metabolizing enzymes in needle biopsies of human liver. Eur J Clin Pharmacol 4:65, 1972
24. Koch-Weser JK, Sellers EM: Drug interactions with coumarin anticoagulants. N Engl J Med 285:487, 1971
25. Kabins SA: Interaction among antibiotics and other drugs. JAMA 219:206, 1972
26. Editorial (Medical News): Risks of drug interactions man exists in 1 to 13 prescriptions. JAMA 220:1287, 1972
27. Goldstein EM: Rx and Malpractice: Drug Interactions. Malpractice X-posure Rep 2:2, 1972
28. Riordan J: An Introduction to Combinatorial Analysis. New York, Wiley, 1958

William S. Beck

2
Enzymatic Mechanisms of the Hematopoietic System

The title originally assigned for this essay was *Enzyme activity in the mechanisms of the hematopoietic system*. However, upon reflection, I concluded that very little is known of the major mechanisms of the hematopoietic system, among which are (a) mechanisms governing the "decision" of a stem cell to become committed to one or another of several cell lines, (b) mechanisms that keep the number of stem cells relatively constant and regulate their interconversion between acting and resting modes, (c) mechanisms by which the "poietin" hormones act, (d) mechanisms that govern the closely scheduled events of several maturation series, and (e) mechanisms that determine the release of newly formed blood cells into the circulating blood. Not only has our understanding of these mechanisms barely reached the descriptive stage, it would be presumption compounded to attempt their explication in terms of "enzyme activity." I chose therefore to modify the title to *Enzyme mechanisms of the hematopoietic system*, which, although still a formidable assignment, will be a more manageable one (when its ultrawide angle has been narrowed) and perhaps more appropriate in the context of this Symposium.

We are here to consider the diverse means by which drugs damage the hematopoietic system. I find it interesting to note how natural it is to assume that the key targets of drug actions are enzymes and enzyme systems. I judge this assumption to have been made by the early appearance of this paper on the program—only a paper on drugs themselves takes precedence—and by the countless published studies on the effect of this or that drug on this or that enzyme. Enzymology, was, of course, an important early chapter in the development of modern molecular biology. I am referring to that branch of biochemistry that can be described only with arrows and whose methodology involves pathway-tracing with labeled compounds and the purification and characterization of enzymes. A brilliant chapter it has been, but for all its success in the making of metabolic

Supported by Grants CA-03728 and AM-06214 from the US Public Health Service, and by the John Phyffe Richardson Fund.

maps, it has not yet succeeded in accounting for such fundamental mechanisms of cell physiology as the active transport of small molecules across membranes, the initiation and completion of mitosis, and other sequential events in the cell life cycle, the regulation of gene expression, malignant transformation, growth, differentiation and, yes, the mode of action of many drugs. Each of these phenomena takes place at a level of biologic organization somewhat higher than that of the enzyme mechanisms themselves, and investigators are ruefully aware of the many impediments to any attempt at explaining complex physiologic behavior in mechanistic terms—that is, in terms of phenomena occurring at lower levels of biologic organization. In part, these difficulties arise from the mutually exclusive nature of the experimental arrangements required for analytic and behavioral investigations. Thus, it may be that all of the insights of modern enzymology are insufficient to account, say, for chloramphenicol-induced aplastic anemia and other of the drug-induced dyscrasias to be discussed in this Symposium.

PROSPECTUS

Having acknowledged the possibility that a discussion of enzymatic mechanisms ought, perhaps, to be at the end of the program rather than at the beginning, I shall proceed by offering certain introductory statements that will have the urgently necessary effect of limiting the scope of these remarks.

Scope of Survey

As much as one would wish to limit discussion to data obtained in studies of the hematopoietic system proper—that is, the blood cell producing components of the bone marrow—knowledge of their enzymatic mechanisms is fragmentary. Since, for reasons to be mentioned later, a coherent literature does not exist in this area, much of the following will deal with the enzymology of circulating blood cells on the not unreasonable assumption that their enzymology and that of their precursors have features in common.

Except for the limited number of glittering and circumscribed examples to be covered later in this Symposium, much of our knowledge of blood cell biochemistry is a catalog of facts without obvious physiologic meaning. This judgment occurs immediately to anyone consulting existing reviews.[1–9] It is noteworthy that most of this literature was written in the context of the leukemia problem (enzymology having also failed thus far to account for leukemia) and that nearly none of it was conceived in the context of the drug reaction problem. We will try, in the following, to pass over most of the well-reviewed facts and to point out wherever possible those enzymatic mechanisms that might be of interest in the latter context.

The fragmentary nature of our knowledge of blood cell enzymology is but a special case of the problem of animal cell enzymology, which lags well behind the field of bacterial enzymology. Similarly, knowledge of the effects of drugs on bacterial cells is often superior to that of drug effects on animal cells. Hence, it will be necessary, in this short essay on the biochemistry of the hematopoietic system, to do some extrapolating from studies on the biochemistry of other animal tissues.

Even a brief glance at the titles of papers to be presented at this Symposium should make it clear that the problem of drugs and hematologic reactions subsumes a large diversity of superficially unrelated topics. Thus, we will hear papers on the interactions of drugs with methemoglobin, with G-6-PD-deficient red cells, with leukocytes, the coagulation reactions, and so forth. One essayist cannot attempt to provide an enzymologic substratum for so many matters. Nor is such background needed, for in many of the cases to be discussed the relevant enzymology is well known and the speakers are able to speak for themselves. I have chosen therefore to keep my remarks largely within the context of the drug-induced hypoplastic disorders, of which so little is known. I shall also focus attention mainly and arbitrarily on mechanisms of DNA synthesis.

Problems and Cautions of Interpretation

Though I am not a pharmacologist, it seems to me that the molecular mechanisms of drugs may be divided into two categories. Though all interact with functionally important molecules in the body, some act by combining with small molecules or ions (e.g., antacids, chelating agents, and so forth) and others act by combining with few or many macromolecules or receptors (e.g., the alkylating agents, cytosine arabinoside, and so forth). In beginning a consideration of the potential toxicity of the latter group, it is useful to recognize that special problems arise in analyzing their effects on the hematopoietic system as a consequence of the arrangements within that system. There are stem cells (and their "microenvironment"); maturation sequences (that early are associated with cell division and later are not); and there is the release of cells into the blood. A drug blocking DNA synthesis wherever it encounters it (as we believe cytosine arabinoside does, for example), will block division in all bone marrow cells capable of dividing and thus have one sort of effect. But a drug that selectively blocks stem cell division, though it combines with fewer receptors, may have a far more devastating effect on the hematopoietic system. In a sense, a useful analogy can be drawn between these considerations and the stoichiometric-catalytic dichotomy of biochemical effects. It should be apparent, in light of this notion, what difficulties might arise in the interpretation of data. Effects of an agent blocking DNA synthesis in marrow by directly compromising an enzyme of the biosynthetic pathway might be difficult to distinguish from those of one diminishing DNA synthesis by damaging stem cells (or their "microenvironment") if the measure of things is the total amount of DNA synthesized. But in the latter case, the decrease in DNA synthesis is not the primary event. In all such studies one would wish to know if an observed biochemical phenomenon was a cause, consequence, or irrelevant accompanient of an abnormal clinical or physiologic picture. I shall refer to this problem again in connection with concrete questions. Suffice it to say that we often lack this knowledge.

Caution should also arise from the possibility that a drug-induced abnormality may be due to effects on cells, tissues, and systems beyond the bone marrow. Abnormal patterns of blood cell proliferation may be the most prominent manifestation of a drug effect, but the disorder could be one of an extramedullary control mechanism best described in quantitative or kinetic terms. In that case, it might leave no clue to its nature within the affected cells.

Much of what has been written on the interpretation of biochemical essentials of the state of malignancy applies to the state of drug-induced abnormality. Cancer is obstensively defined by a pattern of growth behavior exhibited by certain cells within a community of cells and, in the end, it is to this behavioral test that we must put cells to determine whether they are normal or malignant. Obvious difficulties are inherent in such a definition, which establishes dichotomies or sets boundaries between classes of entities. Boutwell,[10] Potter,[11] and others have pointed out that carcinogenesis goes through stages of initiation promotion, and of progression, in which accumulating genetic or epigenetic changes occur—many, no doubt, extraneous to the process of malignant transformation. Though the complex biochemical patterns observed in the fully developed cancer cell may lead to directed chemotherapy, they are unlikely to shed light on the mechanisms of carcinogenesis, since they are diverse, mostly nonessential, and "irrational," i.e., they are not the sensible, selectively advantageous patterns shaped by evolution.

Similar considerations lead one to the intuitive feeling that few, or perhaps none, of the circulating blood cells would be likely to display the significant biochemical changes of a drug-induced abnormality. In part, the problem can be traced to the distinctive arrangements in the hematopoietic system—which include maturation, release, and circulation of mature blood cells. Some circulating cells might be the modified progeny of afflicted cells, but cells bearing the critical biochemical stigmata may repose elsewhere in one or many obscure locations. Hence, it would be difficult to know where to look for useful biochemical evidence on their condition. Thus we must interpret not only the pathophysiologic significance of observed biochemical patterns in the cells found in a dyscrasia, but also the relationship of these cells to the cells altered by primary events. If, in fact, their character bears no meaningful connection with underlying events, biochemical investigation has a rather different reading frame than many think it has.

In the following remarks, I shall briefly discuss the methods used and the methodologic problems arising in the biochemical study of the hematopoietic system. Then I shall attempt to sketch a model of the hematopoietic system as it might be viewed by an enzymologist. Next will be a very brief characterization of the known biochemical properties that set it apart from other systems—with emphasis on nucleic acid metabolism. Finally, I will try to draw certain conclusions about which of these mechanisms seem likely to be useful to students of the drug-induced blood dyscrasias.

METHODOLOGIC PROBLEMS IN STUDIES OF THE HEMATOPOIETIC SYSTEM

For purposes of this discussion, the hematopoietic system consists of the blood-cell producing portions of bone marrow and the mature blood cells of circulating blood. We are not concerned with the lymphoid system or with the mechanism of blood cell destruction, though these would be relevant topics in any comprehensive treatment of untoward drug effects.

Available data on the metabolic and enzymologic properties of bone marrow are astonishingly meager. One notes, for example, that the topic is not treated at all in the large textbooks of hematology that recently became available, though extensive coverage is given to biochemical studies of white cells, red cells, and platelets. Beyond the classic studies of the Warburg school,[12,13] and those that were reviewed by Lajtha some years ago,[5] the literature provides only sporadic data in this area.

The practical reasons for this situation are easily stated: (a) bone marrow is difficult to obtain from living human subjects in substantial quantities, (b) only primitive methods are available for the resolution of the many cell types in marrow into collections of cells homogeneous with respect to morphology and metabolism, (c) wide metabolic differences have been found among the hematopoietic tissues of different species, and (d) confusion has arisen from the fact that certain metabolic data are variably influenced by experimental conditions, such as composition of incubation media, analytical methods, physiologic state (i.e., resting or dividing), cell concentration, and mode of data expression (i.e., dry weight, cell numbers, DNA, protein, or nitrogen).

As noted above, investigators faced with the relative unavailability of bone marrow cells have tended to assume that much of what is true for mature blood cells is true for their immature precursors of bone marrow. Some experimental justification exists for this habit of thought. It was found long ago, for example, that peripheral blood leukocytes have a high aerobic glycolytic rate.[1,12] Suspensions of bone marrow cells have similar properties.[5] Such similarities have led to many problems in the design of experiments, which may be appreciated by recalling the problems of the investigator seeking a control with which to compare a leukemic blast cell. In the design of experiments, should such a cell from blood be compared with a normal blast cell from marrow? If so, how does one obtain a supply of the latter to study?

Yet another problem surrounds the choice of control material. Assuming that alkaline phosphatase is a lysosomal enzyme, would comparison of the amount of enzyme per lysosome be more meaningful in the comparison of different cell populations? If enzyme content per lysosome were the same in two populations but the number of lysosomes per cell were different, observed differences in enzyme level per cell might have a different significance than if the situation were reversed. For one attempting to visualize the chain of events leading to the presence of a given amount of a given enzyme in a given cell, it would be of some moment to know if he were dealing with an abnormal number of normal lysosomes or a normal number of abnormal lysosomes.

AN ENZYMOLOGIST'S MODEL OF THE HEMATOPOIETIC SYSTEM

One would prefer to begin a survey of the biochemical features of the hematopoietic system by examining a detailed working model of that system embodying all of its known properties. Since none is to be found, we must at least try to construct our own. In doing so, we will attempt to identify those features that may be targets for unwanted drug effects.

Physical Properties

Published estimates of the total number of erythroid and myeloid cells in the bone marrow of normal man range from 3.4 to 5.0 $\times$ 10^9 erythrocyte precursor cells per kilogram of body weight and 8.3 to 11.4 $\times$ 10^9 granulocyte precursors per kilogram.[14–16] Taking the means of these ranges as correct working values, the marrow of a 70 kg man would contain about 3 $\times$ 10^{11} erythroid cells and 7 $\times$ 10^{11} granulocyte precursor cells for a total of 10^{12} cells, excluding megakaryocytes and other quantitatively minor cell types. Assuming that 10^{10} cells have a packed wet volume of 6.0 ml,[17] the erythroid and myeloid cells of a normal 70 kg man would by themselves occupy a volume of 600 ml.

The hematopoietic cells are not uniformly distributed in the marrow cavities nor do they fill the cavities. Recent isotope studies of their distribution show them to be most abundant in long bones and vertebrae. Calculations based on total ^{59}Fe uptake show, for example, that the shafts of the femurs contain approximately 12%–16% of the total hematopoietic cells of marrow.

The fine structure of marrow has not been fully elucidated, but it is clear that its function depends significantly on the microanatomy of the vascular network.[18] The arterial supply to the marrow ultimately breaks up into networks of intercommunicating sinuses that permeate parenchymal cords. Few data are available on the possibility that physical segregation appears superficially to be randomly mixed with no specific spatial relationships between the cells. However, indirect evidence suggests that cell-to-cell inductive regulatory processes must be operative in bone marrow. One must agree with Metcalf and Moore[19] that the distribution patterns of various cell types in the marrow are unlikely to be random. Striking segregation is found in the chicken, with granulocytopoietic cells lying in aggregates outside the sinusoids. However, in mammals both granulocytopoiesis and erythropoiesis seems to be entirely extravascular.

The limits of the sinuses and cords are defined by a trilaminar wall that is alternately well developed or attenuated. Weiss pictures the complex of the sinus and intersinal tissue as a responsive system whose two components reciprocally enlarge or diminish according to blood flow, body requirements for hematopoiesis, and other mechanisms. In the critical event in the release of cells into blood, cells traffic between intersinal parenchyma and sinusoidal lumen. The efficient retention of immature cell types within the marrow implies that the exit process is complex and may require active participation of the metabolic processes or surface proteins of a cell that has reached an appropriate stage of maturation. Each of these mechanisms—the "microenvironment" effect, the regulation of development by humoral or cell-to-cell devices, the release at maturity—remains to be explained in biochemical terms.

Kinetic Properties

Differential cell counts on the major cell populations in adult human bone marrow give the following approximate patterns:[20] granulocytes and their precursors, 58%; erythropoietic cells, 16%; lymphocytes, 15%; other cells, 11%.

Thus, granulocytopoietic elements predominate over erythropoietic elements in marrow, though erythrocytes predominate over granulocytes in marrow output. The 10^{12} cells of marrow are responsible for the daily release into the blood (in our 70 kg man) of 2.2×10^{11} erythrocytes and 1.1×10^{11} granulocytes.[21,22] In volumetric terms, 600 ml of bone marrow cells each day generate 22 ml of erythrocytes and 66 ml of granulocytes. The active tissue of marrow is thus expanding by 14.7% each day—red cells accounting for 3.7% and white cells for 11%. This extraordinary rate of activity, matched by few other tissues, is the by-product of unusual biologic arrangements that doubtless depend upon unusual "enzymatic mechanisms."

STEM CELL DIFFERENTIATION

By general agreement, erythrocytes, granulocytes, and thrombocytes originate from a self-perpetuating pool of stem cells that includes both multipotential stem cells and partially differentiated stem cells that are committed to individual cell lines. The early cells also provide a dormant reserve to be activated by incompletely understood signals generated by pools of mature cells. Such signals, probably triggered by a diminution in pool sizes, may be transmitted by cell-to-cell interactions. The early committed stem cells of the several cell lines appear to be cycling continuously, renewing themselves and furnishing cells for further differentiation. The size of the stem cell pool is not known. If the data for mouse stem cells (i.e., 5–30 "CFU's" per 10^5 marrow cells)[19] are applicable to man, a 70 kg man would have $5\text{–}30 \times 10^7$ stem cells—or 0.025–0.15 ml if stem cell volume is equivalent to that of leukocytes—indeed a small volume.

Stem cells are believed to undergo "blast transformation" when exposed to specific "poietins:" erythropoietin for cells committed to erythropoiesis, leukopoietin for cells committed to granulocytopoiesis, and thrombopoietin for cells committed to thrombocytopoiesis. Once committed, the stem cell begins a series of divisions and, at the same time, matures. Some cells die in the marrow.

ERYTHROPOIESIS

Newly formed pronormoblasts undergo three to five mitotic divisions; hence, there is an 8–32 fold multiplication of nuclear units. Meanwhile, cytoplasmic maturation proceeds. Erythropoietic cytoplasmic maturation is a complex process involving (a) an extraction of iron from circulating transferrin by specific surface receptors; (b) the synthesis of heme by processes depending uniquely on mitochondrial integrity, and (c) the fabrication of a single species of protein molecule that comes eventually to account for one-third of the cell's mass. Since much hemoglobin is synthesized after loss of the nucleus—a bizarre and theatrical event—cytoplasm must be endowed with a long-lived variety of messenger RNA.

Nearly mature red cells are released from marrow to begin their long intravascular sojourn some 4–5 days after the start of erythropoiesis.

GRANULOCYTOPOIESIS

In contrast, release of granulocytes and entry into functional pools depend not only on proliferation and maturation in the marrow, but also on the competence of storage compartments in marrow, small blood vessels, and spleen. Ingenious investigators, using diverse quantitative techniques—e.g., labeling by tritiated thymidine (^{3}H-TdR), diisopropylfluorophosphate (DF ^{32}P) and ^{51}Cr, differential counts, mitotic index[22]—have constructed a plausible model,[23] according to which differentiating myeloid cells divide only a finite number of times before a putative cytoplasmic-nuclear interaction causes them to cease cycling.

Two important transitions occur: the "myelocyte → metamyelocyte transition" and the "marrow granulocyte → blood granulocyte transition." In the first, cells labeled in the proliferative or DNA-synthesizing compartment move into the nonproliferating compartment. Cronkite and Vincent have postulated that although serial divisions of myelocytes account for the observed efflux into the nonproliferating compartment, myelocyte divisions become impossible after a time, possibly due to the accumulation of inhibitors in the cytoplasm.[23] In the second transition, labeled cells from marrow become labeled cells in blood. An earlier transition, the initial "stem cell → maturation series" transition, is equally important but not yet accessible experimentally. Nor are the "myeloblast → promyelocyte → transitions," since all three stages are labeled by a pulse of ^{3}H-TdR.

An important recent contribution of the kinetics of granulocytopoiesis is Morley's concept that the periodicity of the blood granulocyte count is controlled by two feedback loops—a slow one that controls entrance of stem cells into the granulocytopoietic pathway and a fast one that controls the release of stored granulocytes from marrow into blood.[24] Preliminary evidence is at hand for a chemical mediator for the fast loop, the release of granulocytes from marrow.[25] I assume we will be hearing, in this Symposium, about the state of the mediator of the slow loop. It may be of incidental historical interest to this Symposium that the concept of release-control derives in part from the 1916 studies of Weiskotten, Schwartz, and Steensland on cell count oscillations resulting from depression of granulocytopoiesis by benzol.[26]

Patt and Maloney have suggested that myelocyte production exceeds the influx of myelocytes into the metamyelocyte compartment.[27] Excess myelocytes die in the marrow, and thus the rate of granulocyte production may, in part, be "death-controlled" by variations in mortality of newly formed myelocytes. Although this model must be validated, it is an attractive notion because it explains how more granulocytes could be quickly provided upon demand. In this view, marrow would respond to demands for granulocytes by (a) dumping of marrow granulocytes into the circulation and (b) increasing production at the myelocyte level. The latter would be achieved by shortening the generation time. This would have no effect on the granulocyte count in blood for, at least, the time needed for transit through the metamyelocyte and band stage. When demand for granulocytes becomes excessive, as it does, for example, in the presence of severe infection or a drug-dependent leukoagglutinin, neutropenia is the inevitable result.

Any model of hematopoietic biochemistry must take into account these kinetic features. The same must be said for the curious morphogenetic features of granulocytopoiesis, among which are the loss of nucleoli and progressive changes in chromatin character, the loss of mitochondria, the development of two types of lysosomal granules in the two faces of the Golgi complex,[28] and the segmentation of the nucleus. Inherited abnormalities of many of these features implies that each is under specific genetic control.

Functional Properties

THE CELL CYCLE

Hematopoietic cells, like all cells, grow by doubling their components between divisions. Balance in such growth requires the continuous maintenance of alignment among all increases in cell elements. Presumably balance is brought about by molecular signals communicating information on the cell's needs for each element. For example, the production of new mitochondria must be governed ultimately by the cell's needs for ATP and the production of new ribosomes by the needs for protein synthesis. We know very little of these regulatory interactions at the cell constituent level.

We do know, however, that such activities are geared to the cell's nuclear cycle of chromosome replication and segregation. These activities define the now familiar periods of the nuclear cycle, i.e., M, G_1, S, and G_2. Data from synchronous cell cultures have greatly expanded understanding in this area. The eventual deciphering of molecular events underlying each of the periods ought to provide a key to understanding cell replication and the actions of factors that inhibit or modify it.

The following events are believed to occur during these periods: M is the brief period of mitosis; G_1, though poorly understood, includes in its terminal phase immediate preparations for the synthesis of DNA, with synthesis of DNA polymerases, thymidylate synthetase, a variety of kinases, and other necessary enzymes. The length of M plus G_2 plus S is relatively constant for proliferating cells. The length of G_1 is the most variable of the four. Prescott, noting the proved expendability of G_1, has characterized it as a time of hesitation or indecision between mitosis and new DNA synthesis.[29]

The S period, the phase of DNA synthesis, is initiated with a burst of protein synthesis. Cells treated with inhibitors of protein synthesis during S undergo a rapid decline in DNA synthesis. This decline may parallel the dependence of bacterial DNA synthesis initiation on new protein synthesis. Alternatively, it might reflect the need for concomitant histone synthesis or for the synthesis of proteins unconnected with initiation. Just how synthesis of individual chromosomes takes place during S is only beginning to be explored. These relationships may not be much different from those seen in prokaryotes. It is interesting to note that Cairns' estimate of the time required to synthesize $20{,}000\mu$ of DNA molecules (one human chromosome), assuming rates similar to those in bacteria, is 6½ hours. This agrees with other data on the duration of the S period of mammalian cells.

The G_2 period includes events that link the end of chromosome replication with those of chromosome segregation. It has been postulated that the cell cycle depends on a temporal sequence of genetic transcriptions that are kept in sequence by the successive dependencies of one transcription on the next. For example, in animal cells in culture, the synthesis of protein needed for assembly of the mitotic apparatus requires prior synthesis of RNA in G_2 and this RNA synthesis depends, in turn, on a prior synthesis of protein.[30] A major task for future research will be to determine the nature of the transcriptions and translations that drive the cell cycle and how these activities produce the ordered chromosomal behavior essential to cell replication.

Other future tasks will be to elucidate the role of extranuclear DNA and its associated structures in the cell cycle. How and when are mitochondria, Golgi apparatus, lysosomes, and other organelles synthesized during the cycle? How many of these contain DNA and what is it coded for? How is its function controlled relative to that of nuclear DNA? What is the source of the ribosomes important to such extranuclear synthesis? Do they come from the nucleus? We will touch on some of these questions later.

DIFFERENTIATION AND MORPHOGENESIS

Differentiation (which occurs in concert with cell division) and maturation and morphogenesis (which do not) are hallmarks of hematopoiesis. Indeed, with the exception of germinal cells of skin and testis, few other systems of body cells make such spectacular developmental displays. In view of the many particular features of hematopoietic differentiation—the synthesis of hemoglobin, so massive quantitatively, the morphogenesis of the myeloid cell nucleus, so unique structurally—one would expect understanding of their mechanisms to be advanced. Alas, it is not.

Until a surprisingly late date, it was believed that the basis of differentiation resides entirely in the cytoplasm. Dividing cells appear to give rise to the equal division of the nucleus between two daughter cells, but the division of cytoplasm is more difficult. It therefore appeared self-evident that chromosomes remain unchanged during differentiation, while large differences arise in cytoplasm. Hence, while the chromosomes in the nuclei were held responsible for the relatively minor pecularities of individuals that we recognize as genetically controlled, differentiation, which is concerned with basic properties common to all members of the species, appeared to originate and to be controlled in the cytoplasm. Then in 1955, King and Briggs provided the first real evidence on the question.[31] By transplantation methods, they managed to replace the nucleus in the fertilized egg of a frog with the nucleus from a cell in a more advanced stage of development. Only nuclei from early stages supported normal development of the egg. Hence, nuclear function changes in the course of differentiation. This experiment now has more historic than probative significance, since later work revealed considerable reversibility in the function of differentiated nuclei. Nonetheless, the concept of nuclear determinism gained acceptance, and new explorations of nuclear differentiation led to the discovery that not all genes are active at all times. Mechanisms exist that induce or repress activities of genes or gene groups. Differential gene transcription provided the conceptual basis for an understanding of how cells with identical genomes can develop unequal specialization modes. It would appear that the attenuation of nuclear function in the course of hematopoiesis is reflected by changes in nuclear shape and chromatin character. In the erythroid series, nuclear modification is complete. The nucleus is eliminated.

Gross has pointed to the difficulties encountered by students of differentiation in distinguishing between the biochemistry of cellular differentiation and the biochemistry of cells that are differentiating.[32] We do not know enough about differentiation to single out one or more pathways of metabolism as having special relevance to the problem. Until a biochemical explanation has been worked out for one example of a "decision" to differentiate and its specific consequences, it will be necessary to assume that everything about the metabolism of a cell is relevant.

Differentiation, then, may be defined as the sum of processes leading to the acquisition of specific metabolic competences that distinguish daughter cells from each other or from the parental cell. Morphogenesis, the acquisition of distinctive shape changes, is a consequence of the acquisition of a distinctive complement of three-dimensional gene products. It reflects a differential chemical composition and a spectrum of enzymes and structural macromolecules. Some have argued that explanations of morphogenesis must include supramolecular forces. But surely the visible components of morphogenesis are consequences of differentiation, which is ultimately to be explained in terms of biochemical controls on biosynthetic pathways and metabolism generally.

Studies of the cell cycle during embryogenesis have shown that the duration of S and G_1 increase progressively. Since the changing durations of DNA synthesis occur upon a background of environmental constancy, they are programmed in some way. Nuclear transplantation data suggest that control of the timing of DNA synthesis resides, at least in part, in the cytoplasm. We are left to speculate on whether the replication of nuclear genomes in hematopoietic cells is under partial control by as yet unidentified cytoplasmic mechanisms.

Biochemical events underlying the differentiation and maturation of bone marrow cells are, of course, poorly understood. We do have certain information on the comparative rates of macromolecular synthesis at the various stages of differentiation and maturation. As noted earlier, the rate of DNA synthesis decreases until the metamyelocyte stage is reached when it ceases completely. It is not known whether the nucleus of the mature granulocyte can be "reactivated." RNA and protein synthesis also decrease during maturation. A major problem in the interpretation of such data stems from the fact that in experiments employing ^{3}H-TdR and other labeled precursors little account has been taken of possible variations in the rate of nucleoside catabolism in cells at different stages of maturity. Conceivably, the fact that mature cells catabolize thymidine more rapidly than immature cells accounts for the lower ^{3}H-TdR incorporation in the more mature cells of the myeloid series.

SURVEY OF BIOCHEMICAL PROPERTIES OF THE HEMATOPOIETIC SYSTEM

An attempt will be made in this section to review, in summary fashion, the enzymatic and metabolic properties of bone marrow that have been: (a) discovered by direct studies of bone marrow and (b) inferred from studies of the normal and abnormal blood cells produced by bone marrow. Major attention will be given to the biosynthesis of RNA* and DNA and their precursors. Detailed bibliographies will be found in cited reviews.[1–9]

* Standard abbreviations for nucleotides, nucleic acids, and other biochemicals have been used in accordance with the approved usage of *The Journal of Biological Chemistry*.

General Characteristics

Bone marrow cells, like other animal cells, possess the major anabolic and catabolic pathways and contain the commonplace constituents, including lipids of diverse types, glycogen, amino acids, nucleic acids, trace metals, and other components. These cells synthesize protein and break it down; synthesize heme and urea and, as we shall presently see, nucleotides and nucleic acids. They actively reduce folic acid and contain the major coenzymes. They also contain many well-known enzymes, published characterizations of which vary in quality and detail.

In addition, these cells have many distinctive biochemical features, among them a rich endowment of lysosomes and their associated hydrolytic enzymes, a relatively high content of zinc, ascorbic acid, and the characteristic enzyme myeloperoxidase, which occurs in granules other than lysosomes. Granulocytes, erythrocytes, and their precursors are relatively poor in mitochondria, and the tricarboxylic acid cycle is correspondingly feeble. Bone marrow cells depend largely on glycolysis for their energy supply. There is a modest Pasteur effect.

Nucleotide and Nucleic Acid Metabolism

CONTENT OF RNA AND DNA

Some years ago we systematically measured certain cellular components in suspensions of normal and abnormal leukocytes in an effort to identify the best reference basis for in vitro metabolic data. The mean results of many assays indicated a DNA content of 70.9 mg per 10^{10} cells and an RNA content of 25.9 mg per 10^{10} cells.[2] Similar results have been reported by other workers in circulating leukocytes and bone marrow cells.[2,6] Because the value for DNA is somewhat higher than that found in other human diploid cells, the myeloid cell has been cited as a possible exception to the rule of DNA constancy in diploid somatic cells.[34] It is difficult to evaluate such a conjecture in the present state of knowledge. There is ample evidence of heterogeneity of DNA content within the circulating leukocyte population, some cells displaying polyploidy and others a seeming hesitancy to synthesize DNA.[35] It is unlikely therefore that mean data from mixed populations will be adequate to resolve the question. Histochemical studies on individual cells are also subject to doubt. Some apparent variations in DNA content of different individual cells may be attributable to unexplained variations in electrovalent dye-binding capacities of the DNA in different cells.

Some reports have suggested that the DNAs of normal and leukemic leukocytes differ in physiochemical properties, such as molecular weight, viscosity, and so forth. Such claims are unaccompanied by data excluding adventitious effects upon isolated DNA by the nucleases in crude extracts.

The foregoing data are interesting in light of the calculations given above of the total numbers of hematopoietic cells. If 10^{10} cells contain 70.9 mg of DNA, 10^{12} cells contain 7.09 g and the turnover due to new cell production each day amounts to 1.56 g for new erythrocytes and 0.78 g for new granulocytes for a total of 2.34 g, a substantial quantity, the precursors of which must be freely available. Degradation of this amount of DNA could potentially give rise each day to some 500 mg of uric acid.

The decrease in cytoplasmic basophilia that accompanies maturation of erythrocytes and granulocytes is a reflection of a progressive decrease in RNA content. Thus, blast cells have higher RNA/DNA ratios than mature granulocytes. Granulocytes contain ribosomal RNA, with sedimentation velocities of 28S and 16–18S, and soluble (4S) RNA. A rapidly labeled polydisperse RNA with characteristics of messenger RNA is also found in granulocytes. It is localized mainly in the nucleus. Its heterogeneity has led to the suggestion that stable and unstable templates for protein synthesis are present. Polyribosomes are also present.

BIOSYNTHESIS OF RIBONUCLEOTIDES

Leukocytes contain all of the usual ribonucleotides, among them NAD, NADP, UDPG (uridine diphosphoglucose), and UDPAG (uridine diphosphoacetylglucosamine). Alternative biosynthetic routes to purine and pyrimidine ribonucleotides exist in most animal cells—de novo pathways, in which simple precursors are fashioned into heterocyclic purines or pyrimidines, and salvage pathways in which preformed purines or pyrimidines, from the environment or from degradative processes within the cell, are converted into ribonucleotides.[36] Although purine ribonucleotides are synthesized by salvage pathways only in unusual circumstances, leukocytes apparently provide such circumstance. Human leukocytes[37] and bone marrow cells[38] cannot negotiate the de novo pathway of purine ribonucleotide synthesis (or do so poorly), though they can synthesize pyrimidine ribonucleotides de novo. The defect appears to be in the early steps of the purine pathway since ^{14}C-glycine is not incorporated into the nucleic acids of leukocytes in vitro; nor is ^{14}C-formate incorporated into nucleic acid purines when intermediates such as aminoimidazole carboxamide or its ribonucleotide are present. Hence, the cells are capable of completing the purine ring.

These indications of substandard de novo synthesis of purine ribonucletides in leukocytes and bone marrow cells imply that synthesis in these cells occurs via salvage pathways. Since these require preformed purines, such moieties would have to be synthesized de novo elsewhere (i.e., in the liver) and transported to the hematopoietic system for salvage and incorporation. Lajtha and Vane have produced evidence for such a scheme in hepatectomized rabbits.[38] These results, in turn, imply the existence of an active capacity for the phosphorylation of preformed purine ribonucleosides.

Several enzymes of the de novo pathway of pyrimidine ribonucleotide synthesis, i.e., aspartate transcarbamylase, dihydroorotase, dihydroorotic dehydrogenase, and orotidylic decarboxylase, have been demonstrated in leukocytes.[39,40] Activities of most decrease with maturity.

BIOSYNTHESIS OF RNA

The "central dogma" of molecular biology—information is transferred from DNA to RNA to protein—appears safe within the human hematopoietic system. Despite technical difficulties in isolating RNA from human material, ample evidence shows that RNA synthesis is directed by DNA in leukocytes. For example: annealing experiments indicate notable complementarity between leukocyte RNA and DNA; RNA synthesis is inhibited by low concentrations of actinomycin D; and leukocyte RNA (unlike the double-stranded product of RNA-directed RNA synthesis), is ribonuclease-sensitive.

According to the current model of RNA synthesis in mammalian cells, RNA polymerase catalyzes the polymerization of ribonucleoside triphosphates into a chain that is a transcript of one of the DNA strands. Probably, only the regions of chromosomal DNA corresponding to euchromatin are transcribed. The nucleolus appears to be a principal site of ribosomal RNA synthesis before its transfer to the cytoplasm where it forms the cytoplasmic ribosomes. Kinetic data indicate a high turnover rate of nuclear RNA. As noted above, a considerable fraction of it is short lived and never reaches the cytoplasm. The basic elements of this scheme of RNA metabolism appear valid for hematopoietic cells, although uncertainties remain about the intracellular loci of the events of RNA metabolism.

Certain features of RNA metabolism in human hematopoietic cells merit comment. We have already noted that blast cells contain more RNA than do differentiated end cells. These cells have high rates of RNA synthesis and turnover than involve ribosomal RNA, 4S RNA, and heterogeneous, rapidly labeled RNA. Mature granulocytes have notable rates of RNA synthesis despite the absence of a well-developed endoplasmic reticulum and nucleolus.

An intriguing and underexplored aspect of RNA metabolism—one that might be a target of drug action—relates to the regulation of ribosome content in animal cells. Such regulation could be achieved by alterations of the rate of synthesis of one or more ribosome components, the rate of ribosome degradation, or both. As we showed some years ago,[41] reticulocytes provide useful opportunities for an approach to this problem. The disappearance of reticulocyte ribosomes during maturation apparently represents a continuance of normal degradative processes that have been unmasked by the termination of ribosome synthesis. Disappearing ribosomal RNA in this system is accounted for by the appearance of extracellular ribonucleosides and other low molecular weight products.

RNA metabolism in differentiated granulocytes is stimulated by phagocytosis. Particle ingestion is followed by increases in the rate of uptake into the cell of labeled RNA precursors and the specific activity of the acid-soluble nucleotide pool. New RNA is formed, and existing RNA is broken down at an accelerated rate. The significance of the increased turnover is not known. Deliberate inhibition of RNA synthesis has no effect on other metabolic changes accompanying phagocytosis.

BIOSYNTHESIS OF DEOXYRIBONUCLEOTIDES

Deoxyribonucleotides, the proximal precursors of DNA, are also fabricated by de novo and salvage pathways. The de novo pathway was discovered recently. Reichard and coworkers, in a series of studies that began in 1960, showed that deoxyribosyl compounds are formed in vivo by direct reduction of the 2′ carbon of ribonucleotides. When the responsible enzyme, ribonucleotide reductase, was purified from *Escherichia coli*, it was found to catalyze the following reaction:[42]

$$\text{ribonucleoside diphosphate} + \text{thioredoxin-(SH)}_2 \rightarrow \text{deoxyribonucleoside diphosphate} + \text{thioredoxin-S}_2$$

Thioredoxin-$(SH)_2$, the hydrogen donor, is a low molecular weight (viz., 12,000) protein that bears two thiol groups. For each molecule of deoxyribonucleotide formed, one molecule of thioredoxin is oxidized. Oxidized thioredoxin is then reduced by NADPH and a flavoprotein called thioredoxin reductase.

A second type of ribonucleotide reductase—one that reduces ribonucleoside triphosphates—was subsequently discovered in the vitamin B_{12} auxotroph *Lactobacillus leichmannii.* The reductase of *L leichmannii,* unlike that of *E coli,* requires demethylbenzimidazolylcobamide coenzyme (DBCC), the active form of vitamin B_{12}. Lactobacillus reductase converts the four major ribonucleoside triphosphates to deoxyribonucleoside triphosphates.[43] Choice of substrate by the enzyme is determined by divalent cations and deoxyribonucleoside triphosphates, each an allosteric effector promoting reduction of a different state of enzyme conformation or subunit aggregation.[44] The resulting network of regulatory effects presumably controls the balance of deoxyribonucleotide synthesis in vivo. Mechanism studies have shown that DBCC is an acceptor-donor of hydrogen that facilitates the transfer of ^3H from ^3H-H_2O (or R-$S^3H)_2$ or DBCC and then to C-2′ of the nucleotide sugar moiety.[45]

There was considerable biologic interest in the fact that ribonucleotide reductase of *E coli,* an organism lacking a vitamin B_{12} requirement, reduces ribonucleoside diphosphates and yet is cobamide-independent. It was unclear what agency in this system serves the hydrogen-transferring function performed by DBCC in the lactobacillus system until the recent discovery of an essential nonheme iron in purified *E coli* reductase.[46]

It remained to be determined which system is present in animal cells. A reductase of the *E coli* type had been found in Novikoff hepatoma,[47] but it was not certain that this tumor system was a protype for vitamin B_{12}-dependent animal tissues, such as bone marrow, until the recent contribution of Hopper suggested that partially purified ribonucleotide reductase of rabbit bone marrow is cobamide-independent.

METABOLISM OF THYMIDYLATE

Special interest is attached to dTMP, the deoxyribonucleotide uniquely associated with DNA synthesis. It, too, arises via de novo and salvage pathways. The de novo pathway of dTMP synthesis in which thymidylate synthetase catalyzes the methylation of dUMP by N^5,N^{10}-methylene tetrahydrofolate, is the major synthetic route. It can be roughly quantified by assaying the incorporation of ^{14}C-formate into DNA thymidine. In leukocytes, considerably more formate is incorporated into DNA thymidine than into purine. Many data have accumulated on the de novo pathway of dTMP synthesis in hematopoietic cells.[7]

In the salvage pathway, dTMP is synthesized by a thymidine kinase-catalyzed phosphorylation of thymidine.[49] Thymidine comes from food sources, from the breakdown of DNA, from the dephosphorylation of intracellular dTMP, from the action of pyrimidine deoxyribosyl transferase, and deoxythymidine phosphorylase on free thymidine, and (in cytokinetics laboratories) from the administration of ^3H-TdR.

The relative importance of de novo and salvage pathways of thymidylate synthesis in myeloid cells has been assessed.[50,51] Thymidylate arises increasingly from exogenous thymidine with increasing exogenous thymidine concentration. With increasing concentrations of exogenous thymidine, incorporation of ^3H-TdR into the dTMP, dTDP, and dTTP pools is considerably greater in leukemic leukocytes than in normal leukocytes.

BIOSYNTHESIS OF DNA

The polymerization of deoxyribonucleotides into DNA is catalyzed by the DNA polymerases. Little is known of this class of enzymes in human hematopoietic cells. A major technical problem in assaying polymerase in crude extracts is the abundance of contaminating deoxyribonucleases and phosphatases that may attack substrate deoxynucleoside triphosphates. Also, it is not known how many DNA polymerases blood cells contain. Precise functions remain to be determined of the three that have been found in *E coli*.[52]

DNA polymerase activity is highest in immature myeloid cells. Levels fall with maturation to barely detectable levels. It is not clear whether the decline in DNA polymerase accounts for the decreased mitotic potential beyond the myelocyte stage of maturation or whether other factors are responsible. The DNA polymerase level of circulating cells from patients with chronic myelocytic leukemia is tenfold higher than the activity of equally immature bone marrow cells from nonleukemic patients. Hence, the increase in polymerase activity may not be attributable solely to cell immaturity.

The recent evidence[53,54] that oncogenic RNA viruses synthesize DNA from an RNA template provides a mechanism for an "antidogma" reversal in the flow of genetic information and new insights into how an RNA virus might affect an animal cell. Recently, Gallo reported the detection of an analogous enzyme in human acute leukemia cells[55] and showed that within the limits of assay sensitivity, activity was not detectable in normal lymphocytes. Partially purified enzyme is inhibited by *N*-dimethylrifampicin. In contrast, DNA-dependent DNA polymerase from normal lymphoblasts is not significantly inhibited. Interpretation of these results is complicated by the fact that RNA-dependent DNA polymerase has been found in nononcognenic viruses. These results raise many interesting issues, to the resolution of which research must now be directed.

MITOCHRONDRIAL DNA

The discovery of recent years that the mitochondrion is a semiautonomous organelle with its own DNA, DNA polymerase, and ribosomes also raises important biologic questions. Is DNA synthesis in mitochondria dependent on an extramitochondrial source of deoxyribonucleoside triphosphates or do mitochondria contain their own enzymes of deoxyribonucleotide metabolism? If they contain a ribonucleotide reductase, is it similar or different from the one that furnishes deoxyribonucleotides for nuclear DNA synthesis? In light of the many findings suggesting that mitochondria are evolutionary descendants of bacteria, can the list be extended to include a bacterial-type reductase system?

It is of interest that mitochondrial DNA consists of several structural forms. One form, a circular dimer, was discovered in leukemic leukocytes but not in normal cells.[56] The conclusion that this finding might relate to the oncogenic process was weakened by the later finding of dimers in L-cells.[57]

In view of the complexity of mitochondrial structure and function, the opportunities seem abundant for abnormalities of both. The possible implication for the cell of mitochondrial abnormalities is a virtually untouched question. Although little is known of the functional significance of mitochondrial DNA, it is vital to eukaryotic cells. Variations in base ratios of mitochondrial DNA indicate that it shares with nuclear DNA the ability to mutate. The presence of multiple copies and the circular structure no doubt confer stability, but mutations would be likely to survive if they promoted an increase in the rate of mitochondrial DNA replication. This situation is believed to account for the petite mutation in yeast.[58] Also of interest is a recent report that antimycin A causes the mitochondria of *Euglena gracilis* to fuse and enlarge.[59] The metabolic consequences of such changes are uninvestigated.

CONSPECTUS

The foregoing brief notes on the biosynthesis of the nucleic acids and their precursors must now be viewed in the context of the problems of drug toxicity. What can we learn about one from consideration of the other?

One has a number of impressions at this point. The first is a relatively simple-minded notion. Any drug that blocks the biosynthesis of DNA or any other essential cell constituent will jeopardize the survival of a cell line. Inhibition of DNA replication will eventually affect the cell's ability to divide. This familiar concept is at the basis of our insistent efforts to block DNA synthesis in leukemic cells or solid tumors with antimetabolites and chemotherapeutic events. To a greater or lesser extent, such drugs inevitably affect DNA synthesis in the bone marrow. Similarly, impairment of DNA synthesis is the basis of bone marrow impairments of megaloblastic anemia,[43] which arise not only from deficiencies of essential vitamins, but from the entrance of drugs that interfere with the metabolism of these vitamins (e.g., methotrexate, diphenylhydantoin, and others). In sum, one whole class of drugs affecting DNA synthesis in bone marrow acts by inhibiting one or another of the steps in the pathways described above. Some are antimetabolites that compete with substrates (e.g., 5-fluorouracil, cytosine, arabinoside, and others). Indeed, such antimetabolites have been useful tools in the elucidation of steps in the pathway of nucleotide metabolism. Others are incorporated into DNA and thereby modify it (e.g., 6-mercaptopurine, 5-azacytidine, 5-bromodeoxyuridine, and others). Others are direct inhibitors of critical enzymes (e.g., hydroxyurea), and so on.

Though familiar, this facet of the drug problem is extremely important. Also, it is one in which it is possible to explicate many toxic drug effects on the basis of well understood "enzymatic mechanisms." Moreover, these effects are manifested almost exclusively in terms of the cell's proliferative capacity. This realization leads to the suspicion that toxic effects of drugs could very well extend beyond proliferative capabilities, even when nucleic acid metabolism is the target. In considering this possibility, I am struck by the fact that much that is interesting in the field of DNA synthesis remains to be discovered. This is clearly indicated by recent reviews[52,60] and by the proceedings of a major symposium held at the last national meeting of the biochemical society.[61] It can be argued, I think, that it is in the unexplored areas where many toxic drug effects will be ultimately explained. I refer to mechanisms such as the initiation of DNA synthesis, mechanisms of chain elongation and chromosome replication (what, for example, is the significance of "repetitive" DNA in animal cell chromosomes?), relations of the cell membrane to DNA replication, the consequences of mutational alteration of enzymes of DNA synthesis, and more. Many of these matters are just now being resolved for bacterial systems. A long journey must be taken before we can extend these concepts to animal cells and then we must elucidate their special features in bone marrow cells.

The field of nucleic acid metabolism was, of course, arbitrarily emphasized in this essay. Quite obviously, drug effects may be mediated through other pathways and systems. However, even within this sphere it seems likely that in the future we will recognize more and more drug effects that involve interactions with nucleic acid biochemistry but that do not grossly impair DNA synthesis and do not manifest themselves primarily as abnormalities of cell divisions. Such actions may be consequences of subtle effects on one or more of the yet-to-be studied facets of nucleic acid metabolism. In a sense, the mutagenic agents, which can alter DNA in diverse ways, presage this category, for the effects of mutation can be greatly amplified and thus far-reaching.

This leads to a closing thought that occult chemicals or pollutants possibly affect the metabolic pathways described above. A cogent example was the discovery, by McKinney and coworkers, that hypoplastic or aplastic anemia can be regularly induced in calves by the single dose or oral administration of a small quantity of S-(1,2-dichlorovinyl)-l-cysteine, a compound that had been discovered as a feed contaminant. Later work by Schultze established that the thymus glands and bone marrow of affected animals acquired a species of DNA that differs in physical and enzymatic properties from normal calf nuclear DNA.[63] In this instance, DNA appears to have been altered as it might have been by an alkylating agent. Of interest to us today is the fact that the apparent result was marrow hypoplasia. In my opinion, this account provides a potential paradigm of the way in which occult chemical substances can exert toxic effects.

Drug-induced cell injury may be affected by many factors—among them the extent of drug entry into the cell, the nature of the "biochemical lesion" produced, the cell's capacity to circumvent this lesion by an alternative pathway, replacement, or repair, and the time permitted for recovery or repair before, by reason of some cellular event, the drug-induced lesion becomes lethal. The "toxicity" of any drug, in the final analysis, is the sum total of its interactions with cell constituents, the potential of these interactions to produce metabolic alterations, and the cell's response to these alterations. As Farber has pointed out,[64] the analysis of the mechanism of toxicity is an important undertaking for both practical and theoretic reasons. Its practical importance stems from the need to interrupt or circumvent the process in the continuing presence of the hazard. The theoretic aspect is the use of "toxic" chemicals as metabolic probes in the analysis of biologic mechanisms on which organisms depend in their responses to environmental hazards.

I have attempted in this essay to point out that the identification of a primary biochemical lesion, though essential, may be insufficient by itself to establish the cell's response and the subsequent course of events. Metazoan cells, like metazoan organisms, have evolved many ways of responding to homeostatic disturbances. A more dynamic understanding of toxic drug effects may have to await a more sophisticated understanding of these response patterns.

SUMMARY

Present knowledge of the enzymatic makeup of the hematopoietic system is limited, and it is possible, only to a meager extent, to explicate fundamental mechanisms of hematopoiesis in terms of enzymatic mechanisms. In part, this limitation is traceable to the fact that knowledge of animal cell metabolism lags behind knowledge of bacterial cell metabolism. In addition, specific problems arise in the application of current knowledge of animal cell metabolism to hematopoietic cells. These problems are considered in some detail.

To place what knowledge we have in the context of the problems of drug effects, an attempt is made to outline some of the physiologic mechanisms and kinetic properties of the hematopoietic system that await biochemical explanation. The system, it is shown, has an unusually high rate of proliferative activity and displays certain unusual biologic properties, which any biochemical model must take into account.

The enzymatic and metabolic properties of the hematopoietic system are briefly reviewed. These include properties that have been discovered in direct studies of bone marrow and those that have been inferred from studies of the normal and abnormal blood cells produced by bone marrow. Major attention is given to the biosynthetic pathways of RNA and DNA and of their nucleotide precursors.

In conclusion, it is suggested that it is perhaps premature to attempt a detailed assessment of the mode of action of many toxic drugs on pathways of nucleic acid metabolism in view of the fact that many important facets of these pathways have not yet been discovered. These include the mechanism by which DNA synthesis is initiated, the mechanism of chain growth, the relations of cell membrance to DNA replication, and so on. In view of this diversity of mechanisms, drugs surely have many targets of opportunity. Those that block the biosynthetic pathway of DNA are already well known. The suggestion is offered that drugs affecting other facets of nucleic acid replication may well manifest themselves in ways unrelated to gross proliferative behavior. Conceivably, some effects may parallel those of the mutagenic agents. Such phenomena may account for the tendency of occult chemicals or pollutants to produce marrow hypoplasia or aplasia.

REFERENCES

1. Beck WS, Valentine WN: The carbohydrate metabolism of leukocytes; review. Cancer Res 13:309, 1953
2. Beck WS: Biochemical properties of normal and leukemic leukocytes, International Symposium on Leukemia-Lymphoma. Edited by CJD Zarafonetis. Philadelphia, Lea and Febinger, 1968
3. Bazin S, Delaunay A: Biochimie des polynucleaires neutrophiles. Rev Franc Etude Clin Biol 1:1019, 1956
4. Cline MJ: Metabolism of the circulating leukocyte. Physiol Rev 45:674, 1965
5. Lajtha LG: Bone marrow cell metabolism. Physiol Rev 37:50, 1957
6. Silber R, Bertino JR: Metabolism of granulocytes, Hematology. Edited by

WJ Williams, E. Beutler, AJ Erslev, et al. New York, McGraw-Hill, 1972, p 575
7. Gallo RC: Synthesis and metabolism of DNA and DNA precursors by human normal and leukemic leukocytes. Acta Haematol 45:136, 1971
8. Cline MJ: Metabolism of RNA in normal and leukemic cells. Acta Haematol 45:174, 1971
9. Beck WS: Leukocyte metabolism. Ser Haematol 1, 4:69, 1968
10. Boutwell RK: Some biological aspects of skin carcinogenesis. Prog Exp Tumor Res 4:207, 1964
11. Potter VR: Biochemical perspectives in cancer research. Cancer Res 24:1085, 1964
12. Warburg O: Uber den Stoffwechsels der Tumoren. Berlin, Springer-Verlag, 1926
13. Burk D: A colloquial consideration of the Pasteur and neo-Pasteur effects. Cold Spring Harbor Symp Quant Biol 7:420, 1939
14. Donohue DM, Reiff RH, Hanson ML, et al: Quantitative measurement of the erythrocytic and granulocytic cells of the marrow and blood. J Clin Invest 37:1571–1576, 1958
15. Patt HM: A consideration of myeloid-erythroid balance in man. Blood 12:777, 1957
16. Suit HD: A technique for estimating the bone marrow cellularity in vivo using ^{59}Fe. J Clin Pathol 10:267, 1957
17. Beck WS: The control of leukocyte glycolysis. J Biol Chem 232:251, 1958
18. Weiss L: The structure of bone marrow. Functional interrelationships of vascular and hematopoietic compartments in experimental hemolytic anemia: an electron microscopic study. J Morphol 117:467, 1965
19. Metcalf D, Moore MAS: Haemopoietic Cells. New York, Elsevier, 1971, p 22
20. Williams WJ: Examination of the bone marrow. p 23
21. Cartwright GE, Athens JW, Wintrobe MM: The kinetics of granulopoiesis in man. Blood 24:780, 1964
22. Perry S: Proliferation of myeloid cells. Ann Rev Med 22:171, 1971
23. Cronkite EP, Vincent PC: Granulocytopoiesis. Ser Haematol 2:3, 1969
24. Morley AA: A neutrophil cycle in healthy individuals. Lancet 2:1220, 1966
25. Katz R, Gordon AS, Lapin DM: Mechanisms of leukocyte production and release. VI. Studies on the purification of the leukocytosis-inducing factor (LIF). J Reticuloendothel Soc 3:103, 1966
26. Weisskotten HG, Schwartz SC, Steenstand HS: The action of benzol. II. The deuterophase of the biphasic leucopenia and antigen-antibody reaction. J Med Res 35:63, 1916
27. Patt HM, Maloney MA: A model of granulocyte kinetics. Ann NY Acad Sci 113:515, 1964
28. Bainton DF, Farquhar MG: Origin of granules in polymorphonuclear leukocytes. Two types derived from opposite faces of the Golgi complex in developing granulocytes. J Cell Biol 28:277, 1966
29. Prescott DM: Sequential events of the cell life cycle, Exploitable Molecular Mechanisms and Neoplasia. Twenty-second Annual Symposium on Fundamental Cancer Research, 1968. Baltimore, Williams and Wilkins, 1969, p 359
30. Tobey RA, Anderson EC, Petersen DF: RNA stability and protein synthesis in relation to the division of mammalian cells. Proc Natl Acad Sci USA 56:1520, 1966
31. King TJ, Briggs R: Changes in the nuclei of differentiating gastrula cells, as demonstrated by nuclear transplantation. Proc Natl Acad Sci USA 41:321, 1955
32. Gross PR: Biochemistry of differentiation. Ann Rev Biochem 37:638, 1968

33. Gurdon JB: On the origin and persistence of a cytoplasmic state inducing nuclear DNA synthesis in frogs' eggs. Proc Natl Acad Sci USA 58:545, 1967
34. Hale AJ: The leucocyte as a possible exception to the theory of deoxyribonucleic acid constancy. J Pathol Bacteriol 85:311, 1963
35. Hale AJ, Cooper EH, Milton JD: Studies of the incorporation of pyrimidines into DNA in single leukaemic and other proliferating leucocytes. Br J Haematol 11:144, 1965
36. Beck WS: The biochemistry of ribonucleotide and ribonucleic acid in normal and malignant cells, Cell Physiology of Neoplasia. Fourteenth Annual Symposium on Fundamental Cancer Research. Austin, University of Texas Press, 1960, p 374
37. Scott JL: Human leukocyte metabolism in vitro. I. Incorporation of adenine-8-^{14}C into the nucleic acids of leukemic leukocytes. J Clin Invest 41:67, 1962
38. Lajtha LG, Vane JR: Dependence of bone marrow cells on the liver for purine supply. Nature (Lond) 182:191, 1958
39. Smith LH Jr, Baker FA: Pyrimidine metabolism in man. III. Studies on leukocytes and erythrocytes in pernicious anemia. J Clin Invest 39:15, 1960
40. Smith LH Jr, Baker FA, Sullivan M: Pyrimidine metabolism in man. II. Studies of leukemic cells. Blood 15:360, 1960
41. Bertles JF, Beck WS: Biochemical aspects of reticulocyte maturation. I. Fate of the ribonucleic acid. J Biol Chem 237:3770, 1962
42. Larsson A, Reichard P: Enzymatic reduction of ribonucleotides. Prog Nucleic Acid Res Mol Biol 7:303, 1967
43. Beck WS: Deoxyribonucleotide synthesis and the role of vitamin B_{12} in erythropoiesis. Vitam Horm 26:413, 1968
44. Beck WS: Regulation of cobamide-dependent ribonucleotide reductase by allosteric effectors and divalent cations. J Biol Chem 242:3148, 1967
45. Abeles RH, Beck WS: The mechanism of action of cobamide coenzyme in the ribonucleotide reductase reaction. J Biol Chem 242:3589, 1967
46. Brown NC, Eliasson R, Reichard P, et al: Nonheme iron as a cofactor in ribonucleotide reductase from *E coli*. Biochem Biophys Res Commun 30:522, 1968
47. Moore EC, Hurlbert RB: Regulation of mammalian deoxyribonucleotide biosynthesis by nucleotides as activators and inhibitors. J Biol Chem 241:4802, 1966
48. Hopper S: Ribonucleotide reductase of rabbit bone marrow. I. Purification, properties, and separation into two protein fractions. J Biol Chem 247:3336, 1972
49. Silber R: Feedback inhibition of deoxyribonucleotide interconversion in human leukocytes. J Clin Invest 43:1248, 1964
50. Cooper RA, Perry S, Breitman TR: Pyrimidine metabolism in human leukocytes, I. Contribution of exogenous thymidine to DNA-thymine and its effect on thymine nucleotide synthesis in leukemic leukocytes. Cancer Res 26:2267, 1966
51. Cooper RA, Perry S, Breitman TR: Pyrimidine metabolism in human leukocytes, II. Metabolism of the thymine nucleotide pools in normal and leukemic leukocytes. Cancer Res 26:2276, 1966
52. Goulian M: Some recent developments in DNA enzymology. Prog Nucleic Acid Res Mol Biol 12:29, 1972
53. Baltimore D: RNA-Dependent DNA polymerase in virions of RNA tumor viruses. Nature (Lond) 226:1209, 1970
54. Temin HM, Mizutani S: RNA-dependent DNA polymerase in virions of Rous sarcoma virus. Nature (Lond) 226:1211, 1970

55. Gallo RC, Yang SS, Ting RC: RNA-dependent DNA polymerase of human acute leukaemic cells. Nature (Lond) 228:927, 1970
56. Clayton DA, Vinograd J: Complex mitochondrial DNA in leukemic and normal human myeloid cells. Proc Natl Acad Sci USA 62:1077, 1969
57. Nass MMK: Reversible generation of circular dimer and higher multiple forms of mitochondrial DNA. Nature (Lond) 223:1124, 1969
58. Carnevali F, Morpurgo G, Tecce G: Cytoplasmic DNA from petite colonies of Saccharomyces, cerevisiae: a hypothesis on the nature of the mutation. Science 163:1331, 1969
59. Calvayrac R, Van Lente F, Butow RA: Euglena gracilis: formation of giant mitochrondria. Science 173:252, 1971
60. Klein A, Bonhoeffer F: DNA replication. Ann Rev Biochem 41:301, 1972
61. Biochemistry Society Symposium: Replication and transcription of DNA. Fed Proc 31:1415, 1972
62. McKinney LI, Weakley FB, Eldridge AC, et al: S-(dichlorovinyl)-L-cysteine: an agent causing fatal aplastic anemia in calves. J Am Chem Soc 79:3932, 1957
63. Bhattacharya RK, Schultze MO: Properties of DNA isolated from tissues of calves treated with S-(1,2-dichlorovinyl)-L-cysteine. Arch Biochem Biophys 145:565, 1971
64. Farber E: Biochemical pathology. Ann Rev Pharmacol 11:71, 1971

Nabih I. Abdou

3

Immunosuppression: Brief Review and Future Hopes

This review of immunosuppression (IS) is a brief and critical discussion of current modes of therapy directed towards suppressing the immune response (IR) in man. It is not intended to be complete but will stress the problems encountered in suppressing a clinical state and will be based on our current and recent knowledge in the field of immunology. Future hopes and current achievements of IS by specific immunologic means will be emphasized. Our goal is to administer the ideal immunosuppressive agent (ISA) which should (a) be specific for the antigen or antibody causing the disease; (b) not be lethal for vital structures, e.g., hemopoiesis and epithelial integrity; and (c) not interfere with established protective immunity or memory.

The review will briefly emphasize four main points: (a) recent advances in the field of immunology as they apply to IS; (b) briefly outline modes of action of current nonspecific ISA, their uses and complications; (c) specific IS by means of antigen, antibodies, or antigen in combination with cytotoxic drugs, describing a few illustrations of successful trials in man; (d) outline of a few promising, but still experimental, approaches that should be considered in the future for specific IS in man.

RECENT BASIC IMMUNOLOGIC CONCEPTS OF RELEVANCE TO IMMUNOSUPPRESSION

Several recent findings in the field of cellular immunology have enhanced our understanding about the cells engaged in IR. The primary IR for most antigens requires the participation of more than one cell type.[1,2] These are

Supported in part by VA grants TR-39 and 642-0030 and by grant AI 00319 from the US Public Health Service.

antigen processing cells, antigen reactive cells, and effector cells that secrete antibody or affect a target tissue or organ. Cell cooperation between thymus dependent (T) and bone marrow dependent (B) cells was shown to be essential for most antigens for antibody production and cell-mediated immunity.[2] Both T- and B-cell systems were postulated to be formed of more than one cell type.[3] The T (T_1, T_2) and B (B_1, B_2) subpopulations represent various degrees of differentiation and/or maturation. Specific markers for each cell type have been described.[4,5] Immunoglobulin molecules (Receptors) were found to be the markers for B cells,[6] and were responsible for the selection of antigen by specific clones of cells.[1] Both theta[5] and transplantation antigens[7] were shown to be the markers for T cells. Successful manipulation of the IR is dependent on (a) cell type against which ISA is directed; (b) class, subclass, and avidity of immunoglobulin secreted by the cells; (c) immunogenicity of antigen and whether it is autoantigen or exogenous antigen; (d) whether ISA is introduced prior to recognition of the antigen and commitment of specific clones of cells, during the proliferative phase of IR or at the efferent phase after the damage of the target organ had occurred.

Table 1 illustrates the current modes used for IS. Combination of one or more of these approaches had been used. There are certain points that have to be answered before immunosuppressive therapy is started. (a) Is there evidence that immune mechanisms play a role in the disease process? If that is the case, what is the nature of antigen(s) and effector mechanism(s) causing the disease? (b) Is IS directed towards an established ongoing IR or will ISA be administered prior to exposure to the antigen? (c) What indices will be taken for adequate IS? (d) Are there adequate measures for close follow-up of patients and early detection of complications?

Table 1
Approaches to Immunosuppression

Specific Agents: Antigen, Antibody
Nonspecific Agents
Drugs
Glucocorticoids
Alkylating Agents: Cyclophosphamide
Antimetabolites: Purine (Imuran), Pyrimidine (5 FU), and Folic Acid Antagonists (Methotrexate)
Antibiotics: Actinomycin-C
Biologic Agents
Antilymphocyte Globulin
Serum Inhibitors: α-2-Macroglobulin
Complement Inhibitors: Epsilon amino caproic acid
Infectious Agents: Measles
Radiation
Whole body or local
Surgical ablation
Thymectomy, thoracic duct drainage

IMMUNOSUPPRESSION BY NONSPECIFIC AGENTS

Immunosuppression by alkylating agents, antimetabolites, steroids, antilymphocyte serum (globulin), radiation, surgical ablation, and various other nonspecific measures had been covered extensively in several recent reviews.[8–10] The points to be emphasized when using these nonspecific approaches are that they are not solely directed against the cell, agent, or humoral factor causing the disease and that their effectiveness in controlling the disease state had not been critically analyzed.[11] In fact, in a long-term study we had shown that administration of azathioprine in therapeutic doses to man does not affect immunoglobulin levels or the immunocompetence of the antigen reactive cell.[12] The drug was, however, partially effective in suppressing cells engaged in the effector phase of the IR.[12] Despite the above criticisms against nonspecific ISA, they are still needed to condition the host or graft or, in their administration in conjunction with specific IS, to induce long-lasting unresponsiveness or IS.[9]

Table 2 illustrates the modes of action of commonly used ISA. It should be emphasized that though several mechanisms had been shown and postulated for IS by cytotoxic drugs, their precise mode of action is still unclear and unsettled.[11] Moreover, due to species differences—results of IS by drugs in animals cannot be extended to man.[10] The continued use of cytotoxic drugs in man is associated by many hazards. These include (a) infections by bacteria, viruses, fungi, and intracellular parasites; (b) irreversible suppression of hemopoietic elements; (c) interference with immune surveillance mechanism, thus leading to proliferation of mutant cells with subsequent neoplasia, the magnitude of which in various disease states has not as yet been carefully studied.[13]

The effectiveness of various ISA needs critical and constructive analysis.[11] Very few adequate double-blind controlled studies had been done. The history of the disease and overall prognosis should be considered. In many trials ISA was started in advanced complicated terminal cases, which makes adequate analysis of drug effectiveness almost impossible. Also, the drugs were given to patients suffering from diseases in which immune mechanisms played no role in the pathogenesis of the disease. In these cases, it is uncertain whether the benefit from the drug would be due to its anti-inflammatory effect or to some unknown mechanism. Therefore, the use of ISA in these diseases should be

Table 2
Immunosuppressive Drugs: Possible Mechanisms of Action

Alkylating Agents
Biologic inactivation of DNA through cross-linkage
Antimetabolites
Incorporation into nucleic acid
Competition of essential enzymatic reaction
Antibiotics
Blocks RNA-dependent DNA synthesis
Steroids
Anti-inflammatory

critically reviewed and the benefits that could be gained should be considered against the many hazards and complications that these drugs cause, including hemopoietic suppression, decreasing host-defense mechanisms against infections, possible chromosomal aberrations, and alteration of the normal immune surveillance mechanism.

SPECIFIC IMMUNOSUPPRESSION

Recent advances in immunology and the realization that the IR is extremely specific and that nonspecific ISA are hazardous, have led several investigators to consider manipulating the IR with specific immunologic agents. This approach has been rewarding in man in several clinical states. Specific antibody, specific antigen, or specific antigen in conjunction with cytotoxic drugs have been used.

Specific Immunosuppression by Antibody

There are general principles that have to be borne in mind when using antibodies for IS:[14] (a) they are effective only if given during the first exposure to antigen and probably only in immune states involving serum antibody of cytotoxic type and not reaginic type; (b) the antibody to be used should be specific to the antigen and of high avidity. There are, however, recent reports indicating that anti-immunoglobulin (antireceptor antibodies) may be valuable in suppressing graft-versus-host reactions[15] and in the recognition of transplantation antigens in vitro, as tested by the mixed leukocyte reaction.[16] One of the most promising approaches in transplantation immunity is the use of enhancing antibodies.[17] Whether these antibodies affect the central or efferent phases of the IR is still unsettled. Their effectiveness is dependent on their efficiency in binding to the antigen(s) prior to its recognition by the host and/or their coating of target tissues, thus preventing them from contact with sensitized cells.[18] The value of anti-Rh antibody in preventing Rh sensitization of Rh negative mothers carrying Rh positive babies is well accepted.[19]

Immunosuppression by Specific Antigens

The mechanisms by which antigens suppress the IR is not the same in all cases. Antigens, when given to immunoincompetent hosts, are capable of inducing specific unresponsiveness, probably by blocking and/or eliminating the specific reactive clones of cells.[20] Solubilized forms of transplantation antigens, prepared from donors of grafts and given to recipients, are promising tools to alleviate graft rejection.[20] The use of aggregate-free horse globulin was found useful in decreasing the incidence of reactions to horse antihuman lymphocyte globulin.[21] The administration of derivatives of penicillin were shown to be effective in specific prevention of reactions due to penicillin.[22] Prolonged administration of ragweed allergen could alleviate symptoms of allergic rhinitis in ragweed-sensitive patients.[23]

Immunosuppression by Antigen and Drugs

Specific elimination of antigen-reactive cells by administering specific antigen and a few hours later a short course of large doses of alkylating agent or antimetabolite had been used with considerable success in ameliorating graft rejection by the host.[24] A similar approach had been used in a few patients with hemophilia and high levels of anti-Factor VIII antibodies.[25] Amelioration of lupus nephritis in NZB/NZW mice by similar approaches, using synthetic RNA as the antigen, was reported.[26] The long-term effectiveness of these approaches needs to be analyzed critically. Moreover, similar modes of therapy in various unwanted immune responses in man with known etiologies should be considered.

RECENT PROMISING APPROACHES FOR IMMUNOSUPPRESSION

The dissection of the immune system into various compartments, and cell types and the demonstration, by various investigators, of cell receptors responsible for the extreme specificity of those cells led to experiments aimed at (a) depleting the host of specific unwanted components of the immune system or (b) manipulating and/or modulating the immune system. A brief outline of these approaches will be discussed.

Exclusion or Depletion of Components Engaged in the Immune Response: Depletion of Specific Clones of Antigen Reactive or Antibody Forming Cells

The discovery of specific recognition units on precursors of antibody forming cells prompted Wigzell[27] and us[4] to pass immunocompetent cells through columns filled with glass beads coated with antigen or with anti-immunoglobulin. In various experimental designs, it was found that the specific cells were retained on the columns. Cells that passed through the column, when tested both in vivo and in vitro, were deficient in cells capable of reacting with the antigen used to coat the glass beads. The concept of specific immunoadsorbents was then extended to include immunofiltration of circulating antigens or antibodies.[28] The elimination of either bone marrow-dependent or thymus-dependent cells by specific antisera was also accomplished.[29]

Modulation of the Immune Response

Specific antibody formation could be prevented or made sluggish by administering antibody prior to the antigen, thus creating feedback inhibition before inducing the immune response. Similar results could be achieved by specific killing of reactive cells. This was accomplished in vitro by administering antigen and then excluding cells that would proliferate in response to that antigen by adding radioactive thymidine with high specific activity or 5-bromodeoxyuridine followed by exposure to ultraviolet rays.[29]

Imbalance between the T and B systems was shown to be associated with certain experimental models of autoimmunity.[30] Manipulating the immune system by augmenting T-cell activity could ameliorate the lupus syndrome in aged NZB/NZW mice.[30]

In conclusion, it could be seen that various modern immunologic concepts have helped the understanding of various modes by which the IR could be suppressed. The rationale for using cytotoxic drugs or nonspecific ISA will very soon find very few supporters. The use of those drugs in combination with various specific approaches is promising and has shown its beneficial effects in bone marrow transplantation and certain abnormal antibody states. If the immune mechanisms involved in the pathogenesis of the disease state is clearly known, treatment with specific immunotherapy is certainly rewarding.

SUMMARY

The various phases of the immune response cannot be suppressed to the same extent by various immunosuppressive agents (ISA). Maximum immunosuppression (IS) could be achieved by giving ISA with or prior to the commitment of specific clones of cells. Various nonspecific ISA are being used. These include alkylating agents, antimetabolites, steroids, antilymphocyte globulin, irradiation, and surgical ablation. All of these agents suppress proliferating cells engaged in various body functions or they interfere with the effector mechanisms of the immune response. They are associated with or followed by many hazards as decreasing host defense mechanisms against various infections and may interfere with immune surveillance.

The ideal ISA should be specific and directed only against the antigen, antibody, immune complex, mediators, or cells causing the disease. It should neither be lethal for vital structures—hemopoiesis and epithelial integrity—nor interfere with protective immunity. Specific IS in man has been achieved in certain cases by specific antibody, specific antigen, or by specific antigen combined with cytotoxic drugs. IS by antibody proved successful in preventing sensitization in Rh disease. Enhancing antibodies have been successful in prolonging allogeneic grafts. Suppression by specific antigens is being evaluated in allergic states due to ragweed and penicillin. Use of solubilized transplantation antigens is being tried to induce tolerance to tissue grafts. Administration of the aggregate-free form of the antigen suppressed reactions to horse antilymphocyte globulin in man. Specific elimination of antigen-reactive cells by administering the specific antigen followed by cytotoxic drugs was successful in prolonging bone marrow grafts, in decreasing circulating anticoagulants in man, and in ameliorating experimental lupus nephritis.

Several recent experimental approaches have been successful in IS. These are (a) elimination of specific cells by passage through antigen-coated glass bead columns or layering on various immunoadsorbents; (b) suicidal exclusion of cells by radioactive antigen or 5-bromodeoxyuridine; (c) compartmental depletion of specific cells by the in vivo exposure to antigens. In conclusion, specific IS with the hope of modulating or manipulating various components of the immune system is rewarding and should be our goal.

REFERENCES

1. Abdou NI, Richter M: Role of bone marrow in the immune response. Adv Immunol 12:201, 1970
2. Miller JFAP, Basten A, Sprent J, et al: Interaction between lymphocytes in immune responses. Cell Immunol 2:469, 1971
3. Greaves MF, Hogg NM: Immunoglobulin determinants on the surface of antigen binding T- and B-lymphocytes in mice. Prog Immunol 1:111, 1971
4. Abdou NI: Immunoglobulin receptors on human peripheral leukocytes II Class restriction of Ig receptors. J Immunol 107:1637, 1971
5. Bianco C, Nussenzweig V: Theta-bearing and complement receptor lymphocytes are distinct populations of cells. Science 173:154, 1971
6. Froland S, Natvig JB: Surface-bound immunoglobulin as a marker of B lymphocytes in man. Nature (New Biol) 234:251, 1971
7. Sprent J, Miller JFAP: Activation of thymus cells by histocompatibility antigens. Nature (New Biol) 234:195, 1971
8. Parker CW, Vaura JD: Immunosuppression. Prog Hematol 6:1, 1969
9. Lance EM: Immunosuppression, Clinical Immunobiology. Edited by FH Bach, RA Good. New York, Academic, 1972
10. Schwartz RS: Immunosuppressive drug therapy, Human transplantation. Edited by FT Rapaport, J Dausset. New York, Grune and Stratton, 1968
11. Skinner MD, Schwartz RS: Immunosuppressive therapy. N Engl J Med 287:221, 1972
12. Abdou NI, Zweiman B, Casella S: Effects of azathioprine therapy on bone marrow dependent and thymus dependent cells in man. Clin Exp Immunol 13:55, 1973.
13. Schwartz RS, Hellstrom K: Routes of escape from surveillance, Immune Surveillance. Edited by RT Smith, M Landy. New York, Academic, 1970
14. Uhr JW, Moller G: Regulatory effect of antibody on the immune response. Adv Immunol 8:81, 1968
15. Riethmuller G, Rieber E-P, Seeger I: Suppression of graft versus host reaction by univalent anti-immunoglobulin antibody. Nature (New Biol) 230:248, 1971
16. Froland SS, Natvig JB: Effect of polyspecific rabbit anti-immunoglobulin antisera on the response of human lymphocytes in mixed lymphocyte culture. Int Arch Allergy 41:248, 1971
17. Feldman JD: Immunological enhancement: a study of blocking antibodies. Adv Immunol 15:167, 1972
18. Voisin GA: Immunological facilitation, a broadening of the concept of the enhancement phenomenon. Prog Allergy 15:328, 1971
19. Clark CA: Prevention of Rhesus isoimmunization. Semin Hematol 6:201, 1969
20. Uhr JW, Cohn M: Speculation on cellular and molecular mechanisms involved in immunological responsiveness and tolerance, Immunological tolerance. Edited by M Landy, W Braun. New York, Academic Press, 1969
21. Weksler ME, Bull G, Schwartz GH, et al: Immunologic responses of graft recipients to antilymphocyte globulin: effect of prior treatment with aggregate-free gamma globulin. J Clin Invest 49:1589, 1970
22. DeWeck AL, Schneider CH: Specific inhibition of allergic reactions to penicillin in man by a monovalent hapten. Int Arch Allergy 42:782, 1972
23. Lichtenstein LM, Norman PS, Winkenwerder WL: A single year of immunotherapy for ragweed hay fever: immunologic and clinical studies. Ann Intern Med 75:663, 1971

24. Santos GW, Owens AH: A comparison of selected cytotoxic agents on the primary agglutinin response in rats injected with sheep erythrocytes. Bull Johns Hopkins Hosp 114:384, 1964
25. Green D: Suppression of an antibody to factor VIII by a combination of factor VIII and cyclophosphamide. Blood 37:381, 1971
26. Steinberg AD, Baron S, Talal N: The pathogenesis of autoimmunity in New Zealand mice I Induction of antinucleic acid antibodies by polyinosinic-polycytidylic acid. Proc Natl Acad Sci 63:1102, 1969
27. Wigzell H: Cellular immunosorbants. Prog Immunol 1:1105, 1971
28. Schwartz RS, Moller G: Modulation of the antibody regulatory mechanism, Immunologic intervention. Edited by JW Uhr, M Landy. New York, Academic, 1971
29. Gowans JL, Dutton RW: Selective removal of lymphocyte subpopulations.[28]
30. Austen KF, Good RA: Approaches to intervention in immunopathologic models.[28]

Thomas G. Gabuzda

4
Drug-Hemoglobin Interactions

Until recently, drugs have been considered chiefly from the point of view of their adverse effect upon hemoglobin. Interest in such toxicity first arose in the last century with the development of the aniline dye industry in Germany and the concomitant awareness that exposed individuals at times developed methemoglobinemia and hemolytic anemia. During recent years the detailed investigation of the structure of hemoglobin and its relation to the proper function of the molecule has launched a new effort to find drugs which will be of therapeutic benefit in patients who suffer pathologic consequences of inherited abnormalities of hemoglobin. Of these, the two most important are homozygous β-thalassemia, in which oxidative damage to unstable globin subunits causes extensive hemolysis, and sickle cell disease, in which patients suffer from the adverse insolubility of deoxygenated abnormal hemoglobin.

Previous reviews of drug-induced methemoglobinemia and oxidative hemolysis have been written by Finch, by Bodansky, and by Jaffe and Heller in 1948, 1951, and 1964, respectively.[1–3]

DRUG-INDUCED METHEMOGLOBINEMIA AND HEMOLYSIS

Hemoglobin—by virtue of its heme iron as well as its thiol groups—is a redox compound. It is bathed in an environment rich in reducing substances. An electron "gap" is maintained which prevents its easy oxidation by the molecular oxygen it must transport. The slow spontaneous oxidation of ferro- to ferrihemoglobin at the rate of about 1% per day is easily reversed by the methemoglobin reductase system. An overwhelming oxidative stress accelerates methemoglobin formation and this is often associated with hemoglobin precipitation into insoluble Heinz bodies, which become attached to the membrane and cause hemolysis.[4,5] Whether the formation of methemoglobin is a necessary precursor to oxidative precipitation is still not known, but the two phenomena are commonly associated. Methemoglobinemia can exist in the absence of hemolysis. The relationship of oxidative hemolysis to methemoglobinemia may be appreciated by examining the structure of the hemoglobin molecule, with the focus directed at its redox properties.

There are ten redox "points" on the normal hemoglobin molecule, one for each of the four heme irons and six for the globin thiol groups, two of which are in each β chain and one in each α chain. The arrangement of these redox points in the molecule and their structural and functional relationships form a starting point for our approach to the problem of hemoglobin oxidation. The heme groups are tucked into clefts in the surface of the much larger globin molecule. These clefts, or "heme pockets," are lined with hydrophobic groupings which exclude water from reaching the heme moiety. Of the six coordinate positions of iron, four are occupied in attaching iron to the tetrapyrole structure. The fifth is bound to the "proximal" histidine, the ninety-second amino acid residue of the β chain and the eighty-seventh of the α chain. Oxygen is reversibly bound between the sixth coordinate position of iron and the "distal" histidine, which is the sixty-third residue in the β chain and the fifty-eighth of the α chain (Figure 1). A molecule of water displaces the oxygen when the iron is in the trivalent state. The precise position of the ferriporphyrin in its hydrophobic den and its suspension between the two histidines is fundamental to its normal reduction to the ferroporphyrin state by methemoglobin reductase. For example: when tyrosine is substituted for the distal histidine, its phenolic group replaces the water molecule and locks the ferriporphyrin into a state resistant to enzymatic

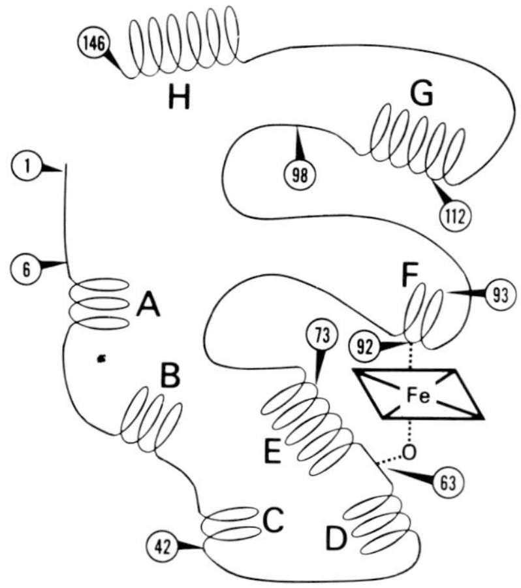

Fig. 1. Diagramatic representation of the β subunit of human hemoglobin. Eight helical regions are designated by the letters A through H. Interhelical regions are represented by letter pairs (e.g., CD). The heme is suspended between the proximal (No. 92) and distal (No. 63) histidines. Thiol groups are shown at No. 93 (reactive) and No. 112 (unreactive). Other numbers show the sites of amino acid substitutions listed in Table 1. The No. 1 and No. 146 represent the N-terminal and C-terminal sites, respectively. (Modified from Giblett ER: Genetic Markers in Human Blood. Oxford, Blackwell, 1969.)

Table 1
Some Abnormal Human Hemoglobins
(Referred to in the Text)

Hemoglobin	Amino Acid Substitution	Clinical Picture
M Saskatoon	β^{63} his → tyr	Methemoglobinemia
M Boston	α^{58} his → tyr	Methemoglobinemia
M Hyde Park	β^{92} his → tyr	Methemoglobinemia
M Iwate	α^{87} his → tyr	Methemoglobinemia
Köln	β^{98} val → met	Unstable hemoglobin; hemolysis
Zürich	β^{63} his → arg	Unstable hemoglobin; drug hemolysis
Hammersmith	β^{42} phe → ser	Unstable hemoglobin; hemolysis & cyanosis
Torino	α^{43} phe → val	Unstable hemoglobin; hemolysis
Sickle	β^{6} glu → val	Sickling
C Harlem	β^{6} glu → val β^{73} asp → asn	Ameliorates sickling
Korle-Bu	β^{73} asp → asn	Ameliorates sickling

reduction (Table 1). The resulting methemoglobinemia is not associated with significant hemolysis. Substitution of tyrosine for histidine at the proximal histidine also causes methemoglobinemia, the most acceptable explanation for which seems to be that the proximal and distal iron binding sites have reversed their usual roles.[6]

Of the six globin thiol groupings, none is readily reactive in the deoxyhemoglobin state while two, those at the β 93 position, immediately next to the proximal histidine, are readily reactive in the oxyhemoglobin state. The remaining thiols—one at each of the β 112 positions and one at each of the α 104 positions—are "masked" and remain unreactive until the molecular structure is unfolded. Thus the β 93 thiols are the first to become oxidized, forming a mixed disulfide of hemoglobin and glutathione, raising the oxygen affinity, and increasing the electrophoretic mobility of hemoglobin. As oxidation proceeds, the remaining thiols are oxidized, the molecules aggregate, and then finally precipitate as insoluble lumps of denatured hemoglobin.[7–9] The high erythrocytic concentration of reduced glutathione serves as its first line of defense against oxidation. Intracellular peroxides are among the most potent oxidative assailants; their oxidative fury is normally spent on reduced glutathione through the mediation of glutathione (GSH) peroxidase, thus protecting the thiol groups on the globin as well as on other cellular structures. If the GSH is overwhelmed either by virtue of the strength of the assault or by virtue of deficient cellular enzymes, globin thiols will be oxidized, as described, a process usually accompanied by some degree of methemoglobinemia. However, since both Heinz bodies and methemoglobin are formed preferentially in old cells, there is a general reciprocal relationship between the severity of hemolysis and the amount of methemoglobin measured in red cells; the older red cells contain most of the methemoglobin and are preferentially destroyed as a consequence of Heinz body formation.[10]

Subtle intramolecular relationships marry the interests of heme with those of the thiol groups on the globin molecule. The resistance of methemoglobin to precipitation in vitro, for example, is markedly enhanced by the insertion of a ligand, such as cyanide, to replace water at the sixth coordinate position of iron.[11,12] The substitution of methionine for valine at position 98 of the β chain loosens the strength of the heme-histidine attachment. Heme loss opens the heme pocket to water and to oxidative precipitation of the heme depleted globin. The resultant clinical syndrome is a Heinz body hemolytic anemia.[13] The substitution of arginine for the distal β 63 histidine (resembling the similar substitution of tyrosine with resultant methemoglobinemia) causes no clinically significant hemolysis until the affected individual is given certain drugs, such as sulfonamides, which cause Heinz body hemolytic anemia. There are approximately 60 points at which the heme molecule comes in contact with globin atoms; amino acid substitution affecting these contact points, as for example at the β 42 or the α 43 position, apparently loosen the position of heme in its pocket, exposing the thiols to oxidation and irreversible aggregation, causing Heinz body hemolytic anemia (Table 1). A large number of other amino acid substitutions scattered at a variety of sites in either the α or β chain also lead to unstable hemoglobin and Heinz body hemolytic anemia. Besides those affecting the heme pocket, a second group affects the region of contact between α and β chains causing these subunits to part easily into a state of unstable dissociation (Figure 2). A third group affects overall molecular configuration by amino acid

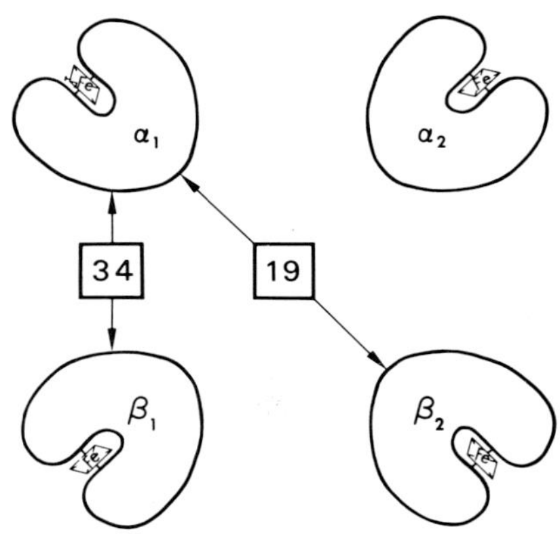

Fig. 2. The association of α and β subunits in the hemoglobin molecule. Heme groups are shown tucked into a hydrophobic pocket in each of the subunits in this diagramatic representation. The symetric pair ($\alpha_1\beta_1$), has extensive contact involving 34 amino acid residues. Mutant hemoglobins affecting this region lead to molecular instability. The asymetrical pair ($\alpha_1\beta_2$) has less extensive contact involving 19 amino acid residues, but this contact is important in the subunit interaction which gives the normal oxygen dissociation curve its sigmoid contour. The binding of 2,3 diphosphoglycerate (DPG) occurs in a "cleft" between the C-terminal groups of the two β chains. The normal Bohr effect is also related to a point on the β subunit near its C-terminal end.

deletion or by disrupting the helical regions of the molecule. Thus, the basic mechanisms whereby mutant hemoglobins are susceptible to oxidative hemolysis are: (a) heme loss, (b) subunit dissociation, and (c) altered overall molecular configuration.[6]

The association of the α with the β chain is a cornerstone of molecular stabilization; separated from one another, the α chains tend to remain in monomeric configuration and are extraordinarily susceptible to oxidative precipitation, while the β chains tend to associate into unstable tetramers, called hemoglobin H when it was first observed clinically in patients with α-thalassemia and Heinz body hemolytic anemia. An important pathogenetic feature of thalassemia is the lack of balance of globin chain synthesis, the excesses of either α subunits in β-thalassemia or the β subunits in α-thalassemia leading to the hemolytic manifestations of these disorders by virtue of their instability to normal oxidative stress. The detailed exploration of the inner workings of molecular stabilization will hopefully evoke new rational and successful pharmacologic approaches to ameliorate the hemoglobin precipitation which characterize these often severe anemias.

The presence of drug-mediated hemoglobin oxidation is detected by measuring methemoglobin and by demonstrating Heinz bodies. Partially oxidized methemoglobin, i.e., with only the α hemes or the β hemes in the ferriporphyrin state, have been demonstrated by minute electrophoretic differences in the four species ($\alpha_2\beta_2$, $\alpha^+{}_2\beta_2$, $\alpha_2\beta^+{}_2$, $\alpha^+{}_2\beta^+{}_2$).[14] Fetal hemoglobin can also exist in a partially oxidized state, with γ chain ferriporphyrin and α chain ferroporphyrin ($\alpha_2\gamma^+{}_2$).[15] Electrophoretically fast moving hemoglobins have been seen in lead-poisoned patients as well as in individuals with diabetes mellitus, but these may represent chemical modifications other than hemoglobin-glutathione mixed disulfides.[16–18] Progressive oxidation of the porphyrin ring splits it open to form "green pigments," variously referred to as verdoglobin, pseudoglobin, choleglobin, or sulfhemoglobin, depending on the specific oxidation method used.[19] The heme lost from the globin molecule in congenital Heinz body hemolytic anemias, and also in thalassemia, is degraded and finally excreted as a dipyrrole in urine, giving it a dark color. This degradative pathway for heme represents a "steal" mechanism with respect to the more usual pathway directed toward bilirubin formation.[5]

OXIDATIVE MECHANISMS OF DRUGS

The oxidative effects of drugs upon hemoglobin commonly produce both methemoglobinemia and Heinz body hemolytic anemia, but the diversity of mechanisms is illustrated by the fact that at the one extreme nitrites produce severe methemoglobinemia without hemolysis, while phenylhydrazine at the other produces severe hemolysis, often with little methemoglobinemia.[20] Some drugs may act directly by virtue of their properties as redox compounds, while others, such as aromatic amines, act indirectly. The oxidative effects of some drugs can readily be demonstrated in vitro, while others appear to produce their oxidative damage only after administration in vivo.[21] Methemoglobin producing drugs include organic compounds, chiefly aromatic amines, inorganic salts, such as chlorate and nitrite (or nitrates which are reduced in the gastrointestinal tract to nitrites), and even heavy metals, such as copper.[21-25] Redox compounds of sufficiently high redox potential establish an electron bridge to permit the flow of electrons from hemoglobin to molecular oxygen. The redox dye dichloroindophenol, for example, has a redox potential (E_m^7) of + 0.216V, and thus will oxidize ferrohemoglobin to ferrihemoglobin, the redox potential of which is + 0.150 V.[26] On the other hand the redox dye methylene blue has a lower redox potential (E_m^7 + 0.011V) than the ferro-ferrihemoglobin redox system and thus will not cause methemoglobin to form.[27] To the contrary, it will cause its reduction by establishing the flow of electrons from intracellular reducing substances of very low redox potential (reduced pyridine nucleotides) to methemoglobin. Cord blood hemoglobin is quite susceptible to methemoglobin formation, but the finding that hemoglobin F has a redox potential about equal to that of hemoglobin A in the physiologic pH range[28] points to another explanation, probably a deficiency in cord blood methemoglobin reductase activity.

The ease with which unstable hemoglobin variants precipitate has impeded direct measurement of their redox potentials. Moreover it is not clear how the redox potential of the ferro-ferrihemoglobin redox couple interrelates with that of the globin thiols. Hemoglobin H, the β chain tetramer, has all eight (two per β chain) of its thiol groups in a readily reactive state. These confer upon the molecule the behavior of an entity of very low redox potential; it undergoes oxidative precipitation by dyes of very low redox potential, for example: neutral red (E_m^7 —0.32V), which is close to that of glutathione itself (E_m^7 —0.34V).[11,29] A hemoglobin with such susceptibility to oxidation unhappily finds itself acting as a "sponge" for oxidants, preempting the role of glutathione. As such, its presence in the same cell with normal hemoglobin spares the latter from oxidation. For example: the addition of dichloroindophenol to an hemolysate containing both hemoglobin H and hemoglobin A will show an extremely rapid reduction of the blue dye which soon is followed by the turbid appearance of hemoglobin H as it undergoes precipitation. The hemoglobin A, however, remains in the oxyhemoglobin state. Addition of the same dye to an hemolysate containing only hemoglobin A will show much slower dye reduction accompanied by the appearance of methemoglobin A. The presence of the unstable hemoglobin thus acts as a buffer protecting hemoglobin A from oxidation. However, such protection is not of physiologic value to the red cell because the insoluble precipitates are detrimental to cell survival. The addition of reduced glutathione immediately after the redox reaction between the dye and hemoglobin H is complete, effectively retards the precipitation of hemoglobin H, indicating that the oxidative damage is reversible within a rather brief period of time (Figure 3).[11]

Nitrites are one of the most potent formers of methemoglobin and yet they spare the globin thiols and do not cause hemolysis.[30] Precisely why the reduced form of this inorganic compound should be such a potent producer of methemoglobin is still not clear. Nitrite apparently forms a complex with heme, the reversibility of which is questionable.[31,32] Possibly the nitrite displaces oxygen from its niche between heme and the distal histidine, thus exposing the heme to oxidation. It does not, however, block the reduction of ferrihemoglobin by methemoglobin reductase or by methylene blue. The binding of nitrite to methe-

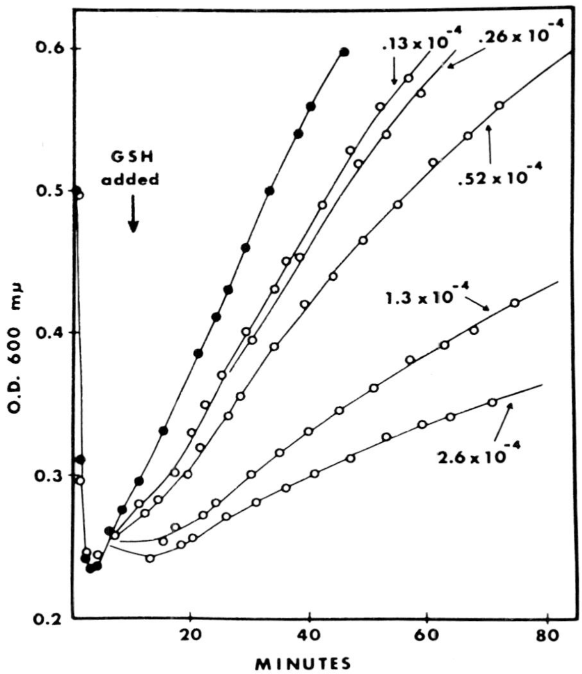

Fig. 3. Oxidative precipitation of Hemoglobin H; its reversible prevention by glutathione. Buffered hemolysate is oxidized by dichloro-indophenol at time 0. Optical density first registers a rapid disappearance of dye color as it is reduced. This is followed in 3 minutes by a rapid increase in optical density produced by turbidity caused by precipitation of the unstable hemoglobin. Glutathione added 10 minutes after hemoglobin oxidation partially reverses the precipitation in a concentration dependent manner. (Closed circles represent control with no added glutathione. Open circles represent reduction in turbidity at various concentrations of glutathione). (Reprinted by permission from Gabuzda, et al from J Lab Clin Med[11]).

moglobin may alter its optical properties and cause error in its estimation by conventional techniques.[31]

Why certain aromatic amines—not redox compound themselves—have the ability to produce oxidative hemolysis and methemoglobinemia has been puzzling, but the explanation appears to be that they have the ability to generate hydrogen peroxide or free peroxide radicals in the cell, measured by special light emission techniques.[19] The oxygen for peroxides is apparently derived from oxyhemoglobin. Phenylhydrazine and phenylhydroxyamine and related derivatives are particularly potent peroxide formers and readily produce oxidative changes in normal erythrocytes. Other less active compounds, such as primaquin, may only be detrimental to enzyme-deficient cells. In the light of the foregoing, it seems no accident of nature that erythrocytes possess glutathione peroxidase to permit rapid glutathione-dependent detoxification of peroxides of high redox potential, a major threat to the maintenance of hemoglobin and other cell thiol groups in the reduced state.

Phenylhydrazine and phenylhydroxyamine are examples of agents active not only in vivo but also in vitro. However, acetophenetidin (phenacetin) does not possess in vitro activity and yet is associated with a syndrome of methemoglobinemia and oxidative hemolysis in certain individuals, usually habitual users, whose red cell enzymes and hemoglobin are otherwise inherently normal.[33,34] This aromatic amine is therefore an example of one that must first be metabolized before its potential as a peroxide former is revealed. The active principle appears to be a phenylhydroxyamine derivative formed in the liver as a minor metabolite (the major metabolite being N-acetyl-*p*-aminophenol).[35,36] Other classes of aniline-derivative drugs are also converted to hydroxylated intermediates which possess greater oxidant properties than the parent compounds.[21,37] Shahidi described an intriguing case of phenacetin-induced hemolysis which appeared to implicate an inherited variation in phenacetin metabolism, the phenylhydroxy amines predominating over N-acetyl-*p*-aminophenol as the major metabolites.[38]

Inherited enzyme defects of the red cell will not be discussed in any depth here, but their importance in the clinical manifestation of oxidative alterations of hemoglobin must receive special emphasis.[39] Heterozygotes for methemoglobin reductase deficiency, not cyanotic under usual conditions, have developed severe methemoglobinemia when given antimalarials, for example.[40] The same agents provoke Heinz body hemolytic anemia in individuals with an inherited deficiency of enzymes affecting the hexose monophosphate pathway and intracellular glutathione metabolism. The rates of absorption and of excretion also modify toxic propensity. Habitual users of phenacetin may develop renal insufficiency secondary to a toxic interstitial nephritis, which will, in turn, aggrevate oxidative hemolysis as the excretory rate of the drug is progressively impaired. Patients thought to have "enterogenous cyanosis"—methemoglobinemia and hemolysis arising from toxic products of bacterial origin in the gastrointestinal trace—are instead likely to be surrepticious users of phenacetin and examination of urine for metabolites of the drug is a worthwhile diagnostic procedure in such cases.[41] Contamination of phenacetin preparations with methemoglobin-forming impurities has also been observed.[33]

PHARMACOLOGIC APPROACHES TO ERYTHROCYTIC SICKLING

The prevalence and severity of sickle cell diseases have recently turned attention toward methods in which drug-hemoglobin interactions might be propitiously applied in therapeutic ways to prevent erythrocytic sickling and thus ameliorate severe vasocclusive and hemolytic manifestations of these disorders. Detailed knowledge of the molecular basis of sickling has been developed sufficiently that a rational foundation now permits the exploration of a variety of pharmacologic approaches to prevent the stacking of hemoglobin S molecules into tactoid shapes that twist and distort the red cell. In hemoglobin S, glutamic acid at position 6 from the N-terminal amino end of the β chain is replaced by valine. This minute change in molecular architecture produces harm only in the deoxy configurational state when the allosteric shifting apart of β chains from one another causes the surface contour of the β chains of one hemoglobin molecule to fit into those of the neighboring α chain, long linear stacks of hemoglobin molecules forming in a state of reversible physical insolubility. There are also cross-linking forces which bind six monomolecular filaments into one twisted coaxial cable-like bundle. The cross-linking forces also produce some degree of sidewise branching of the bundles.

Since sickling is entirely dependent upon the allosteric properties of deoxyhemoglobin S, any agent which increases hemoglobin oxygen affinity will act to inhibit sickling. Increasing intracellular pH, for example, will achieve this by the Bohr Effect.[42,43] However, systemic alkalinization has not proved to be either an effective or safe therapy.[44] The important role that intraerythrocytic 2,3-diphosphoglycerate (2,3-DPG) plays in regulating hemoglobin oxygen affinity opens up the possibility that certain pharmacologic agents might adversely or beneficially influence hemoglobin oxygen affinity through this pathway. Little is known at present of pharmacologic effects upon erythrocyte 2,3-DPG. Propanolol and androgens have been reported to increase 2,3-DPG levels, thus decreasing hemoglobin oxygen affinity.[45,46] Injections of inosine, pyruvate, and phosphate produce a similar action.[47,48] Radiopaque contrast medium, on the other hand, has been found to increase hemoglobin oxygen affinity.[49] In vitro experimental evidence indicates that low molecular weight phosphates, including 2,3-DPG as well as inorganic phosphate, promote the sickling phenomenon in solutions of deoxyhemoglobin S.[50,51] Whether a similar relationship between low molecular weight phosphates and sickling occurs in vivo is not yet known, but somewhat paradoxically, immature erythroid cells have the highest levels of these compounds and yet they are more resistant to sickling, suggesting that other intracellular variables are of even greater importance.

A number of other variables influence sickling, and while they are not of practical therapeutic application at present, they do add to our theoretic understanding of the sickling process. Oxidation of hemoglobin S to the ferrihemoglobin state, introduction of cyanide as a ligand, and ligand formation with carbon monoxide all prevent sickling, presumably through allosteric effects which place these derivatives in the oxyhemoglobin configurational state.[52,53] The presence of other hemoglobins together with hemoglobin S modifies the sickling phenomenon. Hemoglobin C and hemoglobin D interact strongly with it and lead to significant disease states, while hemoglobin A and hemoglobin J interact much less strongly and in combination with hemoglobin S are usually benign.[54] Hemoglobin F appears to interact the least, and its presence with hemoglobin S in the red cell (even as little as 15%–20%) effectively inhibits sickling. The molecular basis of these hemoglobin interactions is not clear, but some recent clues have been observed in patients with mutant hemoglobins. For example: the substitution of asparagine for aspartic acid at the β73 amino acid site results in a hemoglobin which, like hemoglobin F, interacts very weakly with hemoglobin S, suggesting that this point on the surface of the hemoglobin molecule participates in a crucial way in the intermolecular association between hemoglobin molecules which lead to tactoid formation; its alteration deters sickling of deoxyhemoglobin S.[55,56]

Murayama has made important contributions to the theory of sickling. He found that sickling was prevented and even reversed at low temperatures and by such hydrophobic substances as propane. From such experiments he inferred that hydrophobic bonding was important in the sickling of hemoglobin. He hypothesized that an intrasubunit hydrophobic bond was formed between the N-terminal valine and that at the number 6 position of the β chain of hemoglobin S, leading to a configurational change on the surface of the β subunit which set the stage for a β to α chain "lock and key" arrangement between adjacent deoxyhemoglobin molecules.[57] Whether this hypothesis will prove sufficient to explain the complexities of the sickling process just described remains to be determined. Evidence has been advanced that electrostatic and possibly hydrogen bonding are also of importance.

The concept that hydrophobic bonding links hemoglobin S molecules into tactoids led to the suggestion that urea would be therapeutically useful in fracturing these bonds. It was claimed that urea, at concentrations as low as 0.01 M, inhibits erythrocytic sickling,[58] but Segel and associates were unable to demonstrate any effect at concentrations as high as 0.2 M under an atmosphere of 3% oxygen.[53] Indeed, chemical experience would indicate that rather high concentrations of urea—far above the physiologic range—are required to break hydrophobic bonds, a process accompanied by protein denaturation. Cerami and Manning found that 1.0 M urea did inhibit sickling in a reversible manner, but this effect may well have been related to the increase in hemoglobin oxygen affinity produced by urea.[59,53]

The knowledge that solutions of urea spontaneously form cyanate[60] led Cerami and Manning to the observation that 0.01 M cyanate inhibited sickling in an irreversible fashion, suggesting that the hemoglobin itself had in some fashion been permanently altered (Figure 4).[59] They proposed that the N-terminal valine residues of the globin chains were the sole site of modification in a carbamylation reaction. (This site physiologically reacts with CO_2 to form a carbamino linkage).[61] More recent information indicates that the reaction with cyanate occurs with both the β and the α chain without dependence on the specific N-terminal amino acid residue and with a change in electric charge on both globin subunits. The reaction also seems to occur at more than one site on the globin subunit, suggesting that the carbamylation reaction may affect globin amino groups other than those at the N-terminal positions.[62] Carbamyl phosphate has been shown to resemble cyanate in its effect on sickling; presumably it carbamylates the globin chains in a similar fashion.[63,64] Recent reports confirm the initial observation of deFuria, et al that the altered hemoglobin has an increased oxygen affinity and, in addition, purport to demonstrate that the antisickling effect can be entirely explained on this basis without having to postulate that carbamylated residues cause steric hindrance to the stacking of deoxyhemoglobin S molecules.[65–67]

Cyanate treatment of sickle cell erythrocytes in vitro prolongs their life-span significantly after they are reinfused into the patient.[68] Isotopically labeled cyanate taken up by the red cell combines irreversibly with hemoglobin and thus can be used as a tag to measure red cell life span.[69,70] Preliminary reports of acute and chronic toxicity studies in animals are promising, and relatively

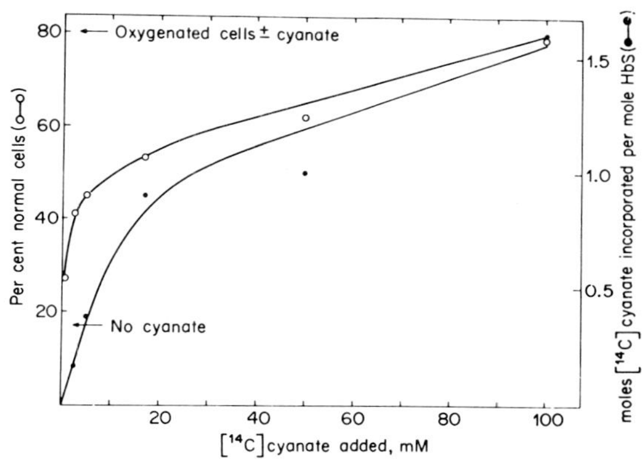

Fig. 4. The reduction of sickling in deoxygenated sickle-cell erythrocytes by treatment with various concentrations of potassium cyanate, expressed as percentage of normal, i.e., nonsickled cells. This value was 80% in the oxygenated state (20% were irreversibly sickled). Upon deoxygenation, only 17% were nonsickled prior to cyanate treatment. Added increments of cyanate incorporated into hemoglobin S is paralleled by a progressive increase in the proportion of normal appearing nonsickled deoxygenated erythrocytes. (Reproduced by permission from Cerami, et al and from Proc Nat Acad Sci, USA[59]).

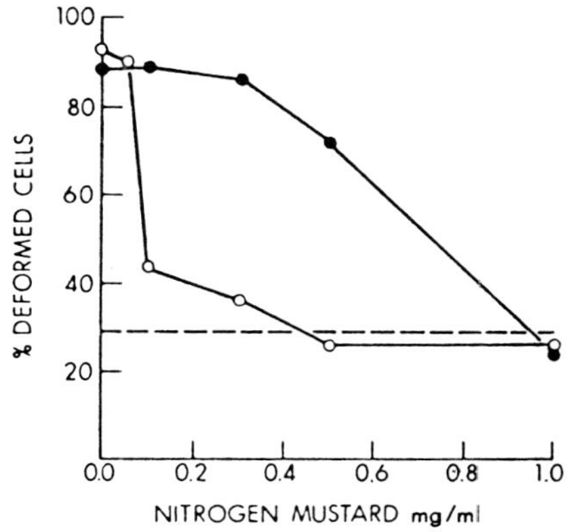

Fig. 5. The reduction of erythrocyte sickling in 1% sodium metabisulfite by treatment of erythrocytes in vitro with nitrogen mustard. Open circles represent washed erythrocytes suspended in buffered saline. Closed circles represent erythrocytes treated as whole blood. The dashed line represents control value of deformed cells present before deoxygenation. (Reprinted by permission from Roth, et al and from Biochem Biophys Res Commun[76]).

short-term observations in patients have not revealed deleterious effects.[71] However, concern surrounds the possibility that irreversible carbamylation of other body proteins in any of a variety of organs may lead to unfavorable long-term consequences. In mice, cyanate appears to impair learning ability and fertility.[72,73] It also inhibits hemoglobin synthesis in reticulocytes.[74] Lens protein becomes carbamylated after cyanate treatment, but whether this protein alteration will lead to cataract formation is unknown.[75]

In this newly developed field, other chemical approaches to the solubilization of deoxyhemoglobin S are being pursued. Alkylation of hemoglobin S by treating intact erythrocytes or solutions of hemoglobin with rather high concentrations of nitrogen mustard inhibits sickling without a significant effect upon the oxygen dissociation curve (Figure 5).[76] The attachment of glutamic acid residues by the treatment of hemoglobin with the N-carboxyanhydride of glutamic acid both increases the negative charge on the molecule and increases its solubility.[77] Such methods are not yet of practical clinical value. However, they may lead to therapy which will be effective and safe in intact erythrocytes as well as in intact patients.

CONCLUSIONS

There has been an immense investment of time, energy, and intellectual curiosity in the determination of the fine structure of the hemoglobin molecule. Contributions from studies of inherited globin chain mutants have added depth to our understanding of the relationship of this fine structure to molecular function. The fruits of this effort are now being examined from a new point of view. Future rewards will hopefully be a more refined appreciation of the nature and prevention of oxidative damage to the molecule and of reversible physical insolubility, leading to successful therapeutic approaches to the symptomatically severe hemoglobinopathies.

SUMMARY

Deleterious actions of drugs upon hemoglobin, occurring as undesirable and sometimes serious side effects of treatment of nonhematologic disease, have dominated investigational interest in this field for almost a century. But more recently, thoughts have been directed to the potential benefits to be derived from drug-hemoglobin interactions, particularly in relation to the treatment of sickle cell disease.

Hemoglobin is a redox molecule. Its heme groups are suspended between histidine groups and lie buried in pockets lined with hydrophobic groups. Hemoglobin stability in the presence of oxidative stresses is related to the symetric association of the $\alpha_1\beta_1$ subunits within the $\alpha_2\beta_2$ tetramer, to the tightness of the heme contact points in their pockets, and to the maintenance of overall molecular configuration.

Some drugs oxidize hemoglobin by virtue of their properties as redox compounds. Many others, such as aromatic amines, are not redox compounds themselves but presumably exert oxidative effects by generating peroxide radicals within the cells. Some aromatic amines are not toxic in vitro but are converted to active metabolites (usually hydroxyl derivatives) in the body. Some drugs, such as nitrites, are potent methemoglobin formers, but cause no hemolysis, while at the other end of the spectrum is phenylhydrazine, a potent hemolytic agent.

Erythrocyte sickling is related to interactions between deoxyhemoglobin S molecules at high concentration, leading to multistranded filamentous structures which grow and distort the red cell. Certain agents influence sickling by changing the oxygen affinity of the hemoglobin. These include agents which alter pH or 2,3-diphosphoglycerate (2,3-DPG) concentrations. Increased concentration of low molecular weight phosphates, including 2,3-DPG and inorganic phosphates, increase the sickling propensity. The search for agents which will inhibit sickling recently focused attention on urea, but this agent is effective in vitro only at high concentrations that preclude its use in vivo. Much lower concentrations of cyanate or carbamyl phosphate are effective antisickling agents, and these agents are currently undergoing experimental tests. They act by carbamylating globin-free amino groups. Their inhibitory effect on sickling appears to be related solely to an increase in hemoglobin oxygen affinity. Alkylation of hemoglobin is another new approach which inhibits sickling without affecting oxygen affinity.

Recent investigations into pharmacologic modification of the hemoglobin molecule following upon elegant descriptions of its fine structure and intimate relation to molecular function and stability will hopefully culminate in the development of effective treatment for the more severe thalassemic and sickle hemoglobinopathies.

REFERENCES

1. Finch CA: Methemoglobinemia and sulfhemoglobinemia. N Engl J Med 239: 470, 1948
2. Bodansky O: Methemoglobinemia and methemoglobin-producing compounds. Pharmacol Rev 3:144, 1951
3. Jaffe ER, Heller P: Methemoglobinemia in man. Progr Hematol 4:48, 1964
4. Necheles TF, Allen DM: Heinz-body anemias. N Engl J Med 280:203, 1969
5. Bunn HF: Erythrocyte destruction and hemoglobin catabolism. Semin Hematol 9:3, 1972
6. Weatherall DJ, Clegg JB: The Thalassemia Syndromes. Oxford, Blackwell, 1972
7. Allen DW, Jandl JH: Oxidative hemolysis and precipitation of hemoglobin, II. Role of thiols in oxidant drug action. J Clin Invest 40:454, 1961
8. Huisman THJ, Dozy AM: Studies on the heterogeneity of hemoglobin. V. Binding of hemoglobin with oxidized glutathione. J Lab Clin Med 60:302, 1962
9. Srivastava SK, Beutler E: Glutathione metabolism of the erythrocyte: The enzymatic cleavage of glutathione-hemoglobin preparations by glutathione reductase. Biochem J 119:353, 1970
10. Brewer GJ, Tarlov AR, Kellermeyer RW, et al: The hemolytic effect of primaquin XV. Role of methemoglobinemia. J Lab Clin Med 59:905, 1962
11. Gabuzda TG, Laforet MT, Gardner FH: Oxidative precipitation of hemoglobin H and its relation to reduced glutathione. J Lab Clin Med 70:581, 1967
12. Rieder RF: Hemoglobin stability: Observations on the denaturation of normal

and abnormal hemoglobins by oxidant dyes, heat, and alkali. J Clin Invest 49:2369, 1970
13. Jacob HS, Brain MC, Dacie JV, et al: Abnormal haem binding and globin SH group blockade in unstable haemoglobin. Nature (Lund) 218:1214, 1968
14. Bunn HF, Drysdale JW: The separation of partially oxidized hemoglobins. Biochim Biophys Acta 229:51, 1971
15. Boi-Doku FS, Pik C: Spontaneous oxidation of the γ-chain of the foetal haemoglobin component of cord blood. Biochim Biophys Acta 115:495, 1966
16. Charache S, Weatherall DJ: Fast hemoglobin in lead poisoning. Blood 28:377, 1966
17. Trivelli LA, Ranney HM, Lai HT: Hemoglobin components in patients with diabetes mellitus. N Engl J Med 284:353, 1971
18. Rahbar S, Blumenfeld O, Ranney HM: Studies of an unusual hemoglobin in patients with diabetes mellitus. Biochem Biophys Res Commun 36:838, 1969
19. Rostorfer HH, Cormier MJ: The formation of "hydrogen peroxide" in the reaction of oxyhemoglobin with methemoglobin-forming agents. Arch Biochem Biophys 71:235, 1957
20. Beutler E, Baluda MC: The role of methemoglobin in oxidative degradation of hemoglobin. Acta Haematol 27:321, 1962
21. Fraser IM, Vessell ES: Effects of drugs and drug metabolites on erythrocytes from normal and glucose-6-phosphate dehydrogenase deficient individuals. Ann NY Acad Sci 151:777, 1968
22. McLean S, Murphy BP, Starmer GA, et al: Methemoglobin formation induced by aromatic amines and amides. J Pharm Pharmacol 19:146, 1967
23. Greenberg MS, Wong H: Methemoglobinemia and Heinz body hemolytic anemia due to phenazopyridine hydrochloride. N Engl J Med 271:431, 1964
24. Salvati AM, Ambrogioni MT, Tentori L: The autooxidation of haemoglobin. Effect of copper. Ital J Biochem 18:1, 1969
25. Carlson DJ, Shapiro FL: Methemoglobinemia from well water nitrates: a complication of home hemodialysis. Ann Intern Med 73:757, 1970
26. Antonini E, Wyman J, Brunori M, et al: Studies on the oxidation-reduction potentials of heme proteins. I. Human hemoglobin. J Biol Chem 239:907, 1964
27. Stossel T, Jennings RB: Failure of methylene blue to produce methemoglobinemia in vivo. Am J Clin Pathol 45:600, 1966
28. Flohe L, Uehleke H: The oxidation-reduction potential of human hemoglobin F. Life Sci 5:1041, 1966
29. Gabuzda TG: Hemoglobin H and the red cell. Blood 27:568, 1966
30. Smith RP, Abbanat RA: Protective effect of oxidized glutathione in acute sulfide poisoning. Toxicol Appl Pharmacol 9:209, 1966
31. Smith RP: The nitrite methemoglobin complex—its significance in methemoglobin analysis and its possible role in methemoglobinemia. Biochem Pharmacol 16:1655, 1967
32. Uchida H, Klapper MH: Evidence for an irreversible reaction between nitrite and human methemoglobin. Biochim Biophys Acta 221:640, 1970
33. Davidson RJL: Phenacetin-induced haemolytic anaemia. J Clin Pathol 24:537, 1971
34. Millar J, Peloquin R, deLeeuw NKM: Phenacetin-induced hemolytic anemia. Can Med Assoc J 106:770, 1972
35. Brodie BR, Axelrod J: The fate of acetanilide in man. J Pharmacol Exp Ther 94:29, 1948

36. Schnitzer B, Smith EB: Effects of the metabolites of phenacetin on the rat. Arch Pathol 81:264, 1966
37. Kiese M: The biochemical production of ferrihemoglobin-forming derivatives from aromatic amines, and mechanisms of ferrihemoglobin formation. Pharmacol Rev 18:1091, 1966
38. Shahidi NT: Acetophenetidin-induced methemoglobinemia. Ann NY Acad Sci 151:822, 1968
39. Jaffe ER: Hereditary methemoglobinemias associated with abnormality in the metabolism of the erythrocytes. Am J Med 41:786, 1966
40. Cohen RJ, Sachs JR, Wicker DJ, et al: Methemoglobinemia provoked by malarial chemoprophylaxis in Vietnam. N Engl J Med 279:1127, 1968
41. Azen EA, Bryan GT, Shahidi NT, et al: Obscure hemolytic anemia due to analgesic abuse. Am J Med 48:724, 1970
42. Greenberg MS, Kass EH, Castle WB: Studies on the destruction of red blood cells. XII. Factors influencing the role of S hemoglobin in the pathologic physiology of sickle cell anemia and related disorders. J Clin Invest 36:833, 1957
43. Greenberg MS, Kass EH: Studies on the destruction of red blood cells. XIII. Observations on the role of pH in the pathogenesis and treatment of painful crisis in sickle cell disease. Arch Intern Med 101:355, 1958
44. Schwartz E, MacElfresh AE: Treatment of painful crisis of sickle cell disease: J Pediatr 64:132, 1964
45. Oski FA, Miller LD, Delivoria-Papadopoulos M, et al: Oxygen affinity in red cells: changes induced in vivo by propanolol. Science 175:1372, 1972
46. Parker JP, Beirne GJ, Desai JN, et al: Androgen-induced increase in red cell 2,3-diphosphoglycerate. N Engl J Med 287:381, 1972
47. Sugerman HJ, Pollock TW, Rosato EF, et al: Experimentally induced alterations in affinity of hemoglobin for oxygen. II. In vivo effect of inosine, pyruvate, and phosphate on oxygen-hemoglobin affinity in Rhesus monkey. Blood 39:525, 1972
48. Miller L, Sugerman H, Cromie W, et al: Pharmacologically induced in vivo alterations of the oxygen-hemoglobin equilibrium curve in man. J Clin Invest 51:65a, 1972
49. Rosenthal A, Litwin SB, Laver MB: Effect of contrast media used in angiocardiography on oxyhemoglobin dissociation. Pediatr Res 6:83, 1972
50. Paniker NV, Ben-Bassat I, Beutler E: Evaluation of sickle hemoglobin and desickling agents by falling ball viscometry. J Lab Clin Med 80:282, 1972
51. Briehl RW: Factors influencing gelation of hemoglobin S. J Clin Invest 51:15a, 1972
52. Beutler E: The effect of methemoglobin formation in sickle cell disease. J Clin Invest 40:1856, 1961
53. Segel GB, Feig SA, Mentzer WC, et al: Effects of urea and cyanate on sickling in vitro. N Engl J Med 287:59, 1972
54. Charache S, Conley CL: Rate of sickling of red cells during deoxygenation of blood from persons with various sickling disorders. Blood 24:25, 1964
55. Bookchin RM, Nagel RL: Ligand-induced conformational dependence of hemoglobin in sickling interactions. J Mol Biol 60:263, 1971
56. Bookchin RM, Nagel RL, Ranney HM: The effect of $\beta 73^{asn}$ on the interactions of sickling hemoglobins. Biochim Biophys Acta 221:373, 1970
57. Murayama M: A molecular mechanism of sickled erythrocyte formation. Nature 202:258, 1964

58. Nalbandian RM: Molecular Aspects of Sickle Cell Hemoglobin: Clinical Applications. Springfield, C C Thomas, 1971
59. Cerami A, Manning JM: Potassium cyanate as an inhibitor of the sickling of erythrocytes in vitro. Proc Natl Acad Sci USA 68:1180, 1971
60. Hagel P, Gerding JJT, Fieggen W, et al: Cyanate formation in solutions of urea. I. Calculation of cyanate concentrations at different temperature and pH. Biochim Biophys Acta 243:366, 1971
61. Kilmartin JV, Rossi-Bernardi L: Inhibition of CO_2 combination and reduction of the Bohr effect in haemoglobin chemically modified at its α-amino groups. Nature 222:1243, 1969
62. Pacheco J, Melvin M, Gabuzda TG: Cyanate-globin reaction independent of specific N-terminal amino acid. Blood 40:929, 1972
63. Kraus LM, Kraus AP: Carbamyl phosphate mediated inhibition of the sickling of erythrocytes in vitro. Biochem Biophys Res Commun 44:1381, 1971
64. *Idem*: Alteration of structure and the sickling phenomenon resulting from carbamyl phosphate modification of hemoglobin S. Fed Proc 31:484, 1972
65. Diederich D. Reissman K: Role of carbamylation in the prevention of the sickling phenomenon. Fed Proc 31:341, 1972
66. May A, Bellingham AJ, Huehns ER, et al: Effect of cyanate on sickling. Lancet 1:658, 1972
67. deFuria FG, Miller DR, Cerami A, et al: The effects of cyanate in vitro on red blood cell metabolism and function in sickle cell anemia. J Clin Invest 51:566, 1972
68. Gillette PN, Manning JM, Cerami A: Increased survival of sickle cell erythrocytes after treatment in vitro with sodium cyanate. Proc Natl Acad Sci USA 68:2791, 1971
69. deFuria FG, Graziano JH, Cerami A: Cyanate-^{14}C: a new method for red cell survivals. J Clin Invest 51:24a, 1972
70. Pacheco JP, Gabuzda TG: Unpublished observation
71. Gilette P, Peterson CM, Manning JM, et al: Decrease in the hemolytic anemia of sickle cell disease after administration of sodium cyanate. J Clin Invest 51:36a, 1972
72. Crist R, Grisolia S, Bettis C, et al: In vivo carbamylation of brain, blood, and liver proteins by carbamyl phosphate and cyanate. Fed Proc 31:231, 1972
73. Graziano JH, Allen TA, Cerami A: The effect of cyanate on the endocrine system. Fed Proc 31:271, 1972
74. Alter BP, Kan YW, Nathan DG: Inhibition of hemoglobin synthesis by cyanate. J Clin Invest 51:4a, 1972
75. Gerding JJT, Koppers A, Hagel P, et al: Cyanate formation in solutions of urea. II. Effect of urea on the eye lens protein α-crystallin. Biochim Biophys Acta 243:374, 1971
76. Roth EF Jr, Nagel RL, Bookchin RM et al: Nitrogen mustard: an in vitro inhibitor of erythrocyte sickling. Biochem Biophys Res Commun 48:612, 1972
77. Kosower EM, Kosower NS, LaCourse PC: The solubilization of deoxyhemoglobin S. Proc Natl Acad Sci USA 57:39, 1967

Allan J. Erslev

5
Pathophysiology of Aplastic Anemia

For many years the term aplastic anemia was used at random to describe pancytopenia, whether it was caused by a reduction in bone marrow volume or function. More recently aplastic anemia has been defined as a pancytopenia caused solely by a reduction and fatty replacement of the functional bone marrow mass. Our current dynamic concept of bone marrow function with self-perpetuating stem cells acting as precursors of differentiated hematopoietic cells has sharpened this definition, and hypoplastic or aplastic anemia is now defined as a pancytopenia caused by a quantitative or qualitative failure of multipotential stem cells.

DISTRIBUTION AND STRUCTURE OF HEMATAPOIETIC TISSUE

In the normal adult, blood cell formation is the exclusive prerogative of bone cavities. These cavities first emerge as hematopoietic organs at about the fifth month of fetal life, when leukopoietic cells appear in the cartilaginous cavities of primordial bones (Figure 1). Initially, the microenvironment here appears to be best suited for granulocytopoiesis, while erythropoiesis passes only slowly from the liver and spleen to bone. However, at birth, the bone cavities have become responsible for the production of all formed elements of blood. Since the ratio between hematopoietic precursor cells and mature circulating cells is constant throughout life, the rapid expansion of blood volume during the first years of life taxes the available space within the bone. This precarious balance forces reactivation of extramedullary foci in the liver and spleen whenever there is an unusual demand for increased blood cell formation. However, at about the age of 4, the growth of bone and bone cavities begin to outstrip the growth

Supported in part by grants H 6374 and H 4612, from the US Public Health Service.

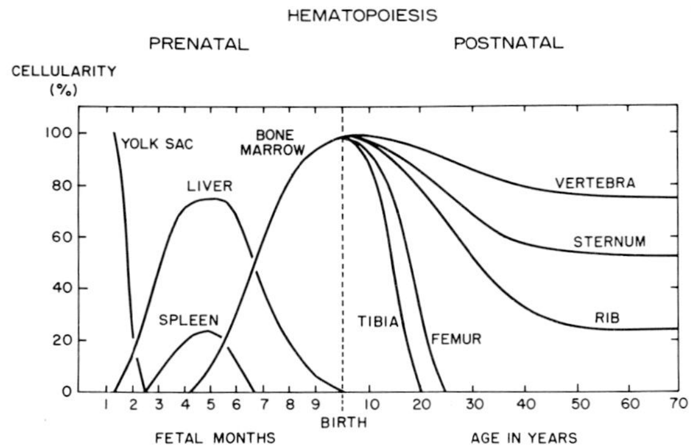

Fig. 1. Expansion and recession of hematopoietic activity in extramedullary sites (redrawn from Ersler AJ[1]).

of the circulating blood cell mass, and reserve space appears in the form of foci of yellow fatty marrow. The fatty replacement occurs first in the diaphysis of long bones then slowly expands centripetally until at about the age of 18 active hematopoietic marrow is found only in the central bones and proximal epiphysis of the femur and humerus. During adult life the expansion of bone marrow space continues, possibly by bone resorption, and there is a gradual increase in the amount of fatty tissue in all bone cavities. Due to the abundant bone marrow space, compensatory reactivation of extramedullary sites rarely takes place in later life, even during periods of prolonged and intense demand for accelerated blood cell production. Extramedullary hematopoiesis during these years usually indicates inappropriate rather than compensatory hematopoiesis.

The size of the hematopoietic organ in the adult is difficult to measure. Estimates based on animal studies suggest that the combined volume of all bone cavities is about 30 to 50 ml per kilogram body weight, or about twice the size of the liver, and that actively hematopoietic tissue occupies 50% of this space.[2,3] This would indicate that the circulating blood cell mass of about 30 ml per kilogram body weight is supported by the same volume of precursor cells, a ratio which seems quite high when compared with current estimates of the number and size of cells in the two compartments. However, normal active bone marrow is not merely a dense accumulation of hematopoietic cells; it is a highly structural, spongy organ arranged around a spoke-like pattern of sinusoids draining into a central vein (Figure 2). The sinusoidal linings are made up by a fenestrated basement membrane covered on both sides by reticular cells. These cells guard the fenestrations, serve as phagocytes, sustain or "nurse" cells in the hematopoietic islands, and can reversibly transform into fat cells. Only little is known of the pathophysiology of the structural cells, but they are undoubtedly as important for hematopoietic function as the hematopoietic precursor cells themselves. The wedge shaped extrasinusoidal compartments, criss-crossed by numerous spurs from the sinusoidal walls, form the immediate microenvironment for hematopoietic cells. These cells emerge from a pool of self-perpetuating stem cells, spend 3–5 days in active proliferation and maturation, stay in the bone

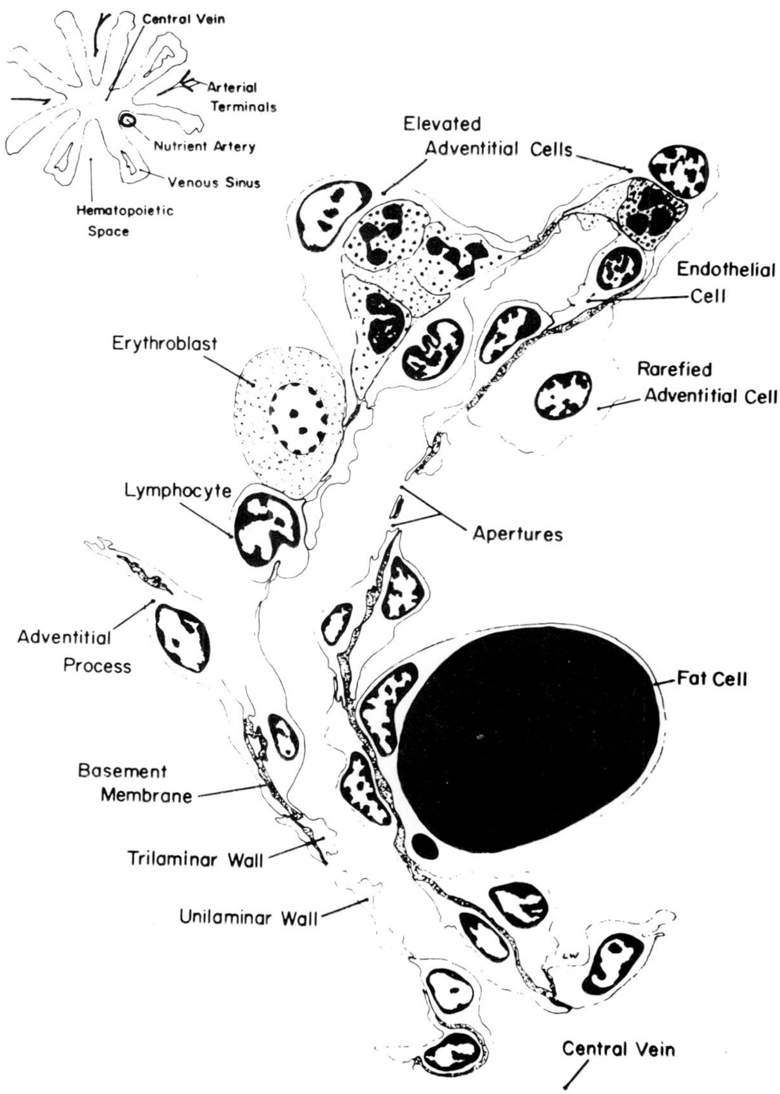

Fig. 2. Small sketch in left upper hand corner depicts vascular pattern of bone marrow as seen in cross section. In large sketch, a sinusoid is depicted with its basement membranes and reticular cells.[4]

marrow for a few days more, and are eventually released through the sinusoidal fenestrations into circulating blood.

A demand for cells may be met initially by enlarging the size of sinusoidal fenestrations, permitting the release of an increased number of maturing cells from hematopoietic compartments. This release may be accelerated through an increase in "population pressure" caused by an accelerated input of early hematopoietic cells from the stem cell pool. However, a sustained and true increase in the release of mature cells have to wait until these newly differentiated cells have finished their orderly process of multiplication and maturation.

The differentiation of stem cells to early hematopoietic cells appears to be governed by specific hormonal "poietins" acting on stem cells committed to single cell lines—erythropoietin on stem cells committed to erythroid cells, leukopoietin on stem cells committed to myeloid cells, and thrombopoietin on stem cells committed to megakaryocytic cells.[5] In addition, there must be poietins and stem cells committed to the T-and B-lymphocytes, which by now are known to be derived from bone marrow.[6]

The morphology of these committed stem cells has not been established, but they may resemble small or large lymphocytes.[7] "Suicide" studies with tritiated thymidine of a lethal specific activity indicate that they are in active cell cycle, regardless of the presence of poietins. It seems likely that one of the daughter cells after each mitotic division either undergoes poietin-induced blast transformation or dies (Figure 3). The other daughter cell must replace the dividing mother cell, since these stem cells are capable of prolonged, unsustained self-perpetuation. It is not known how long they can continue to support the dividing and maturing hematopoietic cell lines without renewal from an earlier compartment. However, under conditions of injury or stress, such a compartment of multipotential stem cells becomes activated and provides an input of new cells into the committed stem cell pools. This process of renewal is best

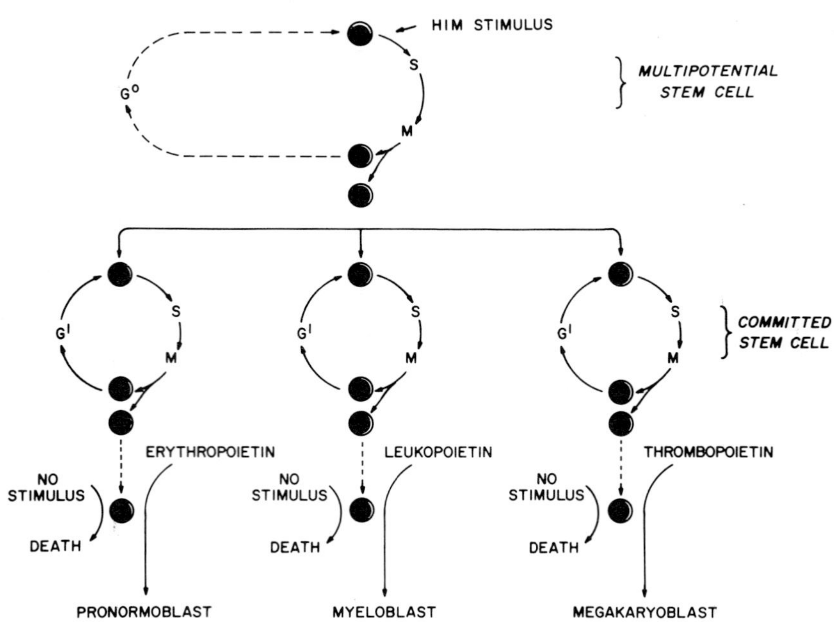

Fig. 3. A hypothetical model of stem cell kinetics. Committed stem cells will undergo continuous mitotic divisions, but their number will not increase since one of the daughter cells will either die or enter the differentiated pools. The multipotential stem cells will be in a resting Go phase unless stimulated to replenish depleted committed stem cell compartments.

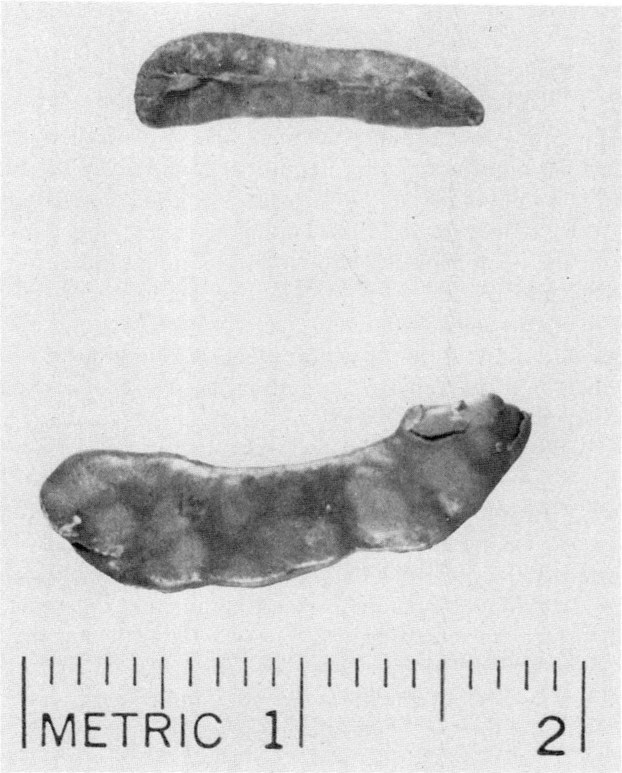

Fig. 4. Bone marrow colonies on the surface of the spleen of a sublethally radiated mouse (bottom). Normal control spleen (top).

observed in mice recovering from an exposure to radiation.[8] Surviving multipotential stem cells in the spleen or bone marrow will become activated, enter into a continuous regenerative cycle, and multiply at a rapid rate for about 4–5 days. At that point, a process of maturation has rendered them responsive to available poietins, and discrete bone marrow colonies appear made up by various mixtures of differentiated hematopoietic cells (Figure 4).

The stimulus generated by the injured tissue and governing the activation of the multipotential stem cells is unknown, but it appears to be a short-range signal, possibly a cell-to-cell interaction. Since the defect in aplastic anemia appears to reside in these multipotential stem cells, it has become extremely important to elucidate the nature of these signals. Studies on the hematopoietic fate of stem cells lodged in various areas of the body have shown that the microenvironment (HIM or Hematopoietic Inductive Microenvironment) is of utmost importance in determining whether the multipotential stem cells will become activated or stay dormant and whether committed stem cells will respond to available poietins.[9] Unfortunately, little or nothing is known about the signals responsible for this interaction between stem cells and HIM.

APLASIA OF HEMATOPOIETIC TISSUE

Demonstration

Hypoplastic anemia and aplastic anemia are interchangeable terms for conditions in which failure of multipotential stem cells cause a reduction in the volume of hematopoietic tissue, a decrease in blood cell production, and a pancytopenia. The diagnosis rests on finding pancytopenia with a low reticulocyte count, on the demonstration of increased amounts of fat in random bone marrow samples, and on ferrokinetic data suggesting decreased erythropoietic activity. Since hematopoietic elements on a smear from bone marrow aspirates often are reduced in number due to dilution, an examination of a sectioned bone marrow specimen may be required to establish that hematopoietic tissue has been replaced by fat. However, a carefully prepared squeeze smear of bone marrow particles obtained by needle aspiration will, in most cases, be diagnostic by revealing the characteristic islands of reticulated stroma surrounded by fatty tissue (Figure 5). In some cases, both biopsy sections and aspirate smears may be misleading, because of a chance-sampling of a "hot pocket" in the bone marrow (Figure 6). These pockets represent remaining hematopoietic tissue involved in intense proliferative activity due to high concentrations of stimulating "poietins." The erythropoietic turnover in such pockets may be so rapid that they, in view of the low reticulocyte count, could suggest a diagnosis of refractory normoblastic anemia or even erythroleukemia. In such cases, it is necessary to

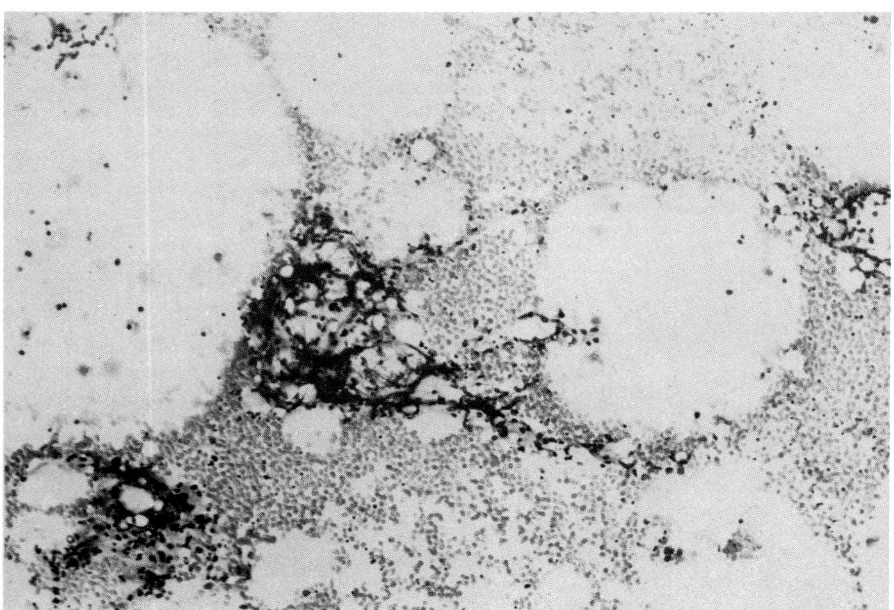

Fig. 5. Hypocellular strands of reticulum cells surrounded by fat particles. A bone marrow squeeze-smear prepared from particles obtained by needle aspiration from a patient with aplastic anemia (McK). Only a few hematopoietic cells are present in reticulum strands and fatty tissue.

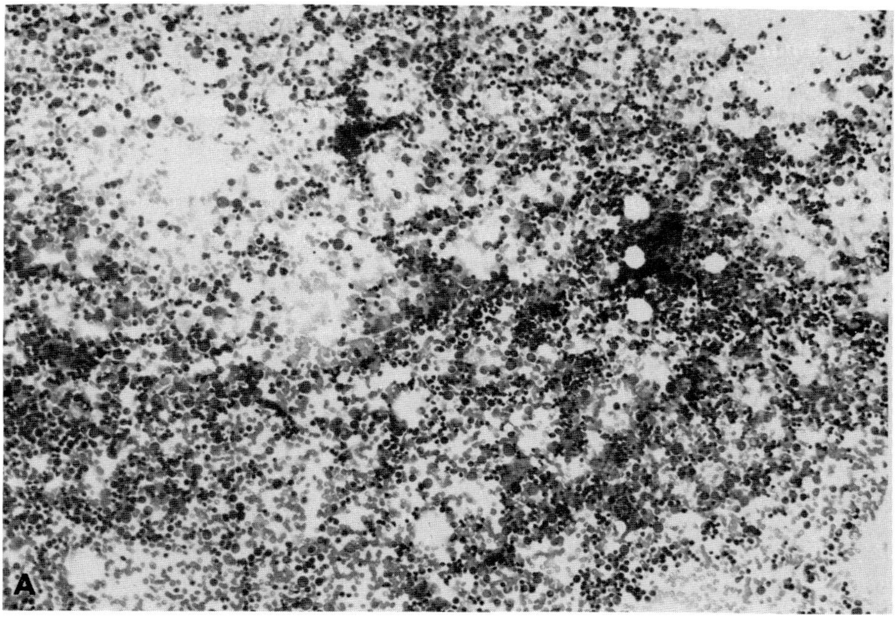

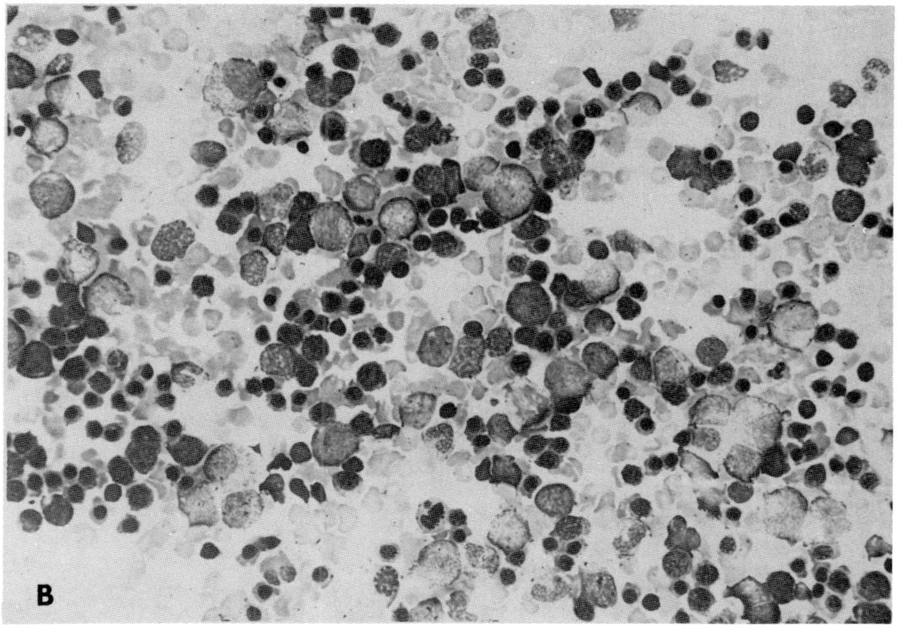

Fig. 6. A "hot pocket" in bone marrow from McK, a patient with aplastic anemia: (**A**) low power, (**B**) high power.

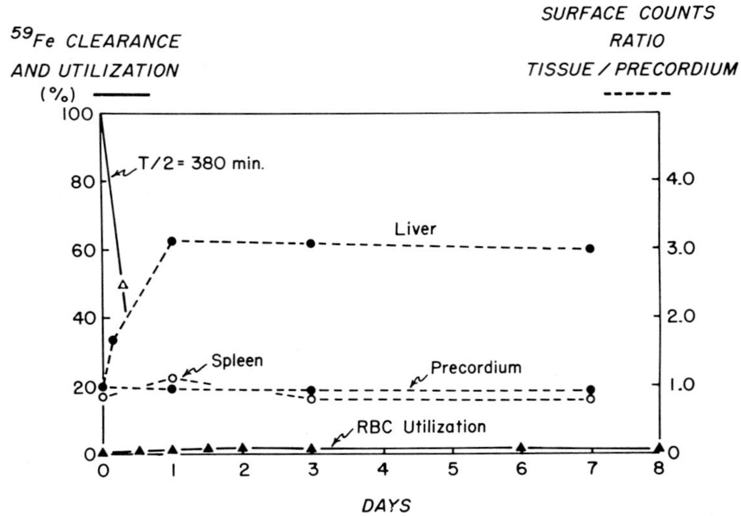

Fig. 7. Ferrokinetics of aplastic anemia: plasma clearance, plasma utilization and organ distribution of radioactive iron in patient McK with aplastic anemia and a "hot pocket" in his bone marrow.

perform not only multiple aspirations but to establish the total size of the erythropoietic tissue through ferrokinetic studies. In aplastic anemia these studies show prolonged plasma clearance of radioactive iron. Due to the prolonged presence of the isotope in plasma, a large part is diverted to other parenchymal tissues, especially the liver, and red cell utilization becomes low (Figure 7). This pattern is distinct from that observed in patients with active but ineffective erythropoiesis. Here red cell utilization is also low, but plasma clearance is rapid, reflecting an expanded but ineffective erythroid marrow (Figure 8). Direct measurements of the size of the hematopoietic tissue by body scanning or by

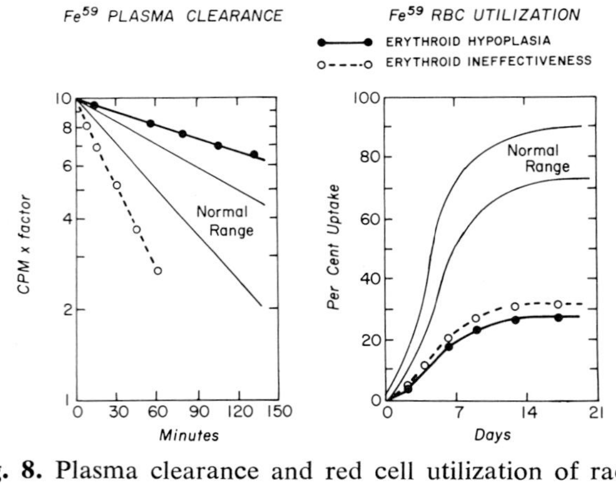

Fig. 8. Plasma clearance and red cell utilization of radioiron in normals, patient with aplastic anemia, and patients with ineffective erythropoiesis. Plasma clearance but not utilization clearly separates them from each other.

special isotope-sensitive cameras are technically feasible, but they still cannot replace more indirect estimates based on ferrokinetic measurements of the total erythroid mass.

Etiology and Pathogenesis

The etiology of stem cell dysfunction resulting in hematopoietic aplasia is completely unknown in about 50% of the cases and only "probable" in the other 50% (Table 1). In some of the idiopathic cases, bone marrow aplasia is constitutional and associated with other congenital abnormalities. There may be chromosomal defects in several cell lines,[10] suggesting a basic dysfunction of a primordial stem cell responsible for the development of a number of tissues. In the acquired idiopathic cases, manifestations and clinical course are so similar to those of secondary cases that the existence of an external etiologic agent has to be assumed, although it cannot be demonstrated. Of the specific pharmacologic agents incriminated in the etiology of secondary cases, chloramphenicol is the most notorious (Table 2). This antibiotic is known to cause mitochondrial injury and reversible bone marrow suppression.[11] However, it has to be conceeded that the relationship between this predictable and reversible effect on bone marrow cells and the capricious and often irreversible bone marrow aplasia is most tenuous. Current studies suggest that a familial susceptibility plays an important part[12] and that a constitutional stem cell sensitivity to chloramphenicol may be more important in the pathogenesis of chloramphenicol-induced aplastic

Table 1
Etiologic Classification of Aplastic Anemia

Idiopathic
Constitutional (Fanconi's anemia)
Acquired
Secondary
Chemical and physical agents
Drugs
Nonpharmacologic chemicals
Radiation
Infectious
Viral: hepatitis
Bacterial: miliary tuberculosis
Metabolic
Pancreatitis
Pregnancy
Immunologic
Antibody
Graft-versus-host
Neoplastic
Myelophthisic anemia
Paroxysmal nocturnal hemoglobinuria

Table 2
Drugs listed by AMA as being associated with the development of aplastic anemia in more than 5 instances[18]

Generic Name	No. of Cases Receiving Drug Alone, or Drug in Combination with Nontoxic Drugs	No. of Cases Receiving Drug in Combination with Potentially Toxic Drug
Acetazolamide	3	7
Chloramphenicol	182	156
Chlordiazepoxide HCI	2	7
Chlorothiazide	2	13
Chlorpheniramine	2	15
Chlorpromazine	3	18
Chlorpropamide	4	2
Colchicine	2	3
Diphenylhydantoin Sodium	3	21
Epinephrine	2	4
Gold Salts	8	2
Mepazine	4	1
Meprobamate	0	15
Penicillin	4	91
Phenacetin	3	31
Phenantoin	9	14
Phenylbutazone	18	22
Potassium Perchlorate	6	4
Primidone	2	6
Prochlorperazine	1	9
Pyrimethamine	2	3
Quinacrine HCL	3	2
Salicylamide	2	3
Streptomycin		31
Sulfadimethoxine	2	4
Sulfamethoxpyridazine	3	11
Sulfisoxazole	3	30
Sulfonamides	4	17
Tolbutamide	7	5
Trimethadione	2	4

anemia than an acquired mitochondrial injury. Both benzene, a potent bone marrow toxin, and radiation energy can cause chromosomal changes in immature hematopoietic precursor cells, presumably rendering the cells sterile and nonproliferative.[13,14] However, how such mitochondrial changes in a few stem cells can cause the elimination of the remaining normal proliferative stem cells is still obscure.

A number of illnesses, especially hepatitis, pancreatitis, and paroxysmal nocturnal hemoglobinuria, have been associated with the development of aplastic anemia. Since some of these diseases involve antigen-antibody reactions, the possibility has been raised that aplastic anemia is another autoimmune disease caused by an immunologic rejection of bone marrow. This possibility has been supported by observations that graft-versus-host reactions occasionally include bone marrow aplasia and that T-lymphocytes are a prominant component of the remaining bone marrow cell population.

Stem Cell Defect

The character of the stem cell dysfunction underlying idiopathic and acquired aplastic anemia is still obscure and it appears that the options are either intrinsic or extrinsic, or, in other words, failure of stem cells or of the microenvironment (HIM). Until recently, it was assumed that the stem cells were defective due to a mutational change caused by environmental agents or by immunologic rejection. However, recent observations on radiation-induced bone marrow aplasia in dogs have suggested that the microenvironment has been altered irreversibly and that stromal changes prevent cellular regeneration.[15] The presence of a similar stromal defect in aplastic anemia in man would have serious implications on attempts to perfect bone marrow transplantation as a treatment for aplastic anemia. However, transplantation of normal bone marrow to identical twins[16] or to HL-A compatible siblings[17] with aplastic anemia has met with some success, and it still looks as if the most likely defect in aplastic anemia resides within the multipotential stem cells themselves.

REFERENCES

1. Erslev AJ: Medullary and extramedullary blood formation. Clin Orthop 52:25, 1967
2. Hudson G: Bone marrow volume in the human foetus and newborn. Br J Haematol 11:446, 1965
3. Mechanik N: Untersuchunger uber das gewecht des Knochenmarkes des Menschen. Z Gesamte Anat 79:58, 1926 (Summarized by Ellis RE: Physiol Med Biol 5:255, 1961)
4. Weiss L: The histology of the bone marrow, Regulation of Hematopoiesis. Edited by AS Gordon. New York, Appleton-Century-Crafts, 1970, p 79
5. Erslev AJ: Feedback circuits in the control of stem cell differentiation. Am J Pathol 65:629, 1971
6. Craddock CG, Longmire R, McMillan R: Lymphocytes and the immune response. N Engl J Med 285:324, 1971
7. Fliedner TM, Calvo W, Haas R, et al: Morphologic and cytokinetic aspects of bone marrow stroma, Hematopoietic Cellular Proliferation. Edited by F Stohlman, Jr. New York, Grune and Stratton, 1970, p 67
8. Porteous DD, Lajtha LG: On stem cell recovery after irradiation. Br J Haematol 12:177, 1966
9. Trentin JJ: Determination of bone marrow stem cell differentiation by stromal hemopoietic inductive microenvironment (HIM). Am J Pathol 65:621, 1971
10. Hirschman RJ, Shulman NR, Abuelo JG, et al: Chromosomal aberrations in two cases of inherited aplastic anemia with unusual clinical features. Ann Intern Med 71:107, 1969

11. Firkin FC: Mitochondrial lesions in reversible erythropoietic depression due to chloramphenicol. J Clin Invest 51:2085, 1972
12. Nagao T, Mauer AM: Concordance for drug-induced aplastic anemia in identical twins. N Engl J Med 281:7, 1969
13. Kissling M, Speck B: Further studies on experimental benzene-induced aplastic anemia. Blut 25:97, 1972
14. Dickle A, Hempelman LH: Morphologic changes in the lymphocytes of persons exposed to ionizing radiation. J Lab Clin Med 32:1045, 1947
15. Knospe WH, Blom J, Crosby WH: Regeneration of locally irradiated bone marrow. Blood 26:398, 1966
16. Pillow RP, Epstein RB, Buckner CD, et al: Treatment of bone marrow failure by isogenetic marrow infusion. N Engl J Med 275:94, 1966
17. Thomas ED, Storb R, Fefer A, et al: Aplastic anemia treated by bone marrow transplantation. Lancet 1:284, 1972
18. Tabulation of reports compiled by the Panel on Hematology of the Registry on Adverse Reactions. Council on Drugs, American Medical Association, May 1965 and June 1967

Nikolay V. Dimitrov
and Viggo Esmann

6

Leukopenia, Phagocytosis, and Infection

The polymorphonuclear (PMN) leukocyte is a cell whose survival depends on its composition, function, and environmental changes. It possesses a cellular control mechanism which is subjected to a variety of injurious factors that result in structural and functional alterations. When the cellular equilibrium of the leukocyte is disturbed, metabolic functions may be increased, decreased, or completely extinguished. The magnitude of these alterations and the compensatory reactions of the leukocyte determine the extent of functional and morphologic reversibility of the cell. If substantial injury is sustained, then the functional capacity of the cell will be diminished or terminated.

LEUKOPENIA

Although a great number of agents are capable of affecting leukocyte function, the fundamental question is to what extent do they damage the regenerative capacity of bone marrow, and consequently, how quickly are quantitative changes in the level of leukocytes in peripheral blood normalized. The quantitative changes do not always parallel qualitative changes in leukocytes. For example, persons with chronic nonfamilial neutropenia have a normal response to stimulation with pyrogen and their leukocytes possess a normal phagocytic function (Figure 1). About 10% of the black population have a neutropenia and most leukopenic individuals respond adequately to pyrogen stimulation.[1] Bone marrow function, the condition of marginal and circulating granulocytic pools, and the phagocytic function of the granulocyte, must be considered seriously in every leukopenic patient. Leukocyte kinetics and their significance are discussed by Stohlman and Quesenberry elsewhere in this book.

It is very important for the clinician to obtain accurate information about the condition of the maturation line in a leukopenic patient. This will allow him to consider whether quantitative changes are due to decreased production in

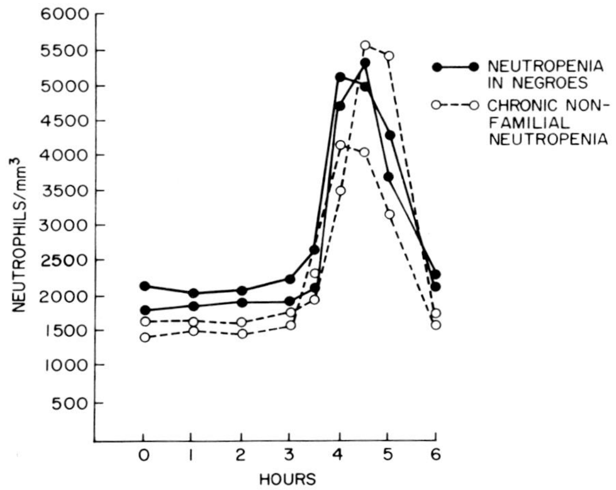

Fig. 1. Graphic presentation of the effect of pyrogen (0.4 ml, intravenously) on neutrophil count during a period of 6 hours in 2 patients with chronic nonfamilial neutropenia and 2 normal black individuals with neutropenia.

bone marrow or increased utilization and destruction somewhere in the peripheral pool. To meet its physiologic responsibility, the functional capacity of bone marrow depends on the ability of its cellular components to multiply and differentiate. If this capacity is in jeopardy, the leukopenic patient is in imminent danger. Many drugs affect granulocyte precursors, thus producing slow regeneration which results in a hypo- or aregenerative leukopenia. The effects of some of these drugs are discussed extensively in the chapter dealing with drugs and leukocytes.

A complete functional classification of the granulocytopenic disorders is given by Finch.[2] This author divides drug-induced granulocytopenia into seven types: (a) cytolytic marrow damage, (b) metabolic interference with granulocyte proliferative pathways, (c) idiosyncratic cessation of granulopoiesis of unknown mechanism, (d) maturation defect of the megaloblastic type, (e) drug-hapten-antibody reaction, (f) production defect and diminished survival, and (g) temporary pseudoneutropenia. In reality, many of these mechanisms could be overlapped, producing enhanced pathophysiologic conditions to accelerate the neutropenic state.

The extent of quantitative and qualitative changes plays an important role in the function of the polymorphonuclear leukocyte (Table 1). Long exposure to myelotoxic agents, such as ionizing radiation, myelosuppressive drugs, chemicals, alcohol, and others produces leukopenia with a significantly diminished functional capacity of granulocytes.[3–6] On the other hand, the granulocytes in genetically determined leukopenia have a normal function and respond normally in case of increased demand (Table 1, Figure 1).

The effects of various agents on the lymphocyte count should also be considered seriously. The interaction between neutrophils and lymphocytes is recognized as an active part of the body's defense mechanism.[7]

Table 1
Comparison of the Quantitative Changes of the Neutrophils and Phagocytic Index in Three Patients with Leukopenia

	Total WBC	Neutrophil Count	Phagocytic Index (%)[37]
Normal Controls (n = 10)	7180±1210*	4360±930	78±11
Black Individual with Leukopenia	3710	1690	74
Patient on Cytoxan Therapy	2960	1320	23
Patient with Acute Alcohol Intoxication	2610	1040	12

* Means ± 1 SD

PHAGOCYTOSIS

One of the most important functions of the PMN leukocyte is its ability to engulf and destroy particulate material and bacteria. These functions are usually combined and referred to as phagocytosis. Many agents, including drugs, are capable of interfering with either one or both functions, thus limiting or eliminating the polymorphonuclear leukocyte as a body defense mechanism. Due to the everlasting fight between micro- and macroorganisms, individuals with functionally incapable leukocytes are prone to infections that frequently cause death at an early age.[8]

Phagocytosis, as mentioned before, consists of two steps, engulfing the microorganisms (real phagocytosis) and a killing effect. Engulfing starts with the movement of granules toward the nucleus[9] and the formation of pseudopods which surround the microorganism. Subsequent swift invagination results in the formation of a plasma membrane-bound phagocytic vacuole (Figure 2a).[10] Factors responsible for the actual engulfment are unknown. It has been shown that the phagocytic process requires glycolytic energy which is furnished by glucose or, in case of glucose depletion, by the breakdown of glycogen.[11]

Following engulfment, the granules fuse with the phagosome (Figure 2b, c, and d), discharging their contents into the vacuole.[9,12] This process is associated with a great increase in both O_2 consumption and hexose-monophosphate shunt activity. In this pathway, glucose-6-phosphate is oxidized to pentose-phosphate with simultaneous formation of reduced nicotinamide adenine dinucleotide phosphate (NADPH) (Figure 3).[11]

It has been proposed that this reaction is followed by NADPH oxidation by means of oxidized glutathione and the enzyme glutathione reductase, which appears to be an immediate response.[11,13,14] Later, further oxidation of NADPH is catalyzed by granular NADPH oxidase, resulting in the formation of hydrogen peroxide (H_2O_2).[15]

The leukocyte granules (lysosomes) contain several proteins (phagocytin,

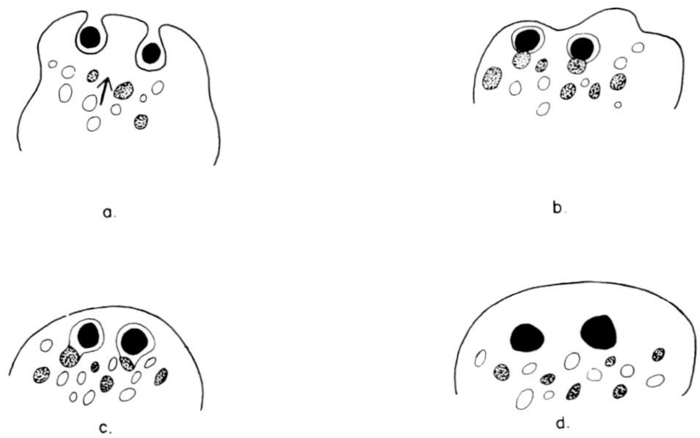

Fig. 2. Schematic presentation of phagocytosis: **a.** Engulfment of particulated material and movement of granules toward the phagocytic invagination. **b.** Adherence of the granules to phagocytic vacuole. **c.** Discharge of the lysosomal material into the vacuole. **d.** Destruction of the phagocytized material.

leukin, and others) which have an antimicrobial effect.[13,14] A number of additional heat-stable cationic proteins exercise this effect by being in contact with the microrganisms when the granules fuse with phagosome. Also, the granules contain a large amount of the enzyme myeloperoxidase which, together with H_2O_2 and halides (iodide, chloride, or bromide), form an extremely potent bactericidal system responsible for the final bacterial killing.[13–16] Since concentrations of chloride are readily attainable, this halide would be the most likely functional factor for myeloperoxidase activity. One possible mechanism is a reaction which involves the formation of a complex (enzyme, H_2O_2, chloride), decarboxylation, and deamination of amino acids to their corresponding alde-

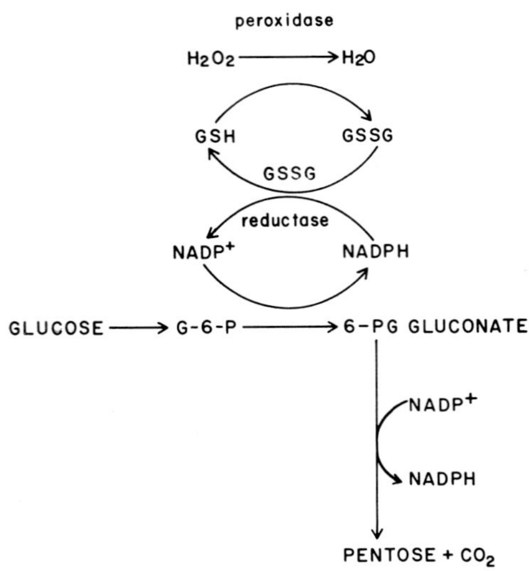

Fig. 3. Metabolic pathways related to stimulation of PMN leukocytes during phagocytosis.

Fig. 4. Probable bactericidal mechanism of PMN leukocytes during phagocytosis.

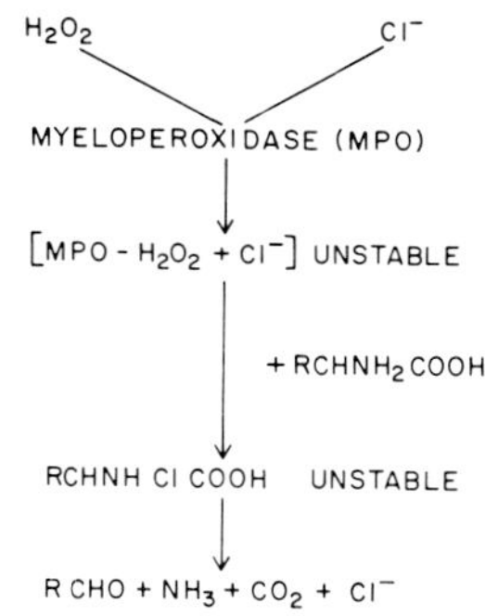

hydes (figure 4).[16] The antimicrobial effect of aldehydes is well known, and the proposal of such a mechanism seems to be acceptable. It has been demonstrated that amino acids are present on the bacterial surface. When the complex of myeloperoxidase, H_2O_2, and chloride reaches the surface or the interior of bacteria, the formation of amino acid chloramine and its conversion to aldehyde will increase antimicrobial activity.[16]

As mentioned before, many drugs could interfere with the proper phagocytic function of the polymorphonuclear leukocyte.[17–21] The main mechanism appears to be the inhibition of various enzymes whose effect is required in the systems involved in producing H_2O_2.[16] All investigations in vitro indicate that, in most cases, the dose of drug required to suppress phagocytosis exceeded the highest therapeutic dose used in humans. The drug effects then include interference with leukocyte movement, chemotaxis, migration of leukocytes from the circulation into tissue, bacterial engulfment, respiration, and bacterial killing.[17,21–25]

Thus, phagocytosis appears to be a process that occurs exclusively in tissue, depending on the state of the circulation, the leukocyte count, the functional and structural integrity of the polymorphonuclear leukocyte, and bacterial potency. Some bacterial secretions could be extremely toxic to the leukocyte. If its important antimicrobial function is eliminated, this will induce bacterial reproduction, leading to fulminant infections. On the other hand, damaged leukocytes, being incapable of killing microorganisms, can harbor and protect them from penetration by and the action of antibiotics and antibodies. This provides a suitable environment for the reproduction of bacteria.

It is well known that opsonization of some bacteria is an essential part of phagocytosis.[26] Drugs that coat the cellular membrane of the granulocyte or interfere with the opsonization of bacteria may depress the engulfing process. There is good evidence for the existence of a phagocytosis-stimulating tetrapeptide (tuftsin) in the gamma globulin fraction of proteins, which has been characterized as a hormone of phagocytosis.[27] The effects of drugs on this tetrapeptide have not yet been investigated. It has been shown that after the spleen is removed, the hormone disappears, and this finding sheds new light on the role of the spleen in the body's defense against infection.

INFECTION

The inflammatory response of tissue to invading microorganisms depends on several factors within the host and the bacterium. The reaction of the host, in general, is quite similar, regardless of the nature of the stimulus—mechanical, thermal, chemical, or bacterial.[28]

Two phases in the inflammatory response have been recognized.[28] The first is of short duration, characterized by a greatly increased blood flow through the affected area due to the dilatation of arterioles and opening of the capillary bed. A slight dilatation of venules, with separation of adjacent endothelial cells, appears to be the anatomic basis for a bulk movement of plasma through slits between cells into the interstitial space. In this period, leukocytes begin to adhere to endothelial cells.[29] This process could be caused by the action of kinins or other agents.[30,31]

The second phase in the inflammatory response lasts for several hours and is associated with leakage of protein through the endothelium and the heavy migration of leukocytes to the extravascular compartment. A diphasic response has been observed in various types of bacterial infections.[31]

In the initial phase of the inflammatory response, histamine, kinins, and epinephrine have been implicated. Histamine is released rapidly in response to a variety of stimuli, and the initial vascular changes have been suppressed successfully by the highly specific antihistaminic drug, mepyramine, or by depleting the test animals of histamine.[32] A suppressive effect of antihistamines on severe or prolonged infections is not to be expected, as tissue stores of histamine are quickly depleted.[33]

The kinins are present in areas of tissue injury and have been found to be capable of inducing inflammatory reactions.[30,31] Bradykinin, in its active form, is formed by several reactions (Figure 5) which begin with the activation of Hageman factor followed by the activation of permeability factor. Activated permeability factor converts plasma prekallikrein to kallikrein, which participates in the conversion of kininogen to bradykinin. Another pathway for the synthesis of bradykinin is through the activation of kininogen, by tissue kallikrein, to kallidin. The latter is catalyzed by the plasma enzyme, aminopeptidase, to

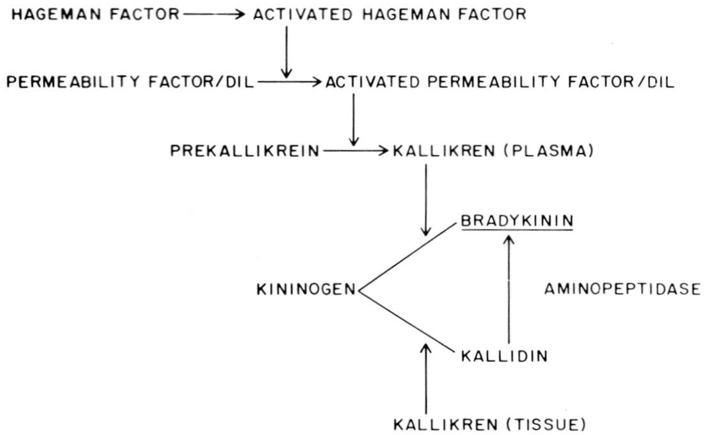

Fig. 5. Schematic presentation of bradykinin formation.

bradykinin. The release of kinins from plasma is inhibited by cortisol in vitro and also in vivo (patients on corticosteroid therapy).[34]

Inflammatory stimuli also release dopa, dopamine, norepinephrine, and epinephrine, which effectively suppress early vascular changes and the exudation of protein.[31] Normally, these vasoactive amines are rapidly degraded, especially by monoamine oxidase which inactivates epinephrine. Activation of monoamine oxidase and the enzymes catalyzing the transformation of tyrosine to epinephrine would thus serve to decrease the inflammatory response. Conversely, monoamine oxidase inhibitors (isocarboxazide and nialamide) definitely increase the concentration of vasoactive amines in different tissues and have been shown to suppress changes in permeability in early experimental inflammation.[31,33] However, the pharmacologic effects of these extremely toxic drugs in man do not include an anti-inflammatory effect.

In bacterial infections, the vascular injury and leakage of protein usually precedes leukocyte migration.[29] The leukocytes make their way through widened slits between endothelial cells and accumulate in large amounts at the site of injury during the following hours. This stage could be associated with leukopenia in peripheral blood as a result of over utilization. Once the cells are out of the bloodstream, they become actively ameboid. Their locomotion depends on the ability of protoplasm to undergo reversible sol/gel transformations and on the presence of microtubular, fibrillar systems. Colchicine, by destroying these cytoplasmic structures, interferes with the motility of the cells.[25,35] The same mechanism may be involved in the effect of caffeine on PMN leukocytes.[23,36] Margination and the adhesive tendency of the leukocytes, as well as diapedesis, have also been affected by cortisol.[33,35]

The directional movement of PMN leukocytes toward the site of injury is caused by chemotactic factors. Recent studies[38] have concentrated on leukotactic factors derived from the complement system. It appears that bacterial proteases are able to generate leukotactic products from C3 and C5. Thus, some factors are present during the late development of inflammation which might be held responsible for the migration of the cells. Chemotaxis is suppressed by some drugs, such as cortisol, chloroquine, and phenylbutazone, which appeared to be granular stabilizing agents.[38]

Normal bone marrow contains large stores of mature PMN leukocytes which are discharged into the bloodstream as they are needed. By impairing leukocyte mobilization, some drugs increase the individual's susceptibility to microbial infection.[23,38] When the drug's effect is added to the already altered production, distribution, extravascular mobilization, and phagocytic function, the entire host defense mechanism will be impaired, with consequent development of progressive infection. This condition could be accelerated when bacterial endotoxins are in effect.

CONCLUSIONS

The use of any drug requires great caution regarding its effect on the hematopoietic system, particularly on PMN leukocytes. This includes not only changes in the leukocyte count, but also on functional cellular alterations. Such precautions will eliminate unnecessary complications which, in some cases, could be fatal. Unfortunately, we have very little knowledge to offer regarding the stimulation of the defense mechanism of the human body. The late George Bernard Shaw in *The Doctors' Dilemma* postulated that nature had provided in leukocytes "a natural means of devouring and destroying all disease germs. There is at bottom only one genuinely scientific treatment for all diseases and that is to stimulate phagocytes. Stimulate the phagocytes. Drugs are a delusion."

In times like ours, when polypharmacy appears to be a fashion, the adverse effects of many drugs on leukocyte function require that the physician pay careful attention to these effects in order to avoid dangerous complications.

REFERENCES

1. Dimitrov NV, Fischer G, Chang H: Neutropenia among the black population. Unpublished data
2. Finch SC: Granulocytopenia, Hematology. Edited by WJ Williams, E Beutler, AJ Erslev, et al. New York, McGraw-Hill Book Co, 1972, p 628
3. Cronkite EP, Bond VP, Conrad RA: The hematology of ionizing radiation, Atomic Medicine. Edited by CR Behrens, ER King, JWJ Carpender. Baltimore, Williams and Wilkins, 1969, p 189
4. Pisciotta AV: Drug-induced leukopenia and aplastic anemia. Clin Pharmacol Ther 12:13, 1971
5. Selvaraj RJ, Sbarra AJ: Effects of x-irradiation on the metabolic changes accompanying phagocytosis. Nature 210:158, 1966
6. Calabresi P, Welch AD: Chemotherapy of neoplastic diseases, Pharmacological Basis of Therapeutics. Edited by LS Goodman, A Gilman. New York, Macmillan, 1970, p 1344
7. Fidalgo BV, Najjar VA: The physiological role of the lymphoid system. III. Leukophilic γ-globulin and the phagocytic activity of the polymorphonuclear leukocyte. Proc Natl Acad Sci USA 57:957, 1967
8. Holmes B, Page AR, Good RA: Studies of the metabolic activity of leukocytes from patients with a genetic abnormality of phagocytic function. J Clin Invest 46:1422, 1967
9. Zucker-Franklin D: Electron microscopic studies of human granulocytes: Structural variations related to function. Semin Hematol 5:109, 1968
10. Hirsch JG: Neutrophil and eosinophil leukocytes, The Inflammatory Process. Edited by BW Zweifach, L Grant, RT McCluskey. New York, Academic, 1965, p 245
11. Karnovsky ML: Metabolic basis of phagocytic activity. Physiol Rev 42:143, 1962
12. Hawiger J, Horn RG, Glenn Koenig M, et al: Activation and release of lysosmal enzymes from isolated leukocytic granules by liposomes. A proposed model for degranulation in PMN leukocytes. Yale J Biol Med 42:57, 1969
13. Klebanoff SJ: Intracleukocytic microbicidal effects. Ann Rev Med 22:39, 1971
14. Klebanoff SJ: Myeloperoxidase-mediated antimicrobial systems, Biochemistry of the Phagocytic Process. Edited by J Schultz. Amsterdam. North Holland, 1970, p 89
15. Sbarra AJ, Jacobs AA, Strauss RR. et al: The biochemical and antimicrobial activities of phagocytizing cells. Am P Clin Nutr 24:272, 1971
16. Sbarra AJ, Paul BB, Jacobs AA, et al: Role of the phagocyte in host-parasite interaction XXXVIII. Metabolic activities of the phagocyte as related to antimicrobial action. J Reticuloendothel Soc 12:109, 1972

17. Crabbe J: The effects of cortisone on the phagocytic activity of rabbit macrophages to staphylococci. Acta Endocrinol 18:251, 1955
18. Crepea SB, Magnin GE, Seastone CV: Effect of ACTH and cortisone on phagocytosis. Proc Soc Exp Biol Med 77:704, 1951
19. Fedorko M: Effect of chloroquine on morphology of cytoplasmic granules in maturing human leukocytes—an ultrastructural study. J Clin Invest 46:1932, 1967
20. Folette JH, Shugarman PM, Reynolds J, et al: The effect of chloramphenicol and other antibiotics on leukocyte respiration. Blood 11:234, 1956
21. Gardner DE, Holzman RS, Coffin DL: Depression of phagocytosis by sulfomethazine. J Bacteriol 96:274, 1968
22. Goldfinger SE, Howell RR, Seegmiller JE: Suppression of metabolic accompaniments of phagocytosis by colchicine. Arthritis Rheum 8:1112, 1965
23. Dimitrov NV, Miller J, Ziegra SR: The effects of caffeine on glucose metabolism of polymorphonuclear leukocytes. J Pharmacol Exp Ther 168:240, 1969
24. Peters WP, Holland JF, Senn H, et al: Corticosteroid administration and localized leukocyte mobilization in man. N Engl J Med 286:342, 1972
25. Caner JEZ: Colchicine inhibition of chemotaxis. Arthritis Rheum 8:757, 1965
26. Rytel MW, Stollerman KH: The opsonic effect of complement on phagocytosis of γ-globulin coated particles. J Immunol 90:607, 1963
27. Najjar VA, Constanopoulos A: A new phagocytosis-stimulating tetrapeptide hormone, tuftsin and its role in disease. J Reticuloendothel Soc 12:197, 1972
28. Zweifach BW: Microvascular aspects of tissue injury.[10] p 161
29. Grant L: The sticking and emigration of white blood cells in inflammation.[10] p 197
30. Kellermeyer RW, Grahm RC Jr: Kinins: Possible physiologic and pathologic roles in man. N Engl J Med 279:754, 1968
31. Wilhelm DL: Chemical Mediators. 1.[10] p 389
32. Spector WG, Willoughby DA: Chemical Mediators.[10] p 427
33. Allison F: Anti-inflammatory agents.[10] p 559
34. Cline MJ, Melmon KL: Plasma kinins and cortisol: a possible explanation of the anti-inflammatory action of cortisol. Science 153:1135, 1966
35. Malawista SE: The action of colchicine in acute gout. Arthritis Rheum 8:752, 1965
36. Hansz J, Dimitrov NV: Effects of caffeine on the metabolic stimulation of polymorphonuclear leukocytes during phagocytosis. Proc Soc Exp Biol Med 137:735, 1971
37. Cline MJ, Lehrer R: Phagocytosis by human monocytes. Blood 32:423, 1968
38. Ward PA: Leukotactic factors in health and disease. Am J Pathol 64:521, 1971

Jack Levin

7
Pathophysiology of Drug-induced Thrombocytopenia

The pathophysiology of drug-induced thrombocytopenia can be better understood by first considering the physiologic mechanisms which produce and maintain normal levels of circulating platelets. Platelets are nonnucleated but are structured pieces of megakaryocytes that enter the circulation after the megakaryocytes mature and demarcation of the cytoplasm into platelets has occurred. Studies of the kinetics of platelet production indicate that cells recognized as megakaryocytes do not replicate and that the megakaryocyte pool is maintained by the entry of new cells from a yet unidentified population of precursor cells.[1,2] However, DNA synthesis in immature megakaryocytes (endoreduplication) results in polyploid cells.[3–6] Recognizable megakaryocytes usually contain a multilobed (or segmented) nucleus,[2–4, 7–9] and have ploidy levels of 8N, 16N, or, 32N (diploid cells are 2N), based on measurements of DNA content.[1,3–5,10,11] Megakaryocytes, at any level of polyploidy, are capable of undergoing cytoplasmic maturation with subsequent production of platelets.[1,2,4,5,8–10] The nonreplicating but polyploid nature of megarkaryocytes makes them unique elements of the bone marrow.

Many experimental studies in rodents and dogs have demonstrated that the production of platelets by megakaryocytes normally reflects the level of circulating platelets. Thrombocytopenia produced either by exchange transfusion or by administration of platelet antiserum is followed by an increased production of platelets; subsequently platelet levels rise to greater than normal ("rebound thrombocytosis").[12–15] Increased platelet production is associated with an increase in the number and size of megakaryocytes,[7,15–17] their rate of maturation,[14,16,18,19] and the influx of precursor cells into the pool of identifiable megakaryocytes.[14,16–18] Conversely, thrombocytosis produced by hypertransfusion

Carried out under Contract COO-3014-6 between the United States Atomic Energy Commission and The Johns Hopkins University, and supported in part by Graduate Training grant TI-AM-5260 from the National Institute of Arthritis and Metabolic Diseases, US Public Health Service.

of platelets is followed by rebound thrombocytopenia, which has been interpreted as secondary to suppression of platelet production.[20–23] Reduction of the number of megakaryocytes 3 to 4 days after the induction of thrombocytosis,[21] and a decrease in the number and size of megakaryocytes after 4 to 10 days of thrombocytosis[7] also suggest decreased thrombopoiesis. Furthermore, that platelet production is suppressed in these circumstances has been suggested by decreases in the rate at which radioactively labeled platelets appear in the circulation after the administration of $Na_2{}^{35}SO_4$ or selenomethionine-^{75} Se(^{75}SeM), isotopes that are incorporated into the cytoplasm of megakaryocytes.[24] It appears that thrombopoiesis is not totally suppressed by sustained thrombocytosis, just as erythropoiesis is not uniformly suppressed by polycythemia.[25–26]

Both stimulation and suppression of thrombopoiesis in rats, after the production of thrombocytopenia or thrombocytosis, respectively, are detectable only after a delay of approximately 24 hours.[15,17,19,21] Adjustment in the rate of thrombopoiesis apparently occurs at the level of megakaryocytic precursors or Stage 1 megakaryocytes,[7,15,17,27] and subsequently a population of megakaryocytes that has been altered in number, ploidy, size, and rate of maturation can be identified in the bone marrow. Maximal rebound thrombocytosis or rebound thrombocytopenia, after the induction of thrombocytopenia or thrombocytosis, occurs approximately 6 days after alteration of the platelet levels of rabbits and rats.[15,21,23] This period of time is that required for two consecutive populations (cohorts) of megakaryocytes to enter the marrow pool, mature, and release platelets.[28,29]

Limited but similar data have been obtained in humans. The administration of ^{3}HTdr to one patient resulted in a gradual increase of the fraction of labeled megakaryocytes in the marrow, with the maximal labeled fraction (50%) occurring at 6 days.[20] The administration of $Na_2{}^{35}SO_4$ or ^{75}SeM to humans resulted in the gradual appearance of labeled platelets in the circulation, with maximal levels reached approximately 6 to 9 days after the isotope was administered.[30–32] This is compatible with the initial incorporation of $Na_2{}^{35}SO_4$ or ^{75}SeM into the cytoplasm of megakaryocytes, maturation of these cells, and then the release of labeled platelets into the circulation. Harker demonstrated alterations in the number and size of megakaryocytes in abnormal hematologic states characterized by thrombocytopenia or thrombocytosis, and has shown a correlation between megakaryocyte mass and platelet turnover,[33,34] except in states of ineffective thrombopoiesis. The average megakaryocyte volume in patients with idiopathic thrombocytopenic purpura was increased, and the magnitude of change was inversely related to the platelet count.[34] In contrast, patients with reactive thrombocytosis had megakaryocytes that were smaller in volume than normal cells.[33] However, Kinet-Denoel, et al[35] and Penington and Weste[36] did not observe increased ploidy in the megakaryocytes of patients with idiopathic thrombocytopenic purpura, and Lagerlöf[11] noted normal or increased ploidy in patients with reactive thrombocytosis.

The observations suggest that there is an effective feedback mechanism by which the rate of thrombopoiesis is affected by the level of circulating platelet mass. Odell, et al[17] and Ebbe, et al[19,37] have suggested that the time lag between the change in platelet levels and the detection of altered megakaryocytopoiesis reflects either mechanisms effective at the level of precursor cells, or a delay in the production of a humoral substance (thrombopoietin) responsible for altered thrombopoiesis, or both. Recent studies in animals and humans have provided evidence for such humoral regulators of platelet production.[23,38–41]

AGENTS WHICH PRODUCE THROMBOCYTOPENIA

There are many mechanisms by which therapeutic agents cause thrombocytopenia. The varied group of substances utilized as antitumor drugs usually act by directly depressing bone marrow functions, in particular, thrombopoiesis. This is presumably the result of depression, not only of cells identifiable as megakaryocytes, but also of megakaryocytic precursors. These toxic effects often provide opportunities to confirm data obtained from experimental studies of platelet production, or to learn new facts about thrombopoiesis in man.

Antitumor Agents

Acute thrombocytopenia, produced by antitumor agents, often is followed by rebound thrombocytosis, with platelet levels occasionally exceeding 1,000,000/mm^3.[42] The administration of cytosine arabinoside by acute intravenous injection is followed by maximal thrombocytopenia 12 days later and by maximal rebound thrombocytosis at 22 days.[43] Folic acid antagonists produce maximal thrombocytopenia 9 to 15 days after administration, with a subsequent rebound thrombocytosis.[44,45] Rebound thrombocytosis, after therapy with amethopterin was started, reached a maximum at about 18 to 22 days, or 7 to 10 days after thrombocytopenia.[45] In contrast, a large dose of mechlorethamine (nitrogen mustard), a noncycle-active agent, although producing maximal thrombocytopenia at 10 to 15 days, was not associated with rebound thrombocytosis.[46] Noncycle-active agents injure cells regardless of their stage in the mitotic cycle (including resting phase, or nonproliferating cells). Cycle-active (or cycle-dependent) drugs are antimetabolic agents that exert their primary effects on cells in a specific stage of the generation cycle.

These data strongly suggest that these agents damage megakaryocytic precursors and megakaryoblasts, thus decreasing the input of new platelets into the circulation. Maximal depression of platelet levels, 10 to 15 days after administration of drug, is compatible with estimations of the life span of human platelets.[47,48] Rebound thrombocytosis approximately 10 days after thrombocytopenia supports the concept of a feedback mechanism in humans, and possibly represents the response to thrombocytopenia of a cohort of megakaryocytes that have been synchronized, as suggested by Lampkin, et al.[49,50]

Some drugs apparently suppress myelopoiesis and thrombopoiesis equally, but this is not always the case. Large doses of mechlorethamine have produced similar degrees of depression of these hematopoietic elements,[46] as has total-body irradiation.[51] However, the administration of small doses of mechlorethamine on alternate days produced thrombocytopenia in only 20 per cent of cases, whereas anemia and leukopenia occurred in 58 to 87 per cent of the patients studied.[52]

Table 1
Effect of Cytosine Arabinoside Upon White Blood Cells and Platelets (222 Trials)

Incidence of Depression			
White Blood Cells/mm³		*Platelets/mm³*	
3,000–5,000	*<3,000*	*50,000–200,000*	*<50,000*
35	31	26	13

Cytosine arabinoside was administered by a single rapid intravenous injection or in a continuous infusion lasting 24, 48, or 96 hours. Hematopoietic suppression increased as the duration of administration was lengthened, and marked leukopenia was more common than thrombocytopenia (modified from Frei, et al.[42]).

Cyclophosphamide, another noncycle-active agent, produces relatively less thrombocytopenia than leukopenia, but, paradoxically, does produce rebound thrombocytosis.[53]

In general, cycle-active agents seem to depress both erythroid and myeloid elements to a significantly greater degree than they do platelet precursors. A striking example of the disparity of the effects of cytosine arabinoside on white blood cells and platelets has been reported by Burke, et al[43] who observed maximal platelet depression at the same time relative leukocytosis occurred, followed by rebound thrombocytosis concomitant with maximal leukopenia. Frei, et al[42] reported greater depression of white blood cells than of platelets in 88 patients given cytosine arabinoside in 1-,2-, or 4-day infusions (Table 1). Single doses of cytosine arabinoside caused slight leukopenia without thrombocytopenia, whereas the same total amount administered in divided daily doses produced greater thrombocytopenia with little additional leukopenia (Table 2).[54] Vincristine, administered intravenously once weekly, produced leukopenia in 25% of the cases, but no instances of thrombocytopenia attributable to the drug were recorded.[55]

Table 2
Effect of Cytosine Arabinoside Upon White Blood Cells and Platelets (8 Trials)

	Maximal Depression	
	Daily	*Single Dose*
WBC/mm³	3,850	4,790
Platelets/mm³	72,300	237,200

Cytosine arabinoside (maximal total dose 50 mg/kg) was administered either daily for 4–10 days, or in a single dose. Repeated daily doses produced significant thrombocytopenia (modified from Talley and Vaitkevicius[54]).

Experimental studies by Morse and Stohlman[56] demonstrated that doses of vincristine that severely depress erythropoietic activity cause little change in the rate of thrombopoiesis. These studies showed no significant changes in the differential counts or morphology of megakaryocytes in rats given vincristine, despite concomitant depopulation of marrow erythroid elements. The continued differentiation of precursor cells into the megakaryocytic pool indicated that vincristine did not halt differentiation of "committed" stem cells into megakaryocytic precursors. The authors therefore concluded that there were different immediate precursor cells for these cell lines. This is supported by observations that erythropoietin does not produce thrombocytosis.[16,22] Amphotericin B also produces anemia without apparent concomitant thrombocytopenia.[57,58]

Studies in animals provide additional understanding of mechanisms by which antitumor agents suppress thrombopoiesis. Incorporation of selenomethionine-^{75}Se(^{75}SeM) into platelets was decreased in rabbits that received mechlorethamine 1, 2, or 4 days before the administration of ^{75}SeM.[23] In each experimental group, there was a delayed increase in the level of ^{75}SeM in platelets, 6 to 10 days after the isotope was administered, which correlated with platelet counts. The increase in percentage of ^{75}SeM associated with platelets, as the platelet count was rising, indicated that a heavily tagged population of new platelets had entered the circulation. Presumably ^{75}SeM, which did not appear in circulating platelets at the usual times (i.e., 2 to 4 days), remained available in the marrow within megakaryocytes or their precursors that were not productive, and subsequently appeared in circulating platelets when megakaryocyte function was reestablished.

Lindell and Zajicek[59] demonstrated that maximal reduction in the number of megakaryocytes in femurs of rats that had received total-body irradition did not occur until 5 to 7 days after irradiation, suggesting that the damage had occurred to megakaryocyte precursors and not primarily to cells that already were in the pool of recognizable megakaryocytes. Furthermore, irradiation of one femur produced the same changes in that area as when animals received total-body irradiation, indicating that during the period of observation the irradiated marrow had not been recolonized by stem cells from nonirradiated areas of the body.[59] Odell, et al[60] reported that the proliferating diploid precursors of megakaryocytes of mice were sensitive to irradiation, in contrast to recognizable megakaryocytes which were radioresistant.

Ebbe and Stohlman[37] have demonstrated that the induction of acute thrombocytopenia either immediately before or after exposure to irradiation partially protects mice against the thrombocytopenic effects of 200 to 400 R of total-body irradiation. Elson reported that production of thrombocytopenia with a rapidly acting nitrogen mustard partially protects animals against the thrombocytopenic effects of subsequently administered busulfan.[51] Both groups[37,51] concluded that bone marrow stimulation, before the maximal depressive action of busulfan or irradiation, had been protective.

Other antitumor agents (e.g., vincristine and vinblastine) may produce thrombocytosis *without* prior thrombocytopenia. This was observed in 13 of 40 cases after weekly intravenous injections of vincristine[55] and also has been reported by Hwang, et al[61] and Robertson and McCarthy.[62] There did not appear to be a significant interval between the time drug therapy was started and the development of thrombocytosis; cessation of the drug seemed to be associated with an immediate drop in the platelet count to pretreatment levels. Thrombocytosis also has been observed in rats after the administration of vincristine.[62–64] Mechanisms which account for these changes are unclear, but it has been suggested that certain dose levels may stimulate thrombopoiesis.[63–65]

Another agent has been shown to result in cyclic changes in levels of some circulating blood cells. Kennedy[66] has reported that patients treated with hydroxyurea may show oscillatory changes in levels of circulating white blood cells and platelets; no changes were observed either in reticulocyte counts or hemoglobin levels. These observations support the suggestion of Morley, et al[67,68] that the kinetics of normal marrow function may be cyclic, and provide additional evidence that committed stem cells of the three hematopoietic cell lines differ significantly from each other.

Other Agents

There are other mechanisms by which drugs or other agents produce thrombocytopenia without suppressing platelet production by megakaryocytes (Table 3). Many drugs, including quinidine, quinine, novobiocin, digitoxin, stibophen, cephalothin, chlorothiazide, and apronalide (Sedormid), have been shown to produce thrombocytopenia secondary to an antigen-antibody re-

Table 3
Production of Acute Thrombocytopenia Without Suppression of Thrombopoiesis

Agent	Mechanism	Reference No.
Quinidine*	Immunologic	81,82
Blood transfusion	Immunologic (post-transfusion purpura)	73,91
Blood transfusion	Intravascular coagulation (hemolytic transfusion reaction)	96,97
Infection	Intravascular coagulation (? endotoxin)	92,93
Malignancy	Intravascular coagulation	93
Blood transfusion	Dilution of circulating platelets	100
Ristocetin	Direct toxic effect on circulating platelets	101

* Many other drugs also produce thrombocytopenia by this mechanism (see text).

action.[69–77] The prerequisite components for this phenomenon include the drug, a plasma protein with which the drug binds, antibody to the drug-protein complex, and platelets. Platelets usually are involved only secondarily by providing a surface to which the antigen-antibody complex can adhere.[73,78] Rechallenge of sensitive individuals with offending drugs results in recurrent thrombocytopenia.[73,74,77,79,80] Agglutination and lysis of platelets from the patient or from normal donors, inhibition of clot retraction, release of platelet factor 3, and complement fixation often can be demonstrated in vitro in the presence of the drug and serum from an affected person that contains the antibody.[73,74,76,77,79–86] The nature of the antibody appears to be the main factor in determining whether thrombocytopenia, leukopenia, or hemolytic anemia is produced in the susceptible patient.[73] The antibody shows a striking specificity for the drug against which it is active, since quinine cannot be substituted for quinidine[82] or digitoxigenin nor digoxin for digitoxin,[74] nor chlorothiazide for hydrochlorothiazide.[87] Immune thrombocytopenia secondary to circulating antibody to a metabolic product of a drug, but not to the drug itself, has been reported.[88,89] In one case, thrombocytopenic purpura was produced by nitroglycerin, but not by closely related erythroltetranitrate.[90] In rare instances, the production of antibodies against *donor* platelets can result in delayed thrombocytopenia (post-transfusion purpura), which takes place when antigen-antibody complexes, containing donor platelets or fragments thereof, adhere to platelets of the recipient.[73,91]

Infection (usually with gram-negative organisms),[92,93] malignancy,[94,95] and hemolytic reactions to blood transfusion[96,97] can result in intravascular coagulation that produces both thrombocytopenia and hypofibrinogenemia. Endotoxin or red cell stroma may be the precipitating triggers of the first and last examples,[93,96,97] but the mechanism by which some tumors produce intravascular coagulation remains unclear. The production of a thromboplastic substance by tumor cells has been suggested as a possible cause.[93] In other instances, turbulent blood flow in vascular tumors is believed to result in sequestration and destruction of platelets sufficient to produce systemic thrombocytopenia.[98,99] The rapid transfusion of large volumes of blood that do not contain viable platelets can produce thrombocytopenia by diluting circulating platelets.[100] Ristocetin, an antibiotic, produces thrombocytopenia in man and rabbits by a direct, dose-related effect on circulating platelets.[101] Lysis of platelets can be demonstrated in vitro by adding the drug to saline suspensions of platelets.[101] It also has been suggested that mithramycin (NSC-24559) causes qualitative changes in circulating platelets (and damages the terminal vascular bed) in addition to thrombocytopenia secondary to hematopoietic depression.[102–104]

The different mechanisms by which thrombocytopenia can be produced without depressing thrombopoiesis should be considered when evaluating any patient who is receiving antitumor agents. Thrombocytosis can be present in patients with malignant disease before therapy.[105,106] The mechanism of thrombocytosis in malignant disease is not understood, and it is not known whether such patients are more resistant to the production of thrombocytopenia by antitumor agents. Harker and Finch[33] have demonstrated overproduction of platelets in patients with thrombocytosis associated with myeloproliferative disorders, suggesting a defective feedback mechanism.

DISCUSSION

The effects of antitumor agents on thrombopoiesis in man and animals strongly support the concept of a feedback mechanism responsive to levels of circulating platelets. Rebound thrombocytosis may be due in part to synchronization of megakaryocytes stimulated by the state of thrombocytopenia during stages of DNA synthesis. Megakaryocytes that mature during a period of thrombocytopenia have increased ploidy and cytoplasmic mass, and probably produce more platelets per megakaryocyte.[3,7,15,27,33,34] The time required for the development of thrombocytopenia and rebound thrombocytosis after the administration of antitumor agents provides additional evidence that the life span of platelets in man is approximately 10 days. A similar, or perhaps shorter, period is required for megakaryoblasts to develop into platelet producing, mature megakaryocytes.

The dissociation between the production of reticulocytopenia, leukopenia, and of thrombocytopenia by antitumor agents[42,55,57,66,104,107,108] is most compatible with the existence of biologically different, committed precursors for these three hematopoietic cell lines, with resultant variations in sensitivity to antitumor agents. Such observations also indicate that an important effect of therapeutic doses of most marrow-suppressive drugs is upon committed stem cells rather than uncommitted or pluripotential stem cells. The administration of ^{75}SeM to rabbits when megakaryocyte function had been severely depressed has provided evidence that megakaryoblasts or their precursors were capable of incorporating and storing this amino acid until function was recovered.[23]

In some studies, single infusions of cytosine arabinoside, a cycle-active drug that blocks DNA synthesis, produced relatively little thrombocytopenia.[42,54] Only megakaryocytic precursors and immature megakaryocytes appear to engage in DNA synthesis[2,5,60]; thus, most of the megakaryocyte population escaped damage because the duration of drug effect was not sufficient to significantly alter the input of new cells into the megakaryocyte compartment. However, when the duration of treatment was extended, significant thrombocytopenia occurred.[54]

Another partial explanation for the relative resistance of megakaryocytes to many antitumor drugs is that the thrombopoietin sensitive cell may be in a resting (or nonsynthetic) state, and therefore is not susceptible to the action of ionizing radiation or drugs that cause similar damage.[37,109] Observations that support this concept are the effects on thrombopoiesis of single doses of irradiation or noncycle-active drugs that affect both proliferating and nonproliferating cells and the increased sensitivity of mice to irradiation after the induction of chronic thrombocytopenia, which presumably increases megakaryocyte flux.[37]

Megakaryocytes are unique in that they are polyploid and do not undergo cellular division. This complex state of high ploidy, in addition to an unknown microenvironment,[110] may account for some of the differences observed. Increased ploidy perhaps alters drug uptake. The large amount of DNA present in megakaryocytes may provide these cells with a reserve capability permitting partial inactivation or loss of DNA or synthetic ability, while retaining the potential to produce some platelets.

Thrombocytopenia also can result from the peripheral destruction of platelets, without the suppression of thrombopoiesis (Table 3). Some drugs produce thrombocytopenia secondary to an immunologic reaction which includes the production of an antibody against the drug or one of its metabolic products. The resultant damage to platelets causes their removal from the circulation. Other mechanisms which result in reduced levels of circulating platelets include intravascular coagulation, dilution by administering large volumes of platelet-poor blood, or a direct toxic effect on platelets.

REFERENCES

1. Odell TT Jr, Jackson CW: Megakaryocytopoiesis, Hemopoietic Cellular Proliferation. Edited by F Stohlman Jr. New York, Grune and Stratton, 1970, pp 278–284
2. Ebbe S: Megakaryocytopoiesis, Regulation of Hematopoiesis. Vol 2. Edited by AS Gordon. New York, Appleton-Century-Crofts, 1970, pp. 1587–1610
3. Odell TT Jr, Jackson CW: Polyploidy and maturation of rat megakaryocytes. Blood 32:102, 1968
4. Paulus J-M: DNA metabolism and development of organelles in guinea pig megakaryocytes: A combined ultrastructural, autoradiographic and cytophotometric study. Blood 35:298, 1970
5. Odell TT Jr, Jackson CW, Friday TJ: Megakaryocytopoiesis in rats with special reference to polyploidy. Blood 35:775, 1970
6. Garcia AM: Feulgen-DNA values in megakaryocytes. J Cell Biol 20:342, 1964
7. Harker LA: Kinetics of thrombopoiesis, J Clin Invest 47:458, 1968
8. de Leval M: Contribution à l'étude de la maturation des mégacaryocytes dans la moëlle osseuse de cobaye. Arch Biol 79:597, 1968
9. MacPherson GG: Development of megakaryocytes in bone marrow of the rat: an analysis by electron microscopy and high resolution autoradiography. Proc R Soc Lond B 177:265, 1971
10. Odell TT Jr, Jackson CW, de Leval M, et al: Cytological analysis of megakaryocyte and platelet kinetics, Platelet Kinetics. Edited by JM Paulus. Amsterdam, North-Holland, 1971, pp. 183–201
11. Lagerlöf B: Cytophotometric study of megakaryocyte ploidy in polycythemia vera and chronic granulocytic leukemia. Acta Cyton 16:240, 1972
12. Craddock CG, Adams WS, Perry S, et al: The dynamics of platelet production as studied by a depletion technique in normal and irradiated dogs. J Lab Clin Med 45:906, 1955
13. Matter M, Hartmann JR, Kautz J, et al: A study of thrombopoiesis in induced acute thrombocytopenia. Blood 15:174, 1960
14. Odell TT Jr, McDonald TP, Asano M: Response of rat megakaryocytes and platelets to bleeding. Acta Haematol 27:171, 1962
15. Ebbe S, Stohlman F Jr, Overcash J, et al: Megakaryocyte size in thrombocytopenic and normal rats. Blood 32:383, 1968
16. Ebbe S: Megakaryocytopoiesis and platelet turnover. Series Haematol 1:65, 1968
17. Odell TT Jr, Jackson CW, Friday TJ, et al: Effects of thrombocytopenia on megakaryocytopoiesis. Br J Haematol 17:91, 1969
18. Odell TT Jr, Kniseley RM: The origin, life span, regulation, and fate of blood platelets. Progress in Hematology. Vol 3. Edited by LM Tocantins. New York, Grune & Stratton, 1962, pp 203–217

19. Ebbe S, Stohlman F Jr, Donovan J, et al: Megakaryocyte maturation rate in thrombocytopenic rats. Blood 32:787, 1968
20. Cronkite EP, Bond VP, Fliedner TM, et al: Studies on the origin, production and destruction of platelets, Blood Platelets. Edited by SA Johnson, RW Monto, JW Rebuck, et al. Boston, Little, Brown, 1961, pp 595–609
21. Odell TT Jr, Jackson CW, Reiter RS: Depression of the megakaryocyte-platelet system in rats by transfusion of platelets. Acta Haematol 38:34, 1967
22. de Gabriele G, Penington DG: Physiology of the regulation of platelet production. Br J Haematol 13:202, 1967
23. Evatt BL, Levin J: Measurement of thrombopoiesis in rabbits using ^{75}selenomethionine. J Clin Invest 48:1615, 1969
24. Levin J: Humoral control of thrombopoiesis, Formation and Destruction of Blood Cells. Edited by TJ Greenwalt, GA Jamieson. Philadelphia, Lippincott, 1970 pp 143–150
25. Stohlman F Jr: Some aspects of erythrokinetics. Semin Hematol 4:304, 1967
26. Schooley JC, Garcia JF: Suppression of erythropoiesis in the plethoric rat by antierythropoietin. Proc Soc Exp Biol Med 133:953, 1970
27. Penington DG, Olsen TE: Megakaryocytes in states of altered platelet production: cell numbers, size and DNA content. Br J Haematol 18:447, 1970
28. Ebbe S, Stohlman F Jr: Megakaryocytopoiesis in the rat. Blood 26:20, 1965
29. Cooney DP, Smith BA: Maturation time of rabbit megakaryocytes. Br J Haematol 11:484, 1965
30. Vodopick HA, Kniseley RM: Sulful-35 studies in man: Platelet survival and plasma and urinary radioactivity assayed by beta liquid scintillation spectrometry. J Lab Clin Med 62:109, 1963
31. Najean Y, Ardaillou N: The use of ^{75}Se-methionin for the in vivo study of platelet kinetics. Scand J Haematol 6:395, 1969
32. McIntyre PA, Evatt BL, Hodkinson BA, et al: Selenium-75 selenomethionine as a label for erythrocytes, leukocytes, and platelets in man. J Lab Clin Med 75:472, 1970
33. Harker LA, Finch CA: Thrombokinetics in man. J Clin Invest 48:963, 1969
34. Harker LA: Thrombokinetics in idiopathic thrombocytopenic purpura. Br J Haematol 19:95, 1970
35. Kinet-Denoel C, Bassleer R, Andrien JM, et al: Ploidy histograms in ITP,[10] pp 280–284
36. Penington DG, Weste SM: Ploidy histograms in ITP.[10] pp 284–287
37. Ebbe S, Stohlman F Jr: Stimulation of thrombocytopoiesis in irradiated mice. Blood 35:783, 1970
38. Penington DG: Isotope bioassay for "Thrombopoietin." Br Med J 1:606, 1970
39. Harker LA: Regulation of thrombopoiesis. Am J Physiol 218:1376, 1970
40. Shreiner DP, Levin J: Detection of thrombopoietic activity in plasma by stimulation of suppressed thrombopoiesis. J Clin Invest 49:1709, 1970
41. Cooper GW, Cooper B, Chung C-Y: Demonstration of a circulating factor regulating blood platelet production using ^{35}S-sulfate in rats and mice. Proc Soc Exp Biol Med 134:1123, 1970
42. Frei E III, Bickers JN, Hewlett JS, et al: Dose schedule and antitumor studies of arabinosyl cytosine (NSC-63878). Cancer Res 29:1325, 1969
43. Burke PJ, Serpick AA, Carbone PP, et al: A clinical evaluation of dose and schedule of administration of cytosine arabinoside (NSC-63878). Cancer Res 28:274, 1968
44. Holland JF: Symposium on the experimental pharmacology and clinical use

of antimetabolites. VIII. Folic acid antagonists. Clin Pharmacol Ther 2:374, 1961
45. Ogston D, Dawson AA, Philip JF: Methotrexate and the platelet count. Br J Cancer 22:244, 1968
46. Sensenbrenner LL, Owens AH Jr.: The effects of mechlorethamine on bone marrow function and iron metabolism in man. Johns Hopkins Med J 121: 162, 1967
47. Aster RH, Jandl JH: Platelet sequestration in man. I. Methods. J Clin Invest 43:843, 1964
48. Shulman NR, Marder VJ, Weinrach RS: Similarities between known anti-platelet antibodies and the factor responsible for thrombocytopenia in idiopathic purpura. Physiologic, serologic and isotopic studies. Ann N Y Acad Sci 124:499, 1965
49. Lampkin BC, Nagao T, Mauer AM: Drug effect in acute leukemia. J Clin Invest 48:1124, 1969
50. Lampkin BC, McWilliams NB, Mauer AM: Cell kinetics and chemotherapy in acute leukemia. Semin Hematol 9:211, 1972
51. Elson LA: Comparison of the physiological response to radiation and radiomimetic chemicals. Patterns of blood response, Advances in Radiobiology. Edited by GC de Hevesy, AG Forssberg, JD Abbatt. Springfield, CC Thomas, 1957, pp 372–375
52. Dameshek W, Weisfuse L, Stein T: Nitrogen mustard therapy in Hodgkin's disease. Blood 4:338, 1949
53. Colvin OM: Unpublished observations
54. Talley RW, Vaitkevicius VK: Megaloblastosis produced by a cytosine antagonist 1–β–D-arabinofuranosylcytosine. Blood 21:352, 1963
55. Carbone PP, Bono V, Frei E III, et al: Clinical studies with vincristine. Blood 21:640, 1963
56. Morse BS, Stohlman F Jr: Regulation of erythropoiesis. XVIII. The effect of vincristine and erythropoietin on bone marrow. J Clin Invest 45:1241, 1966
57. Brandriss MW, Wolff SM, Moores R, et al: Anemia induced by amphotericin B. JAMA 189:663, 1964
58. Butler WT: Pharmacology, toxicity and therapeutic usefulness of amphotericin B. JAMA 195:371, 1966
59. Lindell B, Zajicek J: The effect of whole-body X-irradiation on the megakaryocytic system in rat femur, Advances in Radiobiology. Edited by GC de Hevesy, AG Forssberg, JD Abbatt. Springfield, CC Thomas, 1957, pp 376–381
60. Odell TT Jr, Jackson CW, Friday TJ: Effects of radiation on the thrombocytopoietic system of mice. Radiat Res 48:107, 1971
61. Hwang YF, Hamilton HE, Sheets RF: Vinblastine-induced thrombocytosis (Letter to the editor). Lancet 2:1075, 1969
62. Robertson JH, McCarthy GM: Periwinkle alkaloids and the platelet-count. Lancet 2:353, 1969
63. Robertson JH, Crozier EH, Woodend BE: The effect of vincristine on the platelet count in rats. Br J Haematol 19:331, 1970
64. Robertson JH, Crozier EH, Woodend BE: Vincristine-induced thrombocytosis studied with ^{75}Se selenomethionine. Acta Haematol 47:356, 1972
65. Rak K: Effect of vincristine on platelet production in mice. Br J Haematol 22:617, 1972
66. Kennedy BJ: Cyclic leukocyte oscillations in chronic myelogenous leukemia during hydroxyurea therapy. Blood 35:751, 1970

67. Morley A: A platelet cycle in normal individuals. Australas Ann Med 18:127, 1969
68. Morley A, King-Smith EA, Stohlman F Jr: The oscillatory nature of hemopoiesis, Hemopoietic Cellular Proliferation. Edited by Stohlman Jr. New York, Grune and Stratton, 1970, pp 3–14
69. Harrington WJ: The purpuras. DM July, 1957
70. Weintraub RM, Pechet L, Alexander B: Rapid diagnosis of drug-induced thrombocytopenic purpura. Report of three cases due to quinine, quinidine, and dilantin. JAMA 180:528, 1962
71. Huguley CM Jr: Drug-induced blood dyscrasias. DM October, 1963
72. Crosby WH, Kaufman RM: Drug-induced blood dyscrasias. IV. Thrombocytopenia. JAMA 189:417, 1964
73. Shulman NR: A mechanism of cell destruction in individuals sensitized to foreign antigens and its implications in autoimmunity. Ann Intern Med 60: 506, 1964
74. Young RC, Nachman RL, Horowitz HI: Thrombocytopenia due to digitoxin. Am J Med 41:605, 1966
75. Sheiman L, Spielvogel AR, Horowitz HI: Thrombocytopenia caused by cephalothin sodium. Occurrence in a penicillin-sensitive individual. JAMA 203:601, 1968
76. Karpatkin S, Strick N, Karpatkin MB, et al: Cumulative experience in the detection of antiplatelet antibody in 234 patients with idiopathic thrombocytopenic purpura, systemic lupus erythematosus and other clinical disorders. Am J Med 52:776, 1972
77. Gralnick HR, McGinniss M, Halterman R: Thrombocytopenia with sodium cephalothin therapy. Ann Intern Med 77:401, 1972
78. Shulman NR: Immunoreactions involving platelets. I. A steric and kinetic model for formation of a complex from a human antibody, quinidine as a haptene, and platelets; and for fixation of complement by the complex. J Exp Med 107:665, 1958
79. Day HJ, Conrad FG, Moore JE: Immunothrombocytopenia induced by novobiocin. Am J Med Sci 236:475, 1958
80. Kahn HR, Brod RC: Thrombocytopenia due to stibophen. Arch Intern Med 108:496, 1961
81. Larson RK: The mechanism of quinidine purpura. Blood 8:16, 1953
82. Shulman NR: Immunoreactions involving platelets. IV. Studies on the pathogenesis of thrombocytopenia in drug purpura using test doses of quinidine in sensitized individuals; their implications in idiopathic thrombocytopenic purpura. J Exp Med 107:711, 1958
83. Ackroyd JF: The pathogenesis of thrombocytopenic purpura due to hypersensitivity to Sedormid (allyl-isopropyl-acetyl-carbamide). Clin Sci 7:249, 1949
84. Ackroyd JF: The role of complement in Sedormid purpura. Clin Sci 10:185, 1951
85. Bigelow FS, Desforges JF: Platelet agglutination by an abnormal plasma factor in thrombocytopenic purpura associated with quinidine ingestion. Am J Med Sci 224:274, 1952
86. Gynn TN, Messmore HL, Friedman IA: Drug-induced thrombocytopenia. Med Clin North Am 56:65, 1972
87. Eisner EV, Crowell EB: Hydrochlorothiazide-dependent thrombocytopenia due to IgM antibody. JAMA 215:480, 1971
88. Eisner EV, Shahidi NT: Immune thrombocytopenia due to a drug metabolite. N Engl J Med 287:376, 1972

89. Shulman NR: Immunologic reactions to drugs. N Engl J Med 287:408, 1972
90. Shmushkovich J, Davis E: Thrombocytopenic skin purpura following treatment with trinitrin. Br J Dermatol 67:299, 1955
91. Cimo PL, Aster RH: Post-transfusion purpura. Successful treatment by exchange transfusion. N Engl J Med 287:290, 1972
92. Rosner F, Ritz ND: The defibrination syndrome. Arch Intern Med 117:17, 1966
93. Deykin D: The clinical challenge of disseminated intravascular coagulation. N Engl J Med 283:636, 1970
94. Pittman GR, Senhauser DA, Lowney JF: Acute promyelocytic leukemia. Am J Clin Pathol 46:214, 1966
95. Merskey C, Johnson AJ, Kleiner GJ, et al: The defibrination syndrome: Clinical features and laboratory diagnosis. Br J Haematol 13:528, 1967
96. Krevans JR, Jackson DP, Conley CL, et al: The nature of the hemorrhagic disorder accompanying hemolytic transfusion reactions in man. Blood 12:834, 1957
97. Rock RC, Bove JR, Nemerson Y: Heparin treatment of intravascular coagulation accompanying hemolytic transfusion reactions. Transfusion 9:57, 1969
98. Sutherland DA, Clark H: Hemangioma associated with thrombocytopenia. Am J Med 33:150, 1962
99. Thatcher LG, Clatanoff DV, Stiehm ER: Splenic hemangioma with thrombocytopenia and afibrinogenemia. J Pediatr 73:345, 1968
100. Jackson DP, Krevans JR, Conley CL: Mechanism of the thrombocytopenia that follows multiple whole blood transfusions. Trans Assoc Am Physicians 69:155, 1956
101. Gangarosa EJ, Johnson TR, Ramos HS: Ristocetin-induced thrombocytopenia: Site and mechanism of action. Arch Intern Med 105:107, 1960
102. Koons CR, Sensenbrenner LL, Owens AH Jr: Clinical studies of mithramycin in patients with embryonal cancer. Bull Johns Hopkins Hosp 118:462, 1966
103. Monto RW, Talley RW, Caldwell MJ, et al: Observations on the mechanism of hemorrhagic toxicity in mithramycin (NSC-24559) therapy. Cancer Res 29:697, 1969
104. Kennedy BJ: Metabolic and toxic effects of mithramycin during tumor therapy. Am J Med 49:494 1970
105. Marchasin S, Wallerstein RO, Aggeler PM: Variations of the platelet count in disease. Calif Med 101:95, 1964
106. Levin J, Conley CL: Thrombocytosis associated with malignant disease. Arch Intern Med 144:497, 1964
107. Levin J, Cluff LE: Endotoxemia and adrenal hemorrhage. J Exp Med 121:247, 1965
108. Burke PJ, Owens AH Jr, Colsky J, et al: A clinical evaluation of a prolonged schedule of cytosine arabinoside (NSC-63878). Cancer Res 30:1512, 1970
109. Odell TT Jr, Jackson CW: Megakaryocyte and platelet development and regulation, Blood Cells as a Tissue. Edited by WL Holmes. New York, Plenum, 1970, pp 73–92
110. Stohlman F Jr: Aplastic anemia. Blood 40:282, 1972

PART II

Drug Effects on the Red Blood Cells

William C. Sherwood

8

Incidence of Drug-induced Anemia

One billion two hundred eighty thousand prescriptions were filled by retail pharmacists in the United States in 1970, according to a national prescription audit.[1] This resulted in an average of 17.3 prescriptions per household per year. These drugs were purchased at a total cost of 5.1 billion dollars. Additionally, drugs purchased by hospitals during that year totalled 809.8 million dollars.[1] The leading drug prescribed was phenobarbital; the leading class of drugs prescribed was antibiotics. Tetracycline outranked penicillin by a close margin.

In addition to these total figures, certain trends are significant. The 1970 retail prescription volume reflected a 75% increase over that noted 10 years earlier.[1,2] This increase is compared with a population increase of 14% during the same period.[3]

Of those prescriptions filled in 1970, 53% were refills of a previously written prescription. Only 9% were products prescribed by generic name.[1]

Although these data give an indication of prescription drug usage and the prescribing habits in the United States, only a segment of a much larger issue is observed. Precise data concerning the use of proprietary nonprescription drugs, illicit drugs, and alcohol are not available. It is anticipated that such data would dwarf the prescription drug volume.

Adequate data concerning the adverse effects of drugs are not available. The lack of sufficient data results from the absence of a comprehensive reporting system and poor cooperation in volunteer reporting. Retrospective as well as prospective studies for uncommon adverse drug reactions are severely limited by problems associated with the evaluation of a large sample size. As an example: The National Halothane Study,[4] at a cost of one-half million dollars, examined 850,000 general anesthesia administrations. The study required six years to complete and publish. Although other important data were uncovered, the study could not answer the question as to whether or not halothane might rarely damage the liver.[5] The answer came from the case histories of two anesthesiologists who were repeatedly exposed to small concentrations of the anesthetic.[5]

In spite of the serious misgivings related to sample size and incidence of adverse drug reactions, the field of pharmacogenetics has the potential for developing focus on preselected populations, reducing sample size, and developing meaningful data.

Of importance in the discussion of adverse drug reactions is a definition of the reaction in question. Table 1 provides a simplistic method of classification for clinical use based on three available parameters: laboratory, physiologic, and clinical features. The drug-induced positive direct antiglobulin test provides an excellent series of examples for this scheme.

Drugs may produce reactions in which only laboratory abnormalities are manifest; physiologic changes or clinical features may not be apparent. Such is the case with cephalothin-induced positive direct antiglobulin tests. Although this reaction may appear innocuous, it is important to the patient if he must endure extensive testing to determine the cause or if a compatible crossmatch cannot be found in the blood bank because of a "nuisance" laboratory abnormality.

When physiologic abnormalities arise as adverse drug reactions, the presence or absence of clinical abnormalities generally will be a function of degree. In some patients who are receiving α-methyl DOPA and have a positive direct antiglobulin test, hemolytic disease will occur. However, the hemolytic rate may be sufficiently low to allow adequate bone marrow compensation and anemia may not occur. A positive direct antiglobulin test associated with penicillin therapy is quite rare. However, when it occurs hemolytic disease and anemia are usually present at some point during the course of events.[6]

It is useful to develop a classification of drugs that effect the erythron with regard to type of physiologic change. Again, the presence or absence of clinical features in this scheme will be a function of degree. The term erythron is necessary since it implies all erythroid tissue—early committed erythroid cells as well as mature erythrocytes. Some drugs may effect the erythron in more than one manner, such as alcohol. Additionally, other drugs may affect the erythron only when a preexisting abnormality is present—the effect of "oxidant" drugs on G-6-PD deficient erythrocytes.

Table 2 outlines a classification of drugs that effect the erythron, based

Table 1
Clinical Classification of Adverse Drug Reactions

Laboratory abnormalities without apparent physiologic or clinical abnormalities
- ie: Drug-induced positive antiglobulin test without hemolytic disease—cephalothin

Laboratory and physiologic abnormalities without apparent clinical abnormalities
- ie: Drug-induced positive antiglobulin test with compensated hemolytic disease—alpha-methyl DOPA

Clinical Abnormalities
- ie: Drug-induced positive antiglobulin test with hemolytic anemia

Table 2
Classification of Drugs that Effect the Erythron

Drugs that effect bone marrow function
- A. Underproduction
  - 1. Cellular replication—chloramphenicol
  - 2. Deficiency states—diphenylhydantoin
- B. Overproduction—androgens, cobalt

Drugs that effect erythrocyte survival
- A. Shortened survival
  - 1. Intraerythrocytic effects primaquin, furadantin
  - 2. Extraerythrocytic effects alpha-methyl DOPA, penicillin

Drugs that effect erythrocyte function
- A. Hemoglobin alterations
  - 1. Effects on normal erythrocytes nitrates, inosine
  - 2. Effects on abnormal erythrocytes sulfonamides (methemoglobinemia)

on pathophysiologic events. Three commonly used pathophysiologic features are utilized: (a) changes in red cell production, (b) changes in red cell destruction, (c) changes in red cell function. It is important to note that drugs are in use which may increase as well as decrease red cell production. In addition, drugs are in use which, under certain circumstances, may affect erythrocyte function, altering oxygen delivery to the tissues.

UNDERPRODUCTION—REPORTED INCIDENCES

Fortunately, aplastic anemia is rare. Wallerstein[7] determined that the risk of developing aplastic anemia, from all causes, is approximately 4 per 1 million popultion. He has estimated that half are associated with drug treatment. In that study the incidence of aplastic anemia associated with chloramphenicol was determined to be 1 per 21,000. This association creates a risk 25 times that of the spontaneously occurring disorder.

Of 771 cases of pancytopenia reported to the AMA Council on Drugs, 44% occurred after the use of chloramphenicol.[8] In 46% of these, chloramphenicol was the only drug administered.

In an evaluation of a controlled population of servicemen during World War II, Custer[9] was able to develop incidence data for aplastic anemia associated with quinacrine prophylaxis of malaria—1:50,000.

There are much less data available regarding the incidence of aplastic anemia in association with other drug therapy. The reliability of other incidence figures available—oxyphenylbutazone 1:124,000,[7] potassium perchlorate 1:10,000[10]—is suspect because of the small population samples.

Table 3
Reported Incidences of Adverse Drug Reactions Which Effect the Erythron

Aplastic Anemia		
Chloramphenicol		1:21,000[7]
Quinacrine		1:50,000[9]
Oxyphenylbutazone		1:124,000[7]
Potassium perchlorate		1:10,000[10]
Folic Acid Deficiency		
	Low serum folate	Anemia
Diphenylhydantoin	58%[11]	0.15%–0.75%[11]
Anovulatory drugs	0%–30%[12,13]	Very rare
Hemolytic Disease		
Extraerythrocytic	Direct antiglobulin test	Hemolytic disease
Cephalothin	40%–75%[15,16]	Very rare
Alpha-methyl DOPA	20%[18]	0.2%[18,19]
Penicillin		
	Hemagglutinating antibody general population 3.2%[19] allergic subjects 90%[20]	Very rare
Intraerythrocytic		
Drugs which may effect G-6-PD deficient erythrocytes		Population over 100 million people worldwide[21]

Low serum folate levels have been recognized during treatment with several drugs. Klipstein[11] has reported this phenomenon in 58% of a group receiving diphenylhydantoin. The occurrence of macrocytosis parallels these observations. Anemia, however, appears to be much less common, 0.15%–0.75%.[11]

Subnormal serum folate levels were found in 30% of a clinic population of women taking an estrogen-progesterone contraceptive pill.[12] This association between birth control pills and low serum folate levels could not be confirmed by another group of investigators.[13] However, megaloblastic anemia has been reported to occur rarely in women taking such medications.[14]

OVERPRODUCTION

Both androgens and cobalt act through undetermined mechanisms in this effect.

SHORTENED SURVIVAL—REPORTED INCIDENCES

Positive antiglobulin tests associated with drug therapy are of interest because of their diverse mechanisms and effects. If the implicated drug is necessary as an haptenic moiety of the red cell antigen, then a relationship between the drug and adverse reaction is more certain. Although there is a very high incidence of positive direct antiglobulin tests associated with cephalothin therapy—40%–75%[15,16]—hemolytic disease is rare; when it occurs, it may be associated with a different mechanism.[6]

In addition, a positive antiglobulin test with α-methyl DOPA therapy has been reported to be as high as 20%.[18] In contrast to cephalothin, hemolytic disease occurs with measurable frequency—0.2%.[18,19]

Hemagglutinating antipenicillin antibodies have been found in a large segment of the general population: 3.2%.[19] When subjects who have manifested a penicillin allergy are examined, hemagglutinating antibodies are found in as many as 90% of the samples.[20] The very rare occurrence of hemolytic disease does not appear to be directly related to this commonly recognized antibody.

ERYTHROCYTE FUNCTION

Finally, the incidence of hemolytic disease related to drugs and intraerythrocytic phenomena is a function of both the drug used and the presence and degree of intracellular abnormality. Erythrocyte G-6-PD deficiency is the most common of these abnormalities and will be discussed in detail later in this symposium. Nitrates, inosina and sulfonamides must be considered and compared.

SUMMARY

Drugs may effect the erythron by a number of diverse mechanisms. These may be divided into: (a) drugs that affect bone marrow function, (b) Drugs that affect red cell survival, and, (c) drugs that affect red cell function. There is minimal data available describing the incidence of many of the recognized adverse drug reactions which affect the erythron. Some of the incidence data available is reported and analyzed.

REFERENCES

1. National Prescription Audit—National Hospital Audit, General Information Report. Ninth edition. Dedham, Mass, RA Gosselin and Co Inc, 1970, p 2
2. National Prescription Audit—National Hospital Audit, General Information Reports. First through Eighth edition. Dedham, Mass, RA Gosselin and Co, Inc, 1962–1969
3. Encyclopedic Almanac. The New York Times, 1970, p 202
4. Bunker: The national halothane study: Summary. JAMA 215:1157, 1969
5. Bunker JP: Prospective studies of specific problems, International Conference on Adverse Reactions Reporting Systems October 1970, Washington DC, (abst)
6. van Arsdel PP: Serum antibodies to red cell conjugates in penicillin allergy, Penicillin Allergy. Baltimore, Williams and Wilkins, 1967
7. Wallerstein RO, Condit PK, Kasper KC, et al: Statewide study of chloramphenicol therapy and aplastic anemia. JAMA 208:2045, 1969
8. Williams WJ: Hematology. New York, McGraw-Hill, 1972 p 209

9. Custer RP: Aplastic anemia in soldiers treated with atabrine. Am J Med Sci 212:211, 1946
10. Editorial: Potassium perchlorate and aplastic anemia. Br Med J 1:1520, 1961
11. Klipstein FA: Subnormal serum folate and macrocytosis associated with anticonvulsant drug therapy. Blood 23:68, 1964
12. Shojana AM, Hornady G, Barnes PH: Oral contraceptive and serum folate level. Lancet 1:1376, 1968
13. McLean F, Heine MW, Held B, et al: Relationship between the oral contraceptives and folic acid metabolism. Am J Obstet Gynecol 104:745, 1969
14. Streiff RR: Folate deficiency and oral contraceptives. JAMA 214:105, 1970
15. Gralnick HR, Wright LD, McGuiness NH: Coombs positive reactions associated with sodium cephalothin therapy. JAMA 199:725, 1967
16. Molthan L, Reidensberg MM, Eichman MF: Positive direct Coombs' tests due to cephalothin. N Engl J Med 277:123, 1967
17. Carstairs KC, Breckenridge A, Dollery CT, et al: Incidence of positive direct Coombs' test in patients on alpha-methyl DOPA. The Lancet 2:133, 1966
18. Carstairs KD, Worlledge SM, Dacie JV: Autoimmune hemolytic anemia associated with alpha-methyl DOPA therapy. The Lancet 2:135, 1966
19. Okuno T: Anti-peniciilin antibodies in transfused blood. JAMA 218:95, 1971
20. Schwartz RJ, Vaugh JH: Anti-penicillin antibodies. JAMA 186:1151, 1963

Robert W. Kellermeyer

9
Drugs and G-6-PD Deficiency of Red Cells

It is estimated that 3% of the world population[1] or greater than 100,000,000 people[2] have a deficiency of glucose-6-phosphate dehydrogenase (G-6-PD) in their erythrocytes. Because of this deficiency they are susceptible to a hemolytic reaction after the ingestion of the antimalarial drug, primaquine, or any of more than 30 other therapeutic agents.[3–5] This type of drug-induced hemolytic anemia was first noted, in 1926, after the administration of pamaquine, another 8-aminoquinoline and a potent antimalarial.[6] Fifteen years later, the toxic properties of the 8-aminoquinolines were reevaluated because of their therapeutic effectiveness as antimalarials. During these investigations, it was noted that primaquine, one of the more effective antimalarial agents, induced this hemolysis only in selected individuals. These individuals were called primaquine-sensitive.[7,8] Most of these primaquine-sensitive individuals appear hematologically normal prior to the ingestion of primaquine, as judged by peripheral blood morphology, hematocrit, reticulocyte count, osmotic fragility, mechanical fragility, and Coombs testing.[9]

In 1956, Carson, Alving and coworkers found that the activity of the enzyme G-6-PD in erythrocytes of primaquine-sensitive individuals was only 10% of normal.[10] Before further consideration of this enzyme deficiency or other metabolic defects of the primaquine-sensitive red cell, it will be helpful to digress briefly to relate this enzyme to the overall glucose metabolism of the red cell (Figure 1). After glucose enters the cell, it is phosphorylated to glucose-6-phosphate (G-6-P) and then enters either the glycolytic or the pentose-phosphate pathway. About 90% passes through the glycolytic pathway and is metabolized to lactate, while the remaining 10% goes through the pentose-phosphate pathway.[11] From the glyocytic pathway, the erythrocyte derives ATP, which is essential to the cation pump and other metabolic processes; 2,3-diphosphoglycerate is derived from the Rappaport-Luerbering shunt of this pathway and plays an important role in the binding of oxygen to hemoglobin.[11,12] Glucose-6-phosphate dehydrogenase is the first enzyme in the pentose-phosphate pathway, located within the dotted square of Figure 1. This pathway is responsible for the

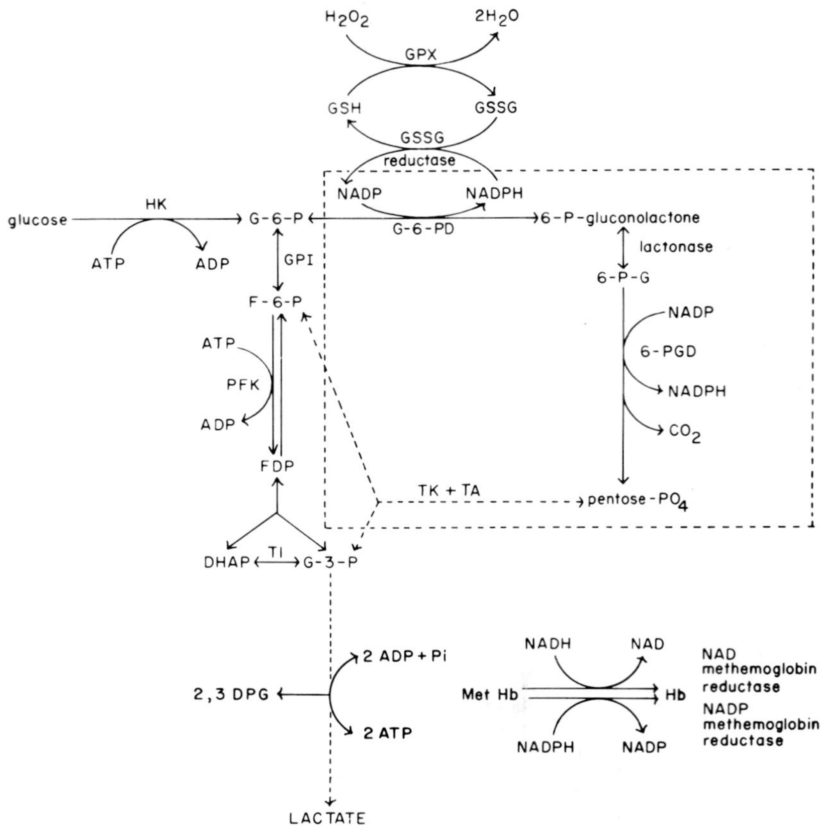

Fig. 1. Abbreviated schematic of glucose catabolism in human erythrocytes: **G-6-P,** glucose-6-phosphate; **F-6-P,** fructose-6-phosphate; **FDP,** fructose-1, 6-diphosphate; **DHAP,** dihydroxy-acetone phosphate; **G-3-P,** glyceraldehyde-3-phosphate; **NAD,** nicotinamide adenine dinucleotide; **NADH,** reduced nicotinamide adenine dinucleotide; **TK,** transketolase; **TA,** transaldolase; **Pi,** inorganic phosphase; **ADP,** adenosine diphosphate; **ATP,** adenosine triphosphate; **2, 3-DPG,** 2, 3-diphospho-glyceric acid; **Met Hb,** methemoglobin; **Hb,** reduced hemoglobin; **6-PGD,** 6-phosphogluconate dehydrogenase; **PFK,** phosphofructokinase; **HK,** hexokinase; **TI,** trioseisomerase; **GPX,** glutathione peroxidase. The hexosemonophosphate shunt is shown within the dotted square.

reduction of nicotinamide adenine dinucleotide phosphate (NADP), to NADPH, which is an important source of reductive power to the red cell, contributing protons and electrons primarily for the reduction of glutathione (GSSG to GSH), also an important source of reductive energy. The deficiency of G-6-PD is sufficient, in primaquine-sensitive erythrocytes, to produce a functional block reflected in diminished NADPH:NADP and GSH:GSSG ratios.[13,14] Although other metabolic abnormalities are recorded, including diminished levels of catalase, diminished content of phospholipid, increased glutathione reductase and adolase activities, and a diminished NADH:NAD ratio,[4] the deficiency of G-6-PD is thought to represent the primary defect.

The deficiency of G-6-PD is genetically transmitted as a sex-linked trait,[15] identical to that found in hemophilia. The hemizygous male and homozygous female represent the fully expressed phenotype, while the female heterozygote has a variable but intermediate expression.[15] Although the defect is present in all red cells of individuals with the fully expressed phenotype, the G-6-PD activity is normal or close to normal in red cells just released from the marrow; this activity falls rapidly as the cell ages, attaining very low levels of activity during the latter stages of the red cell life span.[16] The red cells of the intermediate (heterozygote) can be divided into two populations with respect to G-6-PD activity; one portion will have G-6-PD activity similar to that of normal and the remainder will be identical to those of individuals with full expression of the trait. Whether a cell will have normal or abnormal G-6-PD is dependent on random elimination of one of the X chromosomes, according to the Lyon hypothesis.[17] Because of the random elimination of one X chromosome, mean levels of G-6-PD activity in a large group of heterozygotes will follow a Gaussian distribution, with most having an intermediate level.

Therapeutic doses of hemolytic drugs produce a self-limited hemolysis in most individuals with G-6-PD deficiency (Figure 2).[18] The degree of hemolysis is variable, however, depending on: (a) the blood level of drug which, in turn, is dependent on many factors, such as drug dose, metabolism, excretion, and

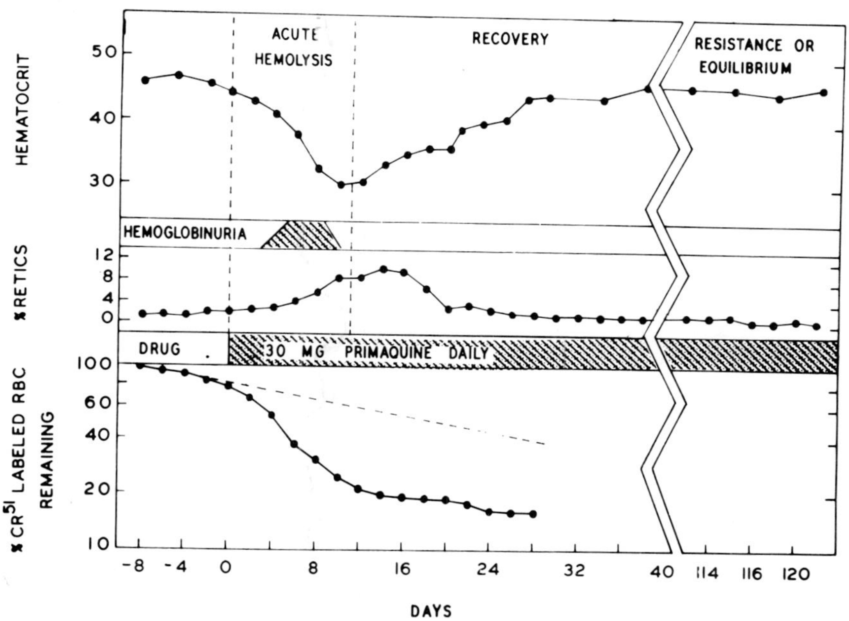

Fig. 2. Clinical course of primaquine hemolysis shown by composite results from 3 healthy males with the fully expressed trait of G-6-PD deficiency (A— type). The hemolysis is self-limited, even though the standard challenge dose of 30 mg daily is continued because the older cells with the lowest level of G-6-PD are most susceptible, leaving the younger red cells and newly formed reticulocytes. The latter are relatively resistant because of a higher level of G-6-PD. A second acute hemolysis can be induced during the "restant" phase if the dose is doubled or quadrupled.

interaction with other agents;[4,5] (b) the quantity and quality of the G-6-PD enzyme activity, ordinarily under genetic control;[15] (c) associated disease states, such as bacterial infections, viral hepatitis, and diabetic acidosis, that can enhance or induce a hemolytic anemia;[4,5,19,20] and (d) other unknown factors, such as those associated with favism.[21,22] The influence of the quantitative degree of the G-6-PD deficiency is demonstrated by the less severe hemolysis that develops in heterozygotes compared to homozygotes receiving the same dose of primaquine (Figure 3).

At the molecular level, several variants of the G-6-PD molecule are recognized. The G-6-PD molecule in erythrocytes of most individuals with the deficiency differs electrophoretically from normal (B type) and is called A− type.[23] In addition to the A− and B types, there are several variant G-6-PD molecules of which the most common is A+. Some of the variants result in markedly deficient activity and either: (a) are associated with a chronic hemolytic anemia even in the absence of drug ingestion or other illnesses, or (b) have a greater susceptibility to drug-induced hemolysis.[24] The A+ and B types have been purified and a single amino acid difference detected.[25] Evidence has been presented to indicate that the total activity of G-6-PD of the A− type is normal, as the reticulocyte leaves the marrow but the specific activity declines much more rapidly than normal to account for the marked decrease in mean activity relative to normal.[17,24] Numerous studies have been done to determine if the G-6-PD is further diminished by primaquine and other drugs similarly hemolytic, but this has never been demonstrated conclusively.[26] Actually, the in vitro

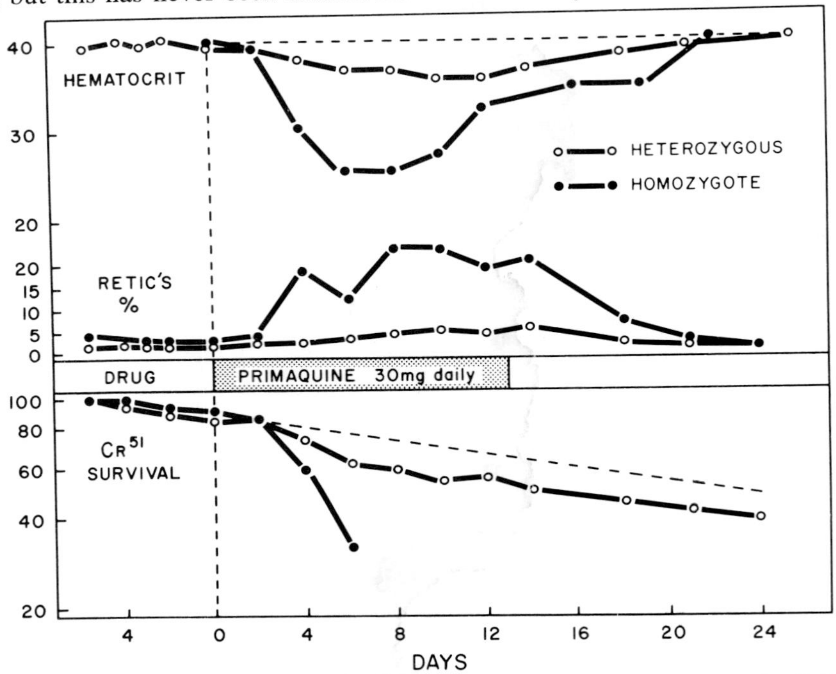

Fig. 3. Clinical course of primaquine hemolysis in a homozygous female (full expression o-o-o) contrasted to composite values obtained from 3 heterozygate females (intermediate expression o-o-o). All 4 individuals were black. The heterozygote has a higher mean level of G-6-PD than the homozygote.

incubation of primaquine with normal or G-6-PD-deficient erythrocytes stimulates the pentose-phosphate pathway,[26] although the increase is less in individuals with G-6-PD deficient erythrocytes.

Glucose-6-phosphate dehydrogenase deficiency is found in all population groups throughout the world; it is most prevalent in the Negroid population (12% of American black males) and in people of Mediterranean extraction; it is rare in most Caucasoid and Mongolid groups.[4] Even before this enzyme deficiency was discovered, several drugs, in addition to primaquine and other 8-aminoquinolines, were recognized to produce hemolysis in primaquine-sensitive individuals;[27] this group of potentially hemolytic drugs has since increased greatly.[3–5] Thus, the clinical importance of this enzyme deficiency and its associated hemolytic susceptibility is accentuated by the widespread distribution of the trait and the large number of commonly used drugs that can induce hemolysis in these individuals.[3–5] This list of drugs includes sulfonamides, sulfones, nitrofurans, 8-aminoquinolines, other aniline derivatives, and a list of miscellaneous drugs (Table 1). The hemolytic potential of these drugs varies, some producing hemolysis only in individuals with certain variants of G-6-PD deficiency.[3]

Table 1
Hemolytic Agents*

Antimalarials	**Sulfones**	**Miscellaneous**
Primaquine	Sulfoxone (Diasone)	Dimercaprol (BAL)*
Pamaquine	2-Amino-5-Sulfanilyl-thiazole (Promizole)	Methylene Blue
Pentaquine	Diaminodiphenylsulfone (DDS)	Naphthalene (Moth balls)
Plasmoquine	**Sulfonamides**	Aminosalicylic Acid
Quinocide (CN1115)	Sulfanilamide	Phenylhydrazine
Quinacrine (Atabrine)†	N-Acetylsulfanilamide	Acetylphenylhydrazine
Quinine (C)	Sulfacitamide (Sulamyd)	Vitamin K (Water soluble analogues)†
Antipyretics and Analgesics	Sulfamethoxypyridazine (Midicil, Kynex)	Chloramphenicol (C)
Acetanilid	Salicylazosulfapyridine (Azulfadine)	Quinidine (C)
Aspirin†	Sulfisoxazole (Gantrisin)	Ascorbic Acid
Acetophenetidin† (Phenacetin)	Sulfamethoxazole (Gantanol)[43]	Naldixic Acid
Aminopyrine (C) (Pyramidon)		Piperizine[44]
Antipyrine (C)		Fava beans and other vegetables
Nitrofurans		Neoarsphenamine (Neosalvarsan)
Nitrofurantoin (Furadantin)		Streptonigrin[43]
Furazolidone (Furoxone)		
Furmethonol (Altafur)		
Nitrofurazone (Furacin)		

(C) These drugs do not produce hemolysis in the Negroid population with G-6-PD deficiency of the A− type.

* Drugs not referenced can be found in references 3, 4, and 5.

† These drugs do not produce significant hemolysis under normal conditions of health and with the usual dosage.

The biochemical reactions induced by primaquine and similarly hemolytic drugs and which lead to cellular alterations and premature death of the red cells are not known. Findings of excessive Heinz body formation, diminished GSH in G-6-PD deficient cells,[28] and a further decrease in GSH by oxidation to GSSG during drug-induced hemolysis in vivo,[29] suggest that the insult to the cells is oxidative. However, the drugs that produce hemolysis are not oxidants per se but are reducing agents. Phenylhydrazine, for example, can reduce methemoglobin in an anaerobic system.[30] Two alternative possibilities have been explored: (a) the drug is converted to an oxidant or (b) the drug induces the formation of an oxidant. Indeed, hydrogen peroxide is produced during the incubation of primaquine or similar drugs with blood and was proposed as a "common denominator" oxidant that induced hemolysis in G-6-PD deficient cells.[31] In addition, there does appear to be a correlation between hemolytic potential of a drug and the ability of that drug to produce hydrogen peroxide in vitro when incubated with blood. Chloroquine, a 4-aminoquinoline, which might be expected to induce hemolysis in G-6-PD deficiency, neither produces hemolysis nor results in hydrogen peroxide formation in vitro when added to blood.[32] Furthermore, phenylhydrazine, an agent much more hemolytic than acetylphenylhydrazine, produces 100-fold more hydrogen peroxide or equivalent free radical as a result of (a) auto-oxidation of the drug or (b) coupled oxidation of the drug or its hydroxylated phenolic derivative with oxyhemoglobin.[30,34] It is of interest to note that bacteriostatic effects of sulfonamides, drugs that produce hemolysis in individuals with G-6-PD deficiency, was attributed to the formation of peroxides prior to the recognition that sulfa drugs inhibited folate synthesis.[35] The peroxides or their equivalent free radicals would cause oxidative damage to the cell or its components only if: (a) the cell were unable to effectively reduce the oxidant, and (b) the pool of antioxidants, such as GSH and vitamin E, had been depleted.

Support is also available for the proposal that the hemolytic drug is converted to a metabolite with oxidant properties. Pamaquine and primaquine are not oxidants nor do the drugs produce hemolysis in vitro, yet catabolites of the 8-aminoquinolines can function as oxidants and produce hemolysis in vitro.[36,37] Urine from patients or dogs who had received an 8-aminoquinoline, produced hemolysis of erythrocytes in vitro.[36,37] The active component in urine has been identified as a 5,6-quinoline-quinone derivative, which is one of the catabolites in the proposed degradative pathway for primaquine (Figure 4),[38–40] that is probably carried out by the hepatic microsomal mixed oxidase system. It is not clear whether the catabolite, however, acts as an oxidant per se or leads to the formation of hydrogen peroxide. One of the suspected catabolites of primaquine, 8-amino-5,6-quinolinediol, causes an increase in mechanical fragility and a decrease in glutathione in G-6-PD-deficient erythrocytes, with a selective effect on the older cells in vitro.[36,41] The mechanical fragility may be a relevant index of a functional but sublytic damage to the membrane, perhaps lipid peroxidation, producing a less deformable cell.

Similarly, acetanilid, a drug that produces both methemoglobinemia and hemolysis in G-6-PD-deficient individuals, can undergo N-hydroxylation to form phenylhydroxylamine (Figure 5) or C-hydroxylation forming *p*-aminophenol.[36,42] Phenylhydroxylamine is a more potent methemoglobin-forming substance than

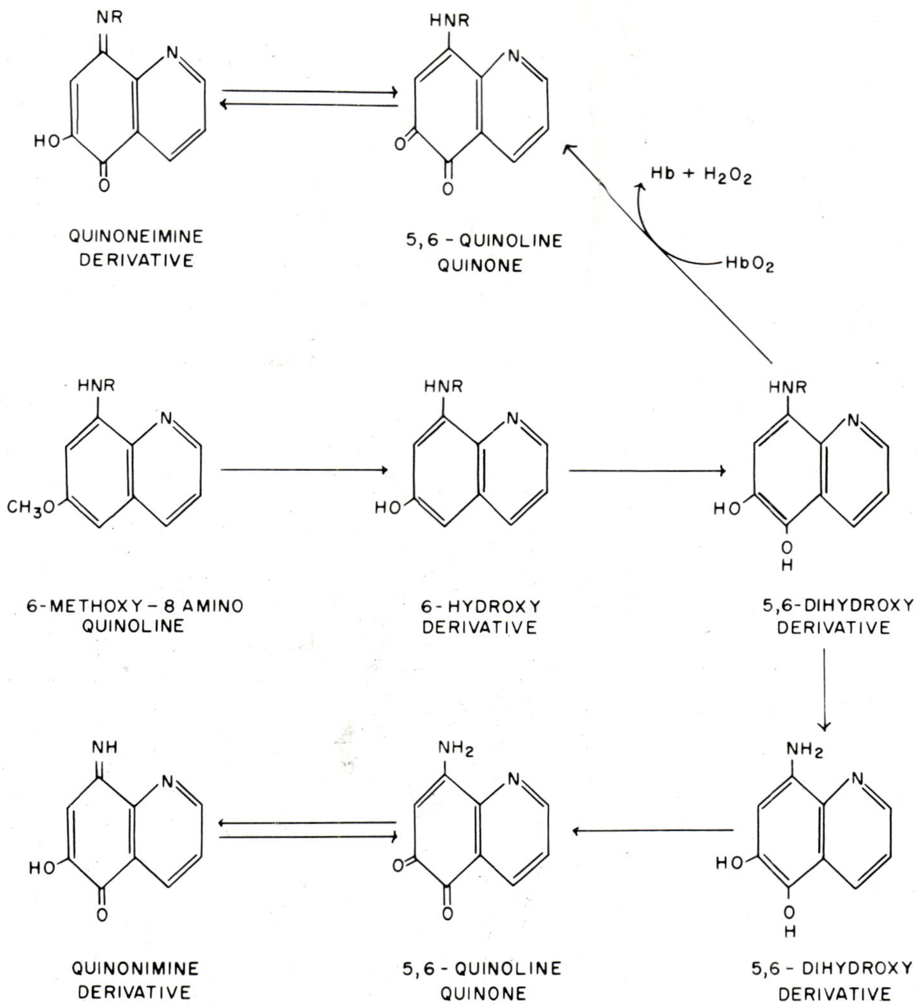

Fig. 4. Suggested pathways for the metabolism of 8-aminoquinolines.[43–45]

p-aminophenol, emphasizing the importance of N-hydroxylation.[42] Phenylhydroxylamine readily interacts with oxyhemoglobin in vitro to produce methemoglobin (Figure 6). Oxyhemoglobin is an essential component of this latter reaction as well as the in vitro formation of Heinz bodies and GSH oxidation by hemolytic drugs. It would seem quite likely that hydrogen peroxide is an active intermediate in this reaction (Figure 6). Furthermore, the nitrosobenzene can be enzymatically reduced back to phenylhydroxylamine by NADPH, which further depletes the erythrocyte of NADPH and reforms phenylhydroxylamine.[42]

Since drug catabolism may vary within a group of individuals, a second pharmacogenetic factor may play a role in the variability of hemolysis associated with G-6-PD deficiency. For example: acetophenetidin has been found to produce significant methemoglobinemia in some members of one family.[43] Excessive methemoglobin formation in these individuals is attributable to a variation in

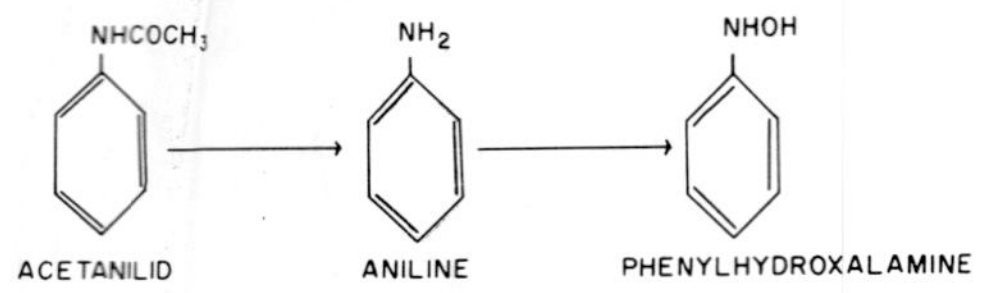

Fig. 5. Formation of phenylhydroxylamine from acetanilid. Other metabolic conversions are possible.[41]

the way in which this drug is metabolized, resulting in a greater quantity of methemoglobin-forming components than normal.

The erythrocyte can neutralize an oxidant stress either directly or indirectly through GSH or NADPH. Low levels of hydrogen peroxide, added exogenously or produced by the addition of hemolytic drugs to erythrocytes in vitro, will be degraded peroxidatically by glutathione peroxidase, with the associated conversion of GSH to GSSG and an increase in the hexosemonophosphate shunt.[44]

It is generally accepted that a low level of hydrogen peroxide produced within human red cells by these drugs is eliminated peroxidatically by the enzyme, a glutothione peroxidase.[44] This enzymatic step requires reduced glutathione. Catalase also destroys hydrogen peroxide and is present in much greater quantity than glutathione peroxidase in human erythrocytes; but because it requires a higher concentration of hydrogen peroxide for effective enzyme activity, catalase is not as important physiologically as glutathione peroxidase.

Nicotinamide adenine dinucleotide phosphate, which serves as a source of protons and electrons for the reduction of glutathione, is derived from the oxidation of G-6-P to 6-phosphogluconate by G-6-PD. Thus, with a deficiency of

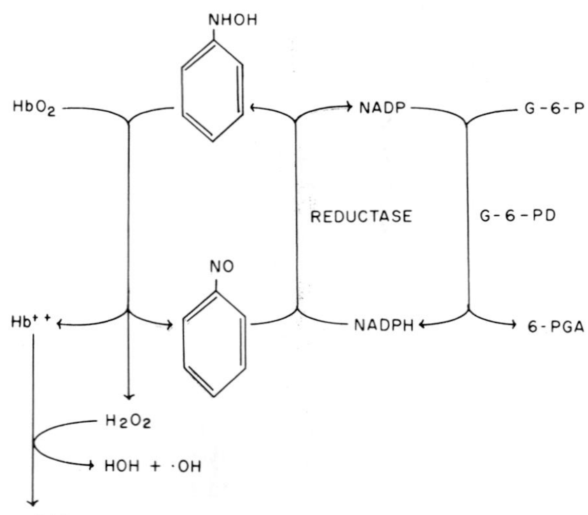

Fig. 6. Interconversion of phenylhydroxylamine and nitrosobenzene[47] coupled to the suggested formation of hydrogen peroxide and the oxidation of ferroheme to ferriheme by peroxide.

G-6-PD, there will be a diminished ability of the cell to produce adequate amounts of NADPH to supply the protons and electrons necessary to neutralize the oxidative effects of hydrogen peroxide.

If the insult that causes premature destruction of G-6-PD-deficient erythrocytes is oxidative and the drugs that produce hemolysis are either converted to oxidants or result in the formation of an oxidizing agent such as hydrogen peroxide, what are the biochemical events that lead to hemolysis? The exact mechanism(s) by which hydrogen peroxide might cause hemolysis is not clear, yet this agent does produce a number of detrimental cellular alterations. If the hydrogen peroxide produced by hemolytic drugs is not neutralized or reduced, it is suggested that the oxidation potential may be directed against: (a) lipids in the cell wall perhaps inducing a process of lipid peroxidation, (b) sulfhydral groups of hemoglobin to produce Heinz bodies, (c) free sulfhydral groups of proteins in the cell wall, and (d) sulfhydral groups of enzymes causing inactivation of enzymes (Figure 7).[2,4,45,46] Which, if any, of the cellular damage listed above is of primary etiologic importance in the drug-induced hemolysis associated with G-6-PD deficiency is not clear.

Lipid peroxidation is thought to play an important role in the hemolysis of erythrocytes deficient in vitamin E[46] and may serve as an example to point up the importance of lipid peroxidation and red cell destruction. Vitamin E is recognized as an agent important to the red cell because of its reducing properties. Therefore, when a red cell is deficient in vitamin E, it is similar to red cells deficient in G-6-PD.

Moderate exposure of erythrocytes deficient in vitamin E to hydrogen peroxide produces an alteration of membrane phospholipids that is termed prehemolytic.[46,47] This alteration of membrane lipids is due primarily to peroxidation of the unsaturated fatty acids of phosphatidyl ethanolamine. These lipids are susceptible to the oxidant stress of the hydrogen peroxide because of the lack of vitamin E and its antioxidant properties. Vitamin E serves as a free radical scavenger, removing free radicals derived from hydrogen peroxides and lipid peroxidation.[45] The formation of lysophosphatidyl ethanolamine by peroxidation and reacylation with saturated fatty acids produces a cell with increased membrane stiffness and rigidity. These latter alterations might not produce hemolysis intravascularly but would alter the surface character and rheologic properties of the red cell, leading to further changes of deterioration while in the

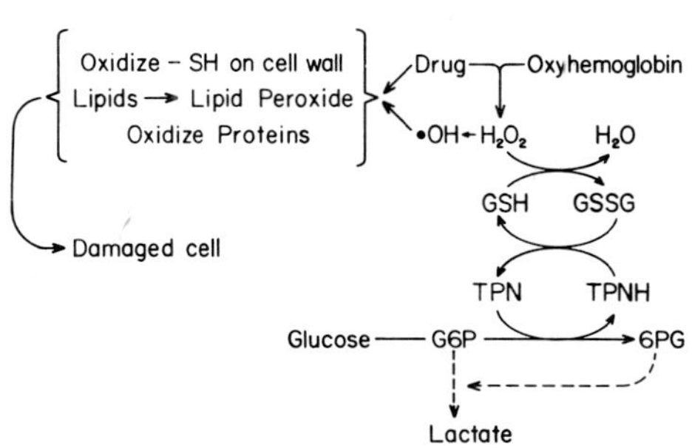

Fig. 7. Summation of proposed oxidant damage to the human erythrocyte.

vascular system and/or premature removal by the reticuloendothelial systems.[46,48] Glucso-6-phosphate dehydrogenase-deficient red cells also have an increased susceptibility to lipid peroxide formation in vitro after exposure to hydrogen peroxide,[49] but not to the same degree as vitamin E-deficient red cells.

The etiologic significance of Heinz bodies in the mechanism of hemolysis in G-6-PD deficiency has been stressed repeatedly.[50] It is suggested that the Heinz body, composed of mixed disulfides of denatured hemoglobin, attaches to the cell wall, producing a less deformable cell that has difficulty in the microcirculation, particularly the spleen, and is further fragmented and eventually removed by the reticuloendothelial system. Recent experiments by Ham and his associates suggest that the development of Heinz bodies may not be so important to the hemolytic process as the conversion of the cell to the pyknocyte,[51,52] a misshapen, poorly deformable erythrocyte whose hemoglobin appears as a condensed eccentric mass with an apron of membrane extending out from it. These cells form during the acute hemolytic phase, as do Heinz bodies, after patients have ingested a hemolytic drug or dogs have been given phenylhydrazine. Yet, the pyknocyte appears to be more closely related to hemolytic mechanism than are the Heinz body, since both Heinz bodies and pyknocytes develop in dogs after a single pulse dose of acetylphenylhydrazine and then clear as hemolysis occurs and recedes (Figure 8). A second dose of acetylphenylhydrazine, 4 weeks later, at a time when no hemolysis is occurring and there is a predominantly young red cell population, produces the same number of Heinz bodies but no pyknocytes and no hemolytic anemia (Figure 8). This strongly suggests that Heinz bodies may reflect the biochemical process producing cellular damage, but it is not the major change that leads to cell destruction. It is not clear whether the cellular damage resulting in pyknocyte formation is due to alteration of the membrane, of the hemoglobin, or both.

What does one do when this type of hemolysis is encountered in clinical practice? There is not recognized specific therapy which will prevent this hemolysis. An appreciation of the self-limited nature of the drug-induced hemolysis in most individuals with G-6-PD deficiency may be of assistance in managing these cases, but removing the initiating cause of hemolysis, and if the hemolysis is severe the transfusion of blood with normal G-6-PD activity, are the only means of treating this entity. Perhaps the best way to treat this type of problem is to have a high degree of suspicion when you are using potentially hemolytic drugs in a population group that has a greater incidence of hemolytic susceptibility. The case of the individual with G-6-PD deficiency and chronic hemolytic anemia, jaundice, and splenomegaly requiring chronic blood transfusion may benefit from splenectomy, yet this is not nearly as satisfactory as in hereditary spherocytosis. In experimental animals, the concomitant administration of xylitol diminished the hemolysis induced by acetylphenylhydrazine.[1] This therapeutic maneuver is presumed to be effective because it would supply more NADPH as the xylitol is oxidized to xylulose by xylitol dehydrogenase. In a similar type of experiment, an increase of glutathione reductase activity associated with the administration of riboflavin offered some protection to GSH in red cells after exposure to oxidant drugs.[53] These are interesting experimental approaches.

In conclusion, the data summarized in the preceding discussion indicate that the "oxidant" drugs causing hemolysis in G-6-PD deficiency are not oxidants

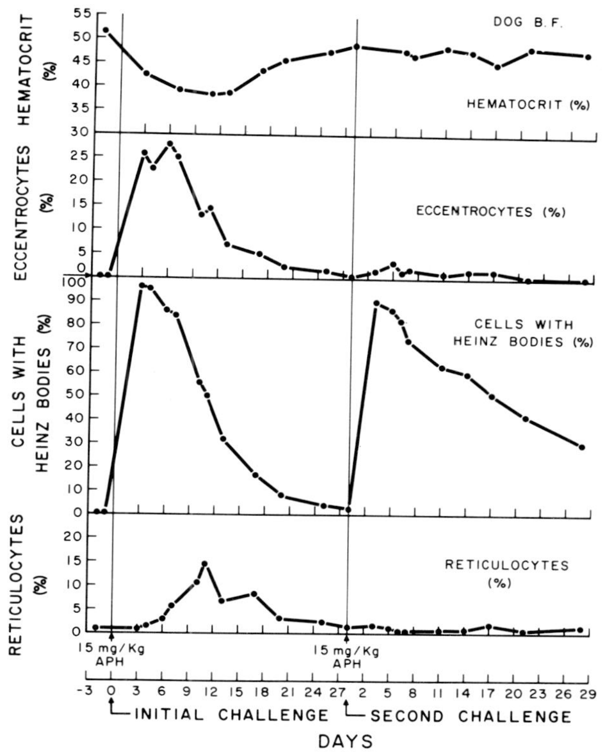

Fig. 8. The relationship of Heinz body formation to pyknocyte formation in a dog given two hemolytic doses of acetylphenylhydrazine (APH) 27 days apart. Note the marked increase in Heinz bodies after both doses of APH, yet hemolysis and pyknocyte formation did not occur after the second challenge.[52]

per se. They may either be converted to oxidant metabolites or the drug (or drug metabolite) undergoes a coupled oxidation with oxyhemoglobin, producing hydrogen peroxide or equivalent free radicals. If the cell fails to effectively neutralize these oxidants, the oxidants will oxidize vital components of the cell, perhaps membrane sulfhydral groups and/or lipids that lead to intravascular destruction of the cell or diminished deformability, resulting in fragmentation and removal by the reticuloendothial system. An adequate supply of NADPH is crucial if the erythrocyte is to survive in the presence of oxidant substances. Therefore, patients with G-6-PD deficiency are relatively more susceptible than normal to hemolysis induced by "oxidant" drugs.

SUMMARY

Deficiency of glucose-6-phosphate dehydrogenase (G-6-PD) in erythrocytes is associated with an acute hemolytic anemia after the ingestion of a large number of therapeutic drugs, including sulfonamides, nitrofurans, sulfones, and the antimalarial 8-aminoquinolines. Although the hemolysis induced by these drugs is usually self-limited and benign, the hemolytic anemia may be severe. Variability of the hemolytic process is dependent on (a) the quantity and quality of G-6-PD in erythrocytes; (b) the blood level of active hemolytic components of drug which, in turn, will depend on dosage, metabolism, excretion, and drug interaction; (c) the presence of other disease processes, such as diabetic acidosis and viral hepatitis; and (d) the chemical nature of the drug ingested. The drugs produce oxidant damage to the red cell, manifest during hemolysis by oxidation of glutathione, Heinz body formation, and lipid peroxidation. The mechanism of this damage is related to the G-6-PD deficiency, and the consequent diminished ability of red cells to generate reductive energy in the form of NADPH and reduced glutathione to neutralize the oxidant stress of the drugs or disease processes. The drugs that induce hemolysis, however, are not oxidants per se but are metabolized to oxidizing substances and/or lead to the formation of an oxidant such as hydrogen peroxide. These oxidants, if not effectively reduced, damage membrane or intracellular components, causing the cell to be removed from the circulation prematurely.

REFERENCES

1. Wang YM, Patterson JH, van Eys J: The potential use of xylitol in glucose-6-phosphate dehydrogenase deficiency anemia. J Clin Invest 50:1421, 1971
2. Carson PE: Glucose-6-phosphate dehydrogenase deficiency in hemolytic anemia. Fed Proc 19:995, 1960
3. Beutler E: Drug-induced hemolytic anemia. Pharmacol Rev 21:73, 1969
4. Tarlov AR, Brewer GJ, Carson PE, et al: Primaquine sensitivity. Arch Intern Med 109:209, 1962
5. Kellermeyer RW, Tarlov AR, Brewer GJ, et al: The hemolytic effect of therapeutic drugs: clinical considerations of primaquine type hemolysis. JAMA 180:388, 1962
6. United Fruit Co, Medical Department: Observations on the toxic effect of plasmochin. Sixteenth Annual report, 1927 p 64
7. Hockwald RS, Arnold J, Clayman CB, et al: Status of primaquine: IV. Toxicity of primaquine in negroes. JAMA 149:1568, 1952
8. Dern RJ, Weinstein IM, LeRoy GV, et al: The hemolytic effect of primaquine: I. The localization of the drug-induced hemolytic defect in primaquine sensitive individuals. J Lab Clin Med 43:303, 1954
9. Buetler E, Dern RJ, Alving AS: The hemolytic effect of primaquine: III. A study of primaquine sensitive erythrocytes. J Lab Clin Med 44:177, 1954
10. Carson PE, Flanagan CL, Ickes CE, et al: Enzymatic deficiency in primaquine-sensitive erythrocytes. Science 124:484, 1956
11. Murphy JR: Erythrocyte metabolism: II. Glucose metabolism and pathways. J Lab Clin Med 55:286, 1960
12. Benesch R, Benesch RE: Intracellular organic phosphates as regulators of oxygen release by haemoglobin. Nature 221:618, 1969
13. Schrier SL, Kellermeyer RW, Alving AS: Coenzyme studies in primaquine-sensitive erythrocytes. Proc Soc Exp Biol Med 99:354, 1958
14. Srivastava SK, Beutler E: Oxidized glutathione levels in erythrocytes of glucose-6-phosphate dehydrogenase deficient subjects. Lancet 2:23, 1968

15. Childs B, Zinkham W, Browne EA, et al: Genetic study of a defect in glutathione metabolism of the erythrocyte. Bull Johns Hopkins Hosp 102:21, 1958
16. Marks PA, Johnson AB, Hirshberg E: Effect of age on the enzyme activity in erythrocytes. Proc Natl Acad Sci 44:529, 1958
17. Davidson RG, Nitowsky HM, Childs B: Demonstration of two populations of cells in human female heterozygous for glucose-6-phosphate dehydrogenase variants. Proc Natl Acad Sci (US) 50:481, 1963
18. Dern RJ, Beutler E, Alving AS: The hemolytic effect of primaquine: II. The natural course of the hemolytic anemia and the mechanism of its self-limited character. J Lab Clin Med 44:171, 1954
19. Kattarnis CA, Tjortjatou F: The hemolytic process of viral hepatitis in children with normal or deficient glucose-6-phosphate dehydrogenase activity. J Pediatr 77:422, 1970
20. Gellody AM, Greenwood RD: G-6-PD hemolytic anemia complicating diabetic acidosis. J Pediatr 80:1037, 1972
21. Kantor SZ, Argesman CE: Serologic studies on favism. J Allergy 30:114, 1959
22. Piomelli S, Puca F, Sinascalo M: Possibli variazoni individuali nell assorbimento del principio attivo delle fave in rapporto, al favism clinico. Atti Assoc Genet Ital, Pavia 8:99, 1963
23. Boyer SH, Porter IH, Weilbacher RG: Electrophoretic heterogeneity of glucose-6-phosphate dehydrogenase and its relationship to enzyme deficiency in man. Proc Natl Acad Sci (US) 48:1868, 1962
24. Beutler E, Mathai CK, Smith JE: Biochemical variants of glucose-6-phosphate dehydrogenase giving rise to congenital nonspherocytic hemolytic disease. Blood 31:131, 1968
25. Yoshida A: Human glucose-6-phosphate dehydrogenase: Purification and characterization of negro type variant (A+) and comparison to normal enzyme (B+). Biochem Genet 1:81, 1967
26. Welt SI, Jackson EH, Kirkman HN, et al: The effects of certain drugs on the hexose monophosphate shunt of human red cells. Ann NY Acad Sci 179:625, 1971
27. Dern RJ, Beutler E, Alving AS: The hemolytic effect of primaquine: V. Primaquine sensitivity as a manifestation of multiple drug sensitivity. J Lab Clin Med 45:30, 1955
28. Beutler E, Dern RJ, Flanagan CL, et al: The hemolytic effect of primaquine: VII. Biochemical studies of drug-sensitive erythrocytes. J Lab Clin Med 45:286, 1955
29. Flanagan CL, Schrier SL, Carson PE, et al: The hemolytic effect of primaquine: VIII. The effect of drug administration on parameters of primaquine sensitivity. J Lab Clin Med 51:600, 1958
30. Rostorfer HH, Cormier MJ: The formation of "hydrogen peroxide" in the reaction of oxyhemoglobin with methemoglobin-forming agents. Arch Biochem Biophys 71:235, 1957
31. Cohen G, Hochstein P: Glucose-6-phosphate dehydrogenase and detoxification of hydrogen peroxide in human erythrocytes. Science 134:1756, 1961
32. Cohen G, Hochstein P: Primaquine-induced generation of hydrogen peroxides in erythrocytes. Blood 20:785, 1962
33. Cohen, G: On the generation of hydrogen peroxide in erythrocytes by acetylphenylhydrazine. Biochem Pharm 15:1775, 1966
34. Lemberg R, Legge JW, Lockwood WH: Coupled oxidation of ascorbic acid and hemoglobin. III quantitative studies on choleglobin formation, estimation of hemoglobin, and ascorbic acid oxidations. Biochem J 35:339, 1941

35. Henry J: The Mode of Action of Sulfonamides. New York, Josiah Macy Foundation, 1944
36. Fraser IN, Vesell ES: Effects of drugs and drug metabolites on erythrocytes from normal and glucose-6-phosphate dehydrogenase-deficient individuals. Ann NY Acad Sci 151:777, 1968
37. Brodie BB, Udenfriend S: Metabolites of pamaquine in urine. Proc Exp Biol Med 74:845, 1950
38. Alving AS, Powell RD, Brewer GJ, et al: Malaria, 8-aminoquinolines and hemolysis, Drugs, Parasites, and Hosts. Edited by LG Goodwin, RH Nimneo-Smith. London; Churchill, 1962
39. Smith CC: Metabolism of pentaquine in the rhesus monkey. J Pharmacol 116: 67, 1956
40. Elderfield RC, Smith LL: On the physiological disposition of pentaquine. J Am Chem Soc 75:1022, 1953
41. Fraser IM, Tilton BE, Vesell ES: Alterations in normal and G-6-PD deficient human erythrocytes of various ages after exposure to metabolites of hemolytic drugs. Pharmacology 5:173, 1971
42. Kiese M: The biochemical production of ferrihemoglobin-forming derivatives from aromatic amines and mechanisms of ferrihemoglobin formation. Pharmcol Rev 18:1091, 1966
43. Shahidi NT: Acetophenetidin-induced methemoglobinemia. Ann NY Acad Sci 151:822, 1968
44. Mills GC: The purification and properties of glutathione peroxidase on erythrocytes. J Biol Chem 234:502, 1959
45. Hochstein P: Glucose-6-phosphate dehydrogenase deficiency: mechanisms of drug-induced hemolysis. Exp Eye Res 11:389, 1971
46. Shohet SB: Hemolysis and changes in erythrocyte membrane lipids. N Engl J Med 286:577, 1972
47. Lubin BH, Shohet SB: Alterations in membrane fatty acids (FA) turnover in vitamin E deficient erythrocytes (E-RBC) during exposure to hydrogen peroxide. Pediat Res 4:466, 1970
48. Danon D, Marikovsky Y, Skutelsky E: On the sequestration of old red cells and extruded nucleii, Clinical Aspects of Red Cell Structure and Metabolism. Edited by B Ramot. New York, Academic, 1970
49. Stocks J, Kemp M, Dormondy TL: Increased susceptibility of red-blood cell to autoxidation in hemolytic states. Lancet 1:266, 1971
50. Rifkind RA: Heinz body anemia: an ultrastructure study. II. Red cell sequestration and destruction. Blood 26:433, 1965
51. Ham TH, Dunn RF, Murphy JR: Pyknocytes in drug-induced hemolytic anemia. Clin Res 17:464, 1969
52. Ham TH, Graull JA, Dunn RF, et al: Physical properties of red cells as related to effects in vivo. IV. Oxidant drug producing abnormal intracellular concentration of hemoglobin (pyknocytes) with a rigid red cell hemolytic syndrome. J Lab Clin Med (in press)
53. Flatz G: Effect of riboflavin supplementation on erythrocyte glutathione stability. Klin Wochenschr 48:746, 1970
54. Allen SD Jr, Wilkerson JL: The importance of glucose-6-phosphate dehydrogenase screening in urologic practice. J Urol 107:304, 1972
55. Buchanan N, Cassel R, Jenkins T: G-6-PD deficiency and piperizine. Br Med J 2:110, 1971

Scott N. Swisher

10
Antibiotics and Red Blood Cells

The topic assigned for this paper is designed to bring attention to an important group of general mechanisms of drug-related blood cell injury, namely those mediated by drug-induced immune reactions. Antibiotics provide some of the best understood examples of these reactions, which, because antibiotics are so widely used, are encountered clinically, relatively frequently. Before considering the specific role of antibiotics in relation to red blood cells, it might be appropriate to review briefly several known immune mechanisms involved in these reactions so to establish the background for this and several related papers included in this Symposium. As hemotoxic drug reactions not yet understood are considered, it is reasonable to keep these mechanisms in mind, for they may have broader applicability than is now recognized.

DRUG-RELATED IMMUNE MECHANISMS OF BLOOD CELL INJURY

There appear to be at least three identifiable mechanisms by which drugs interact with the immune system to induce hemolytic anemias characterized by a positive antiglobulin test.[1]

The Haptenic Mechanism

Here, the drug binds firmly to the red cell and acts as an antigen as well. If antibodies of certain classes of immunoglobulins are induced after initial exposure to the drug, second exposures to the same agent will result in sensitization of erythrocytes, subsequent interaction with antibody, and hemolysis of variable severity. Penicillin acts by this mechanism, and is probably the most common drug-related immunohemolytic state. Hemolysis usually occurs after high doses of penicillin, although it is not a common complication even in this situation.

Immune Complex Formation

Red blood cell damage produced by this mechanism has also been referred to as the "innocent bystander phenomenon," a designation possibly more colorful than enlightening. Although hemolytic anemias induced by this mechanism have been observed and well documented, as in the Fuadin-induced hemolysis in the classic studies of Harris,[2] our understanding of the details of the mechanism itself has largely derived from studies of drug-induced thrombocytopenia, particularly those studies of Shulman.[3,4] Here, the immunogenic drug interacts with the antibody, usually of the IgM type, in vivo on second exposure, thus forming an immune complex capable of attaching complement (C′) to the cell membrane. In the case of the red cell, this results in a positive anti-C′ antiglobulin test, with negative anti-γ reactions.

In this situation, the drug-antibody complex appears to have high affinity for the cell membrane, but the drug alone has a lesser affinity for the membrane than it does for its corresponding antibody.[5] The binding of complement, particularly C_3, may be involved in the dissociation of the immune complex. The ultimate mechanism of red cell destruction is not entirely clear. Complement injury may be involved, but it is not possible to reproduce regularly a classic C′ hemolytic mechanism in vitro. Fragmentation of red cells may be involved in vivo.[6]

Autoantibody Induction By Drug Administration

The discovery, in 1966, that a substantial proportion of patients receiving α-methyldopa for hypertension developed positive anti-γ antiglobulin tests, and that hemolyses occurred in some of these patients, uncovered still another mechanism of drug-related immune red cell injury.[7,8] This mechanism, since it was found to be induced by a number of other agents such as L-dopa, mefenamic acid, and chlordiazepoxide,[9] was distinctly different from the known mechanisms previously described, in that the presence of the drug was not required in the interaction of immunoglobulin and red cell in vitro. Furthermore, the immunoglobulin eluted from the red cells of antiglobulin-positive patients is commonly of the IgG type and displays many of the serologic characteristics associated with autoantibodies similarly recovered from patients with spontaneous warm-reacting autoimmune hemolytic disorders (AHD), including failure to react with so-called "Rh null" red cells. In spite of intensive study of this problem, the mechanism of this reaction is still not understood.

Cephalothin-induced Coombs' Tests

Cephalothin or cephaloridine, administered in large doses, particularly to patients with renal insufficiency in whom very high blood levels are reached, may also produce positive antiglobulin tests.[10] Hemolysis is irregularly associated with positive antiglobulin reactions and is frequently difficult to relate to drug administration, since these patients tend to be severely ill with multiple problems in which mild hemolysis may be a clinical feature. There is great variability in the reported proportion of patients receiving these drugs who become Coombs positive, a problem which will be discussed in some detail later. Although hemolysis by itself seems infrequently, if ever, related, the phenomenon is significant as a possible source of diagnostic confusion, particularly when transfusing such patients.

ANTIBIOTIC INTERACTIONS WITH ERYTHROCYTES

The interactions between antibodies and red blood cells of principal interest belong to the first and last categories outlined. The titles employed for these two mechanisms may be somewhat misleading. With regard to the first category, the so-called "haptenic mechanism," it is not clear whether penicillin acts as an immunogen in the sense of a classic hapten, that is, active only if bound to a protein carrier. If indeed it is a true hapten by this definition, it is even less clear whether the protein carrier is derived from the red cell membrane. Thus, the final immunologic reaction in which we are interested, that which occurs between the antibiotic-derived antigenic determinant group now bound to red cell membrane proteins and the corresponding antibody, may not be directly related to the immunizing event.

The title of the last category is even more misleading. It is now clear that cephalosporin antibiotics occasionally induce immune red cell injury by the haptenic mechanism in which they do become bound firmly to the red cell membrane.[11] Furthermore, it is also probable that the more common type of interaction of cephalosporins with red cells, which results in a type of antiglobulin reactivity of the cells, is not immunologic in the sense that a specific immune response is involved. Although no other drug in common therapeutic use is known to mediate this type of red cell membrane alteration leading to nonimmune absorption of immunoglobulins, several in vitro models of such reactions have been well studied. The effects of multivalent metal ions are one example, well studied by Jandl and colleagues over 15 years ago.[12] A more appropriate title for the last category might be "drug-induced nonimmune immunoglobulin absorption," although it is likely that reactions of this type will be called "Keflin-type" for a long time.

The immunologic mechanisms involved in antibiotic-induced immunohemolytic anemias are summarized in Figure 1A and B. Penicillin, as a potent immunogen for man, was first recognized by Ley and colleagues in 1958. These authors demonstrated, in their blood bank, that red cells, stored for serologic use and to which penicillin had been added to inhibit bacterial growth, reacted in patterns not explainable by donor-recipient blood group incompatibilities when they were treated with sera from many recipients in crossmatch tests.[13] From these observations, a huge literature has grown which can only be summarized for its pertinence to penicillin-induced immune hemolysis. Large numbers of patients, and, indeed, Americans selected at random, have antibodies specific for penicillin antigenic determinants; Levine, et al have demonstrated such antibodies in over 90% of randomly selected patients.[14,15] It is probable that therapeutically administered penicillin (or at least penicillin administered with therapeutic intent, if not reason!), was responsible for this immunization, although other routes of immunization are probably operating since about a

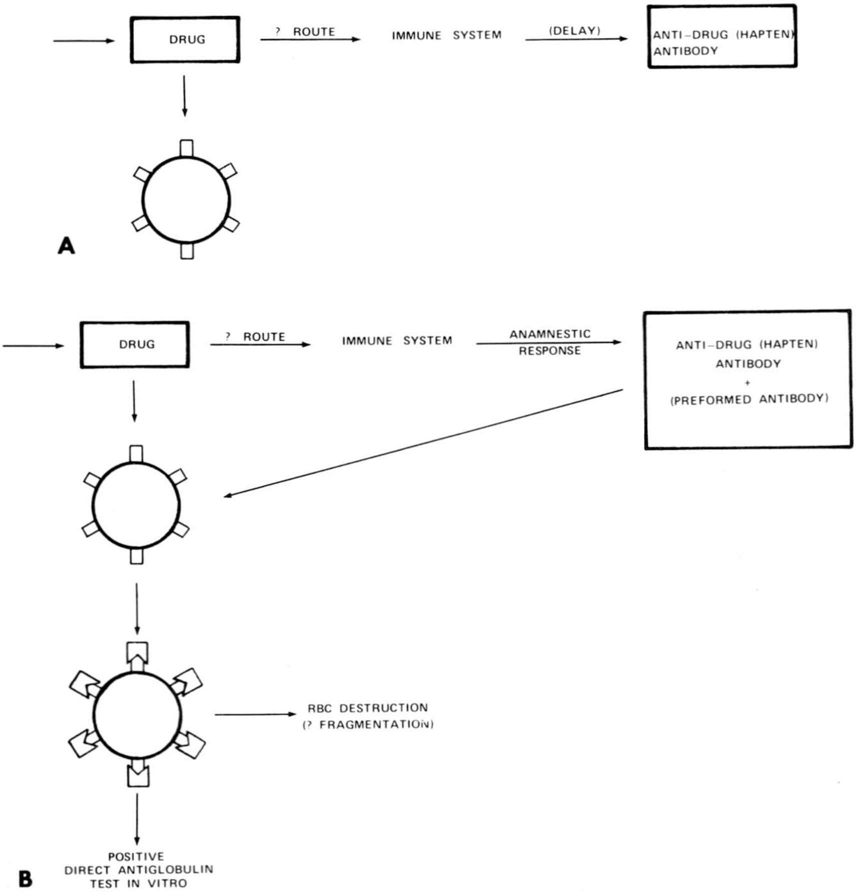

Fig. 1. Haptenic mechanism of drug-induced immune hemolysis. (**A**) First exposure. (**B**) Second exposure.

fourth of these subjects denied medical exposure to penicillin. The great majority of such antibodies belong to the IgM class of immunoglobulins, and it is surprising that they have not been implicated in any significant way in the clinical phenomena of penicillin sensitivity or the immunohemolytic process.[16,17] Penicillin antigenic determinants, specifically the benzyl penicilloyl group (BPO), are strongly bound to the red cell membrane, a fact of key significance in the pathogenesis of immune hemolysis. Levine, et al have shown that penicillin treated red cells do not decrease in titer against anti-BPO antibodies after 15 to 25 washes.[14] Since penicillin has been shown to bond covalently with amido groups of proteins, a high energy bond, it seems reasonable that a similar bond is formed between the penicillin antigenic group and an unknown protein of the red cell membrane. The strength of this bond appears to bind antipenicillin antibodies firmly to the red cell membrane and prevent the dissociation of antigen-antibody complex from the cell surface, as seems to occur in the "innocent bystander" type of mechanism.

It has been observed clinically that penicillin sensitization of red cells in vivo is dependent upon the duration and dosage of drug. Immune hemolysis is usually associated with high doses and prolonged treatment. In the preparation of penicillin-coated red cells for use in serologic tests, Spath, et al have described optimal conditions for this reaction in vitro.[17] They have found that carrying out the sensitization reaction at pH 10 results in a marked increase in titer of cells against a standard antibody, as compared with pH 7.3. It is of interest that sensitization of erythrocytes with cephalothin was not significantly enhanced by alkaline pH.

More than one antigenic determinant grouping derived from penicillin is involved in these immune responses. Stereoisomeric BPO specificities occur and BPO degradation products, benzyl penamaldic acid, benzyl penicillanic acid, benzylpenaldyl-propylamine, and penicillamine disulfides are all minor determinants.[14] The work of Levine and colleagues, carried out over the last 10 years, has clarified this complex problem.[19–21]

By contrast to the common occurrence of IgM antipenicillin antibodies, antibodies responsible for immunohemolytic anemia are usually of the IgG class. It is unclear why IgG antipenicillin antibodies have the capacity to induce this reaction, whereas other classes of immunoglobulin rarely do. But, it may be related to the strength of the antigen-antibody bond which permits the red cell to accumulate a critical, bound globulin load that, in turn, results in a positive direct antiglobulin test and activation of the mechanism of red cell destruction in vivo. Steric considerations may also be involved. Relatively little investigation has been done in patients with overt hemolytic processes to determine exact specificities of penicillin derived hapten or quantitative aspects of the immunochemical reaction. It is still possible that, as yet, unrecognized specificities or immunoglobulin characteristics may be involved.

With regard to the mechanisms of hemolysis activated by these immune reactions, much of what we think happens is inferred from more detailed studies of other immunohemolytic disorders. Observations of several such patients in our laboratory suggest that microfragmentation of globulin-coated cells causes these cells to lose membrane material in excess of their intracellular contents, become rigid, ultimately spherocytic, and then removed in the microcirculation. This process may reflect, in part, the decrease in zeta charge of coated cells, as well as immunoglobulin-mediated interactions with fixed phagocytic cells which pluck off small bits of membrane.[22] Evidence for this can be seen in blood smears of these patients; they exhibit varying degrees of spherocytosis, elongated projections of membrane, and identifiable red cell fragments.

Although the mechanism just described is classically associated with penicillin therapy, it is also now clear from reports of a number of well-investigated cases, such as that of Gralnick and colleagues,[11] that cephalothin is also capable of mediating the same reactions. This is not surprising in view of the chemical structural relationships between these two drugs and similarities in their clinical use. These workers showed that an IgG anticephalothin antibody was found in the sera and eluates of 2 patients with hemolysis and positive direct antiglobulin tests. Antipenicillin antibody activity was also demonstrated in 1 patient, but the contribution of cross-reactivity between penicillin- and cephalothin-derived antigenic determinants to either in vitro or in vivo phenomena is not clear. Nesmith and Davis have shown that cephalothin-treated red cells have shortened survival in a patient who had a hemolytic process after penicillin administration.[23] The relationships between these several antigenic determinants as immunogens and in the induction of immune hemolysis remains to be defined.

Cephalothin and related cephalosporin antibiotics have a second more frequent but less well-understood interaction with red blood cells. In 1967, Molthan and colleagues,[10] and Gralnick and colleagues[24] observed positive direct antiglobulin tests in a group of patients who were generally receiving large doses of cephalothin, were seriously ill, and frequently had renal failure of some degree. Hemolysis did not appear to be a significant feature of this clinical picture and, if present, might also be ascribed to the underlying disease process. As additional similar observations were made, it became apparent that a different mechanism was involved in this reaction, and that the anticephalothin antibodies demonstrated in serums from these and other patients were probably not involved in producing the positive antiglobulin tests. From these observations was generated the hypothesis that cephalothin administration, under certain undefined circumstances, produces alterations of the red cell membrane which lead to nonimmune uptake of immunoglobulins.

Subsequently a large literature dealing with this phenomenon has appeared which, in general, confirms the hypothesis and, to some extent, elucidates responsible mechanisms. A question not clarified thus far by these publications is the frequency with which positive antiglobulin tests are encountered in patients receiving these antibiotics. Table 1 shows a variety of figures for this incidence, arranged by increasing frequency.

The author's experience with this problem supports the lower group of figures of incidence. Clearly positive antiglobulin tests, due to this cause, were very infrequent in a series of patients examined in our laboratory, including a number of patients receiving large doses of cephalothin with and without renal insufficiency.[28] In our laboratory, antiglobulin reactions are not read microscopically, and at least 1+(weak) reactions, demonstrable on repetition with appropriate negative controls employing saline and absorbed normal rabbit serum, are required before the test is called positive. It is unclear how much of the reported

Table 1
Frequency of Positive Direct Antiglobulin Tests in Patients Receiving Cephalosporin Antibiotics

Investigators	Date	No. of Patients	DCT positive (%)	Comment
Spath, et al[25]	1971	97	4.0	320 tests
Petz, et al[26]		146	3.4	Includes cases above
Fass, et al[27]	1970	75	8.0	Cephalordine
Ferrone, et al[28]	1971	42	12.0	
Perkins, et al[29]	1968	143	38.0	
Gralnick, et al[24]	1967	20	40.0	
[11]	1971	150	65.0	
Molthan, et al[10]	1967	31	75.0	

difference in incidence may be due to different standards of test interpretation or to other technical factors, such as the time and temperature of incubation of the test and the amount of centrifugation employed before reading the results. Our tests were centrifuged lightly immediately after assembly, read, resuspended, and incubated at room temperature for 1 hour, centrifuged, and reexamined.

Possible differences in the specificity and strength of antiglobulin reagents employed may also be a factor. Several sera of broad antihuman γ-globulin specificity were employed in our laboratory, in both high and low dilutions, to avoid prozone phenomena and to detect participation of all classes of immunoglobulin. Other sera also detecting bound C_3 and C_4 and their derivatives were also employed. Differences in the way in which antiglobulin reagents have been absorbed may also influence the patterns of reaction obtained. For example: Abraham, et al have shown that a large proportion of sera obtained from normal hospital workers who received penicillin in the remote past contain "spontaneously occurring" anticephalothin antibodies.[26] If such a phenomenon were to occur, as a result of environmental antibiotic exposure, in the serum of even a single rabbit, pooled to prepare antiglobulin serum, a reaction not truly antiglobulin in nature might be encountered when cephalothin-exposed cells were tested. Unfortunately, it is not clear, from several of the publications cited, if adequate controls for such phenomena were employed.

These differences cannot be explained at present. It is of interest that this phenomenon is not recognized with any significant frequency in our blood banks, although it was first encountered in this setting. The ultimate resolution of the problem would depend upon an appropriate exchange of reagents, methods, and test samples among investigators working on the matter.

The biochemical and biophysical mechanisms responsible for this phenomenon, as distinguished from those cases in which cephalothin acts as a hapten, are still unclear. The mechanism is presumably nonimmunologic, and by implication involves an undescribed change in the red cell membrane ultrastructure which leads to the relatively firm adsorptive binding of serum proteins.[31] Spath, et al have shown that cephalothin-sensitized red cells still absorb serum proteins, including albumin, after all traces of anticephalothin antibodies have been absorbed. Similarly, such cells will take up the third component of serum complement (C_3) from EDTA-treated plasma in which immunologic C' fixation is inhibited.[25]

A membrane change in antiglobulin-positive red cells of patients treated with cephalothin is inferred, in part, from metabolic, structural, and functional studies of such cells. Perkins, et al found osmotic fragility, autohemolysis, ATP levels, and glycolytic rates normal in monkey cells that had become antiglobulin positive after being treated with cephalothin.[29] Ferrone and colleagues studied this problem intensively, and in a series of brief papers reported several intriguing observations. The survival of red cells rendered antiglobulin positive by treatment in vitro and then labeled radioactively is essentially normal in vivo.[32] Studies of in vitro conditions required to induce a positive antiglobulin test when cephalothin is added to whole blood or artificially assembled blood samples show an inverse relationship between the concentration of serum proteins present, principally the γ-globulins. The concentration of cephalothin required to induce the reaction at serum γ-globulin concentrations of 100 mg per 100 ml is about 1.0 mg per milliliter, whereas at 7000 mg per 100 ml γ-globulin, only 0.096 mg per milliliter is required.[33] Of a number of biochemical and enzymatic activities studied, Ferrone, et al reported a decrease of acetylcholinesterase activity, and decreased oxygen uptake in the presence of methylene blue in red cells treated in vitro. The effects were related to drug dosage and appeared before a positive antiglobulin test could be demonstrated.[34] Similar findings did not appear in 5 patients whose positive antiglobulin test was acquired in vivo.[28] Herz, et al published similar in vitro findings.[35] Morphologic studies by scanning electron microscopy revealed small irregular membrane protuberances of the type Brecher and Bessis recently classified as echinocyte alterations;[36,37] unfortunately a high degree of specificity cannot be assigned to these findings.

The phenomenon of cephalothin-induced positive antiglobulin tests remains to be explained mechanistically, although it is clear that it is not associated with hemolysis in the same sense as in true immunologic reactions. Its principle clinical importance lies in the possible source of confusion positive antiglobulin tests of this type may provide in either blood bank serology or in the investigation of hemolytic disorders of other etiology.

One final point should be made on the basis of these experiences with the interactions of red blood cells and antibiotics. It would be wise to carry out systematic antiglobulin tests on initial groups of patients receiving new antibiotics or any new drug for that matter. Antibody responses to such drugs should also be searched for systematically, and in vitro evidences of drug-red cell interactions should also be a part of such new drug evaluations. There is good reason to believe that the reactions discussed here are protypes of problems that will be encountered as our therapeutic armamentarium enlarges.

REFERENCES

1. Croft JD Jr, Swisher SN, Gilliland BC, et al: Coombs' test positivity induced by drugs. Mechanisms of immunologic reactions and red cell destruction. Ann Intern Med 68:176, 1968
2. Harris JW: Studies on the mechanism of drug-induced hemolytic anemia. J Lab Clin Med 47:760, 1956
3. Shulman NR: Mechanism of blood cell damage by adsorption of antigen-antibody complexes. Third International Symposium on Immunopathology. Edited by P Grabar, P. Miescher, Basel, Schwabe, 1963, p 338
4. *Idem*: A mechanism of cell destruction in individuals sensitized to foreign antigens and its implications in autoimmunity. Ann Intern Med 60:506, 1964
5. *Idem*: Mechanism of blood cell destruction in individuals sensitized to foreign antigens. Trans Assoc Am Physicians 76:72, 1963
6. Mollison PL: Destruction of incompatible red cells in vivo in relation to antibody characteristics, Mechanism of Cell and Tissue Damage Produced by Immune Reactions. Second International Symposium on Immunopathology. Edited by P Grabar, P Meischer, Basel, Schwabe. 1962, p 267
7. Carstairs KC, Breckenridge A, Dollery CT, et al: Incidence of a positive direct Ccombs' test in patients on alpha-methyldopa. Lancet 2:133, 1966

8. Worlledge SM, Carstairs KC, Dacie JV: Autoimmune haemolytic anaemia associated with alpha-methyldopa therapy.[7] p 135
9. Dacie JV, Worlledge SM: Autoimmune hemolytic anemias, Progress in Hematology. Sixth edition. Edited by FEB Brown, CV Moore. New York, Grune and Stratton, 1969, p 82
10. Molthan L, Reidenberg MM, Eichman MF: Positive direct Coombs' tests due to cephalothin. N Engl J Med 277:123, 1967
11. Gralnick HR, McGinniss M, Elton W, et al: Hemolytic anemia associated with cephalothin. JAMA 217:1193, 1971
12. Jandl JH, Simmons RL: The agglutination and sensitization of red cells by metallic cations: interactions between multivalent metals and the red cell membrane. Br J Haematol 3:19, 1957
13. Ley AB, Cahan A, Mayer K: A circulating antibody directed against penicillin, Proceedings of the Seventh Congress of the International Society of Blood Transfusion. Rome, 1958. Bibl Haematol 10:539, 1959
14. Levine BB, Fellner MJ, Levytska V: Benzylpenicilloyl-specific serum antibodies to penicillin in man. I. Development of a sensitive hemagglutination assay method and haptenic specificities of antibodies. J Immunol 96:707, 1966
15. Levine BB, Fellner MJ, Levytska V, et al: Benzylpenicilloyl-specific serum antibodies to penicillin in man. II. Sensitivity of the hemagglutination assay method, molecular classes of the antibodies detected and antibody titers of randomly selected patients.[14] p 719
16. VanArsdel PP Jr, Tobe AD, Pasnick LJ: Association of hemagglutinating antibodies with skin sensitivity in penicillin allergy. J Allergy 34:526, 1963
17. Thiel JA, Mitchell S, Parker CW: The specificity of hemagglutination reactions in human and experimental penicillin hypersensitivity. J Allergy 35:399, 1964
18. Spath P, Garratty G, Petz L: Studies on the immune response to penicillin and cephalothin in humans. II. Immunohematologic reactions to cephalothin administration. J Immunol 107:860, 1971
19. Levine BB: Studies on the mechanism of the formation of the penicillin antigen. II. Some reactions of D-benzylpenicillenic acid in aqueous solution at pH 7.5. Arch Biochem Biophys 93:50, 1961
20. Levine BB, Ovary Z: Studies on the mechanism of the formation of the penicillin antigen. III. The N-[-α-benzyl-penicilloyl] group as an antigenic determinant responsible for hypersensitivity to penicillin G. J Exp Med 114:875, 1961
21. Levine B, Redmond A: Immunochemical mechanisms of penicillin induced Coombs' positivity and hemolytic anemia in man. Int Arch Allergy 21:594, 1967
22. Weed RI, Reed CF: Membrane alterations leading to red cell destruction. Am J Med 41:681, 1966
23. Nesmith L, Davis JW: Hemolytic anemia caused by penicillin. Report of a case in which antipenicillin antibodies cross-reacted with cephalothin sodium. JAMA 203:27, 1969
24. Gralnick HR, Wright LD Jr, McGinniss MH: Coombs' positive reactions associated with sodium cephalothin therapy. JAMA 199:725, 1967
25. Spath P, Garratty G, Petz L: Studies on the immune response to penicillin and cephalothin in humans. I. Optimal conditions for titration of hemagglutinating penicillin and cephalothin antibodies. J Immunol 107:854, 1971
26. Abraham GN, Petz LD, Fudenberg HH: Immunohaematological cross-allergenicity between penicillin and cephalothin in humans. Clin Exp Immunol 3:343, 1968

27. Fass RJ, Perkins RL, Saslow S: Positive direct Coombs' tests associated with cephaloridine therapy. JAMA 121:3, 1970
28. Ferrone S, Zanella A, Scalamogna M: Red cell metabolism in positive direct Coombs' test after cephalothin therapy. Experientia 27:194, 1971
29. Perkins RL, Mengel CE, Saslow S: Direct Coombs' test reactivity after cephalothin or cephaloridine in man and monkey. Proc Soc Exp Biol Med 129:397, 1968
30. Swisher SN, Trabold N: Unpublished Observations
31. Davis WC, Douglas SD, Petz LD, et al: Ferritin-antibody localization of erythrocyte antigenic sites in immunohemolytic anemias. J Immunol 101:621, 1968
32. Ferrone S, Sirchia G: Survival of cephalothin treated erythrocytes. JAMA 206: 378, 1968
33. Ferrone S, Mercuriali F, Scalamogna M: Cephalothin positive direct Coombs' test. Relationship to serum immunoglobulin concentration. Experientia 27:193, 1971
34. Ferrone S, Zanella A, Mercuriali F, et al: Normal human blood treated in vitro with cephalothin. Relationship between serologic and metabolic abnormalities of red blood cells. Experientia 26:1255, 1970
35. Herz F, Kaplan E, Sevdalian DA: Loss of acetylcholinesterase activity in human erythrocytes treated with cephalothin. Acta Haematol (Basel) 41:94, 1969
36. Ferrone S, Lambertenghi-Deliliers G, Ranzi T: Normal human red cells treated in vitro with cephalothin. A scanning electron microscope study. Acta Haematol (Basel) 245, 1971
37. Brecher G, Bessis M: Present status of spiculed red cells and their relationship to the discocyte-echinocyte transformation: a critical review. Blood 40:333, 1972

Adel A. Yunis

11

Effects of Chloramphenicol on Erythropoiesis

Many drugs are capable of causing some form of bone marrow injury resulting in blood dyscrasias ranging from single cytopenias to complete bone marrow aplasia and pancytopenia. The pathogenic mechanisms involved are not completely understood. Among the various potential bone marrow toxins, chloramphenicol continues to head the list as a cause of aplastic anemia in man. It is not surprising therefore that this drug is the most extensively studied in this regard. While much remains to be learned about the pathogenesis of chloramphenicol-induced aplastic anemia, a great deal of progress has recently been made in our understanding of the biochemical mechanisms by which this drug affects erythropoiesis. This review will summarize this progress and discuss its relevance to the general problem of drug-induced bone marrow injury.

SALIENT CLINICAL FEATURES OF CHLORAMPHENICOL TOXICITY

Chloramphenicol produces two types of toxic effect in bone marrow:[1,2] the first is a dose-related reversible lesion characterized by (a) ferrokinetic changes,[3] including increased plasma iron, increased saturation of iron-binding globulin, delayed clearance of ^{59}Fe from the plasma, and decreased iron utilization; (b) morphologic bone marrow changes in the form of maturation arrest and vacuolization in early erythroblasts and less frequently in early myeloid precursors;[4–8] and (c) reticulocytopenia and occasionally mild anemia, leukopenia, and thrombocytopenia. This lesion has two important features: (a) it is dose related and can be produced at will if large enough doses are given and (b) it has always been reversible without known exceptions. The occurrence of erythroid suppression correlates with CAP blood levels, signs of toxicity developing in most patients at serum drug concentrations of 35 μg per milliliter.[9]

The second type of toxicity is a rare but devastating complication characterized by a late clinical onset (3–6 weeks after the last drug dose), lack of dose-effect relationship, bone marrow hypoplasia or aplasia, pancytopenia, and, in most cases, a fatal outcome from hemorrhage and/or infection. The most important question regarding these two types of lesion is whether they are related clinically or pathogenetically. This question was dealt with in a detailed analysis of 95 reported cases of incidental CAP toxicity.[1] It was concluded from this study that the erythropoietic lesion and bone marrow aplasia from CAP were unrelated. The erythropoietic lesion must be regarded as a pharmacologic effect of CAP and must not be construed as a warning of impending aplastic anemia. Further support for this statement is derived from biochemical studies and will be dealt with below. The clinical implications of this conclusion are clear: one should not be deluded into believing that by discontinuing CAP as soon as early evidence of bone marrow suppression appears the development of aplastic anemia will be prevented. It also follows that monitoring blood counts, although it may be a sensible approach in patients receiving CAP, is without proven value as a preventive measure for aplastic anemia.

PATHOGENESIS

Any discussion of pathogenetic mechanisms of CAP toxicity should take into consideration the two types of lesions that the drug produces. Although biochemical mechanisms underlying aplasia from CAP are not well understood, a great deal of progress has been made in elucidating the molecular basis of CAP-induced reversible erythroid suppression. For a clearer understanding of this problem, let us consider briefly the biochemical effects of CAP in microorganisms and mammalian cells.

Effects in Microorganisms Compared with Mammalian Cells

In sensitive bacteria, CAP is a specific inhibitor of protein synthesis.[10,11] This action is related to the stereospecific binding of CAP to the 50 S ribosomal subunit;[12–14] binding is prevented by CAP analogues with antibacterial activity but is unaffected by isomers which lack such activity.[15] Chloramphenicol blocks peptide bond formation,[16] probably by direct inhibition of peptidyl transferase,[17] an enzyme which is an integral part of the 50 S ribosomal subunit.[18]

Until recently, extensive in vitro studies have failed to uncover a metabolic parameter in mammalian cells, which is sensitive to therapeutic concentrations of CAP. Thus, drug concentrations well above 100 μg per milliliter are needed to inhibit leukocyte respiration,[19] heme synthesis,[20] or DNA or RNA synthesis in human bone marrow cells.[21] The dramatic and specific inhibitory effect of CAP on bacterial protein synthesis does not occur in the mammalian cell.[22] Although antibody response may be inhibited by CAP,[23,24] there is no evidence that this results from a direct inhibition of ribosomal protein synthesis. Indeed, working with mouse myeloma cells in tissue culture, Hartman, et al[25] noted a decrease in the total amount of globulin synthesized in the presence of CAP, but the rate of synthesis per cell was unchanged, suggesting that the drug inhibited cell proliferation. From our studies, carried out simultaneously in sensitive bacteria and in mammalian reticulocytes,[22] we concluded that protein synthesis, both in whole mammalian cells and in a cell-free system prepared from them, was, in contrast to bacterial protein synthesis, resistant to CAP. The failure of CAP to inhibit ribosomal protein synthesis in mammalian cells may be explained by the lack of binding of the drug to mammalian ribosomes.[15,26]

Extensive studies on mammalian cell mitochondria in recent years have clarified many uncertainties regarding the metabolic activities of these organelles. Among these was the finding that mitochondria are capable of independent protein synthesis. Subsequent investigations showed that mammalian mitochondrial protein synthesis was exquisitely sensitive to CAP.[27–30]

MECHANISM OF REVERSIBLE ERYTHROID SUPPRESSION BY CAP

The characteristics of the erythropoietic lesion suggest strongly a direct toxic effect of CAP on bone marrow cells, which is reversible. The exquisite sensitivity of mitochondrial protein synthesis to CAP led us to a series of investigations aimed at establishing a relationship between this metabolic effect of the drug and its myelotoxicity.[31–35] In our initial study, we demonstrated that CAP, in a concentration of as little as 10 μg milliliter had a profound inhibitory effect on protein synthesis in mitochondria from rabbit and human bone marrow.[31] This effect was not secondary to the inhibition of mitochondrial respiration or oxidative phosphorylation, since these were not affected by the drug concentrations employed. In comparable concentration, drugs not known to be myelotoxic, such as penicillin, streptomycin, and erythromycin, had no significant effect on mitochondrial protein synthesis. Although tetracycline was equally as inhibitory as CAP, its inhibition was blocked by the addition of magnesium. Furthermore, while CAP inhibited mitochondrial protein synthesis in vivo, tetracycline had no effect. Thus the absence of inhibition by antibiotics, which are not associated with the occurrence of the erythropoietic lesion, provided indirect evidence of a relationship between the inhibition of mitochondrial protein synthesis by CAP and its myelotoxicity.

The second line of evidence for this relationship was derived from detailed electronmicroscopic studies of bone marrow cells derived from patients receiving CAP.[32,33] The drug produced ultrastructural modifications in the mitochondria resulting in an increase in the density of mitochondrial matrix. The extent of these changes correlated strikingly with serum CAP levels and they were no longer demonstrable 2 months after the drug was discontinued. Mitochondria of bone marrow cells from patients receiving tetracycline exhibited the orthodox configuration. It was thus clear that CAP produced a mitochondrial lesion, which, like reversible erythroid suppression, occurred concurrently with drug therapy, was directly related to CAP blood levels, and was likewise reversible.

Our attention was directed next to the question of the apparent vulnerability of erythroid cells. If the inhibition of mitochondrial protein synthesis by CAP is not tissue specific, why then do erythroid cells appear to be particularly susceptible. The apparent vulnerability of erythroid cells to CAP must reside in some specific property of these cells. The inhibitory effect of CAP in mitochondria is directed primarily at the synthesis of membranous proteins.[36–38] Tissues with a high mitotic index and rapid rate of mitochondriogenesis would be particularly susceptible, and bone marrow cells may fall in this category.

On the other hand, in considering what might constitute a target for CAP in erythroid cells, one must first consider heme synthesis, their primary function. Two steps in heme synthesis are known to occur in mitochondria: the synthesis of ALA catalyzed by ALA synthetase and the coupling of iron with protoporphyrin catalyzed by the enzyme ferrochelatase or heme synthetase. Recently, ferrochelatase has been demonstrated to be tightly bound to the inner mitochondrial membrane;[39,40] hence, the possibility that CAP might inhibit the synthesis of ferrochelatase itself or a binding site for the enzyme on the inner mitochondrial membrane. This question was examined in our next study carried out in dogs,[35] and the results were as follows: (a) CAP at a dose of 100 mg/kg/day resulted in a decrease in bone marrow ferrochelatase activity to 5%–35% of control values; (b) accompanying this fall in enzyme activity there was a rise in erythrocyte-free protoporphyrin and an accumulation of stainable iron in bone marrow, findings consistent with a block in the final step of heme synthesis; (c) ferrochelatase activity and free erythrocyte protoporphyrin were found to be normal 8 weeks after CAP was discontinued; (d) 2 of 3 dogs developed significant reticulocytopenia; (e) enzyme activity remained normal in dogs receiving tetracycline or sucrose; (f) CAP did not inhibit ferrochelatase activity in vitro. These results indicated that CAP profoundly suppressed ferrochelatase activity accompanied by a block in heme synthesis and depressed erythropoiesis, all reversible when the drug was discontinued.

It thus appears that suppression of ferrochelatase activity offers a reasonable explanation for the apparent vulnerability of erythroid cells to CAP. It should be pointed out, however, that this is by no means the only factor underlying reversible bone marrow suppression from CAP, and that there are undoubtedly additional factors involved. Other important mitochondrial membranous proteins, enzymes, or otherwise, are also probably suppressed by CAP. Recently, Firkin[41] reported depletion of cytochromes $a + a_3$ and b from mitochondria of rabbits receiving CAP and was able to correlate this with erythropoietic depression. Other mitochondrial effects of CAP will likely be found as we learn more about mitochondrial membranous proteins and their individual roles in cell metabolism.

PATHOGENESIS OF BONE MARROW APLASIA FROM CAP

Much less is known about the mechanism by which CAP causes bone marrow aplasia. Our working hypothesis here is that aplasia results on the basis of an individual biochemical predisposition probably genetically determined. This complication occurs only in the occasional individual who receives CAP, and the lack of a dose-effect relationship is consistent with this hypothesis. In vitro metabolic studies have provided strongly suggestive experimental evidence for this proposed mechanism.[2,42] Our findings can be summarized as follows: (a) CAP in concentrations of 25–50 μg per milliliter caused a 25%–30% inhibition of formate uptake into DNA of bone marrow from patients who recovered from CAP-induced aplastic anemia; (b) in each of 2 cases a similar effect was noted in the father's bone marrow; (c) a concentration of CAP over 100 μg per milliliter was needed to exert significant inhibition of DNA synthesis in bone marrow from random control subjects. These findings suggest a biochemical predisposition involving the pathway of DNA synthesis. It is of interest that the pattern of inhibition of DNA synthesis in bone marrow from these subjects appears to be biphasic,[1] suggesting that the small degree of inhibition at the low CAP concentration may represent a selective effect of the drug on a susceptible cell population. We believe this may be the stem cell compartment, but this is uncertain at present.

We have recently made some observations with a CAP analogue which could have profound clinical and pathogenetic implications. The analogue is called thiamphenicol and differs from CAP by substitution of the paranitro group with a methylsulfonyl group (CH_3–SO_2⋞). Thiamphenicol is currently being used extensively in Europe. It is estimated that over 10 million people have received this drug without a single reported case of aplastic anemia. Even more intriguing is that thiamphenicol produces reversible erythroid suppression as readily as does CAP. Clearly, comparative metabolic studies might provide an important clue to the pathogenesis of CAP-induced aplastic anemia. The results of our studies to date may be summarized as follows: (a) thiamphenicol in comparable concentrations was equally potent as an inhibitor of mitochondrial protein synthesis as CAP; (b) when given to dogs, thiamphenicol caused a comparable suppression of ferrochelatase activity without affecting the activity of ALA synthetase; (c) progressive inhibition of DNA synthesis occurs at CAP concentrations above 100 μg per milliliter, approaching 60% at 320 μg per milliliter (10^{-3} M); thiamphenicol had little effect (Table 1). Thus, chloramphenicol appeared to possess the distinct property of being an inhibitor of DNA synthesis when used in high concentrations. Our findings would lend support to the following: (a) reversible erythroid suppression is a lesion distinct clinically and pathogenetically from aplasia; (b) reversible erythroid suppression by CAP results from the inhibition of mitochondrial protein synthesis and suppression of ferrochelatase activity; (c) bone marrow aplasia from CAP is related to the distinct ability of this drug to inhibit DNA synthesis; the paranitrogroup may be a key structural feature responsible for this property. Clearly, further studies on thiamphenicol and other analogues might shed further light on this problem.

Table 1
Effect of CAP and TAP on the Incorporation of Formate-^{14}C into DNA or Dog Bone Marrow

Concentration of Drug (M)	CPM/100 μg DNA (In Duplicate)
0	6229, 6112, 6166*
CAP–6×10^{-4}	3178, 3364
CAP–1.2×10^{-3}	1896, 1482
TAP–6×10^{-4}	4601, 5132
TAP–1.2×10^{-3}	4778, –

* In triplicate

SUMMARY

Chloramphenicol produces two types of bone marrow lesions: a common dose-related reversible erythroid depression and a rare complication characterized by lack of a dose-effect relationship, bone marrow aplasia, pancytopenia, and usually a fatal outcome. There is no evidence that the two lesions are related clinically or pathogenetically. Reversible erythropoietic depression from chloramphenicol is due to the inhibitory effects of the drug on mitochondrial protein synthesis, and its suppression of ferrochelatase activity. Other enzymes associated with the mitochondrial membrane probably are also affected. Bone marrow aplasia probably occurs on the basis of a genetically determined biochemical predisposition involving the pathway of DNA synthesis, but further studies are needed to establish this mechanism beyond doubt.

REFERENCES

1. Yunis AA, Bloomberg GR: Chloramphenicol toxicity: clinical features and pathogenesis. Progr Hematol 4:138, 1964
2. Yunis AA: Drug-induced bone marrow injury. Adv Intern Med 15:357, 1969a
3. Rubin D, Weisberger AS, Botti RE, et al: Changes in iron metabolism in early chloramphenicol toxicity. J Clin Invest 37:1286, 1958
4. Rubin D, Weisberger AS, Clark DR: Early detection of drug-induced erythropoietic depression. J Lab Clin Med 56:453, 1960
5. Rosenbach L, Caviles A, Mitus WJ: Chloramphenicol toxicity; reversible vacuolization of erythroid cells. N Engl J Med 263:724, 1960
6. Saidi P, Wallerstein RO, Aggeler PM: Effect of chloramphenicol on erythropoiesis. J. Lab Clin Med 57:247, 1961
7. Jiji RM, Gangarosa EJ, Dela Macorra F: Chloramphenicol and its sulfamyl analogue. Arch Intern Med 111:70, 1963
8. Gussof BD, Lee SL: Chloramphenicol induced hematopoietic depression: a controlled comparison with tetracycline. Am J Med Sci 251:8, 1966
9. Scott JL, Finegold SM, Belthin GA, et al: A controlled double-blind study of the hematologic toxicity of chloramphenicol. N Engl J Med 272:1137, 1965
10. Gale EF, Folkes JB: The assimilation of amino acids by bacteria. XV. Actions of antibiotics on nucleic acid and protein synthesis in *Staphylococcus aureus*. Biochem J 53:493, 1953
11. Wissman CL, Jr, Smadel JE, Hahn FE, et al: Mode of action of chloramphenicol. I. Action of chloramphenicol on assimilation of ammonia and on synthesis of proteins and nucleic acids in *Escherichia coli*. J Bacteriol 67:662, 1954
12. Wolfe AD, Hahn FE: Mode of action of chloramphenicol. IX. Effects of chloramphenicol upon a ribosomal amino acid polymerization system and its binding to bacterial ribosomes. Biochim Biophys Acta (Amst) 95:146, 1965
13. Vazquez D: Binding of chloramphenicol to ribosomes. Biochim Biophys Acta (Amst) 114:227, 1966
14. Hurwitz C, Braun CB: Measurement of binding of chloramphenicol by intact cells. J Bacteriol 93:1677, 1967
15. Vazquez D: Uptake and binding of chloramphenicol by sensitive and resistant organisms. Nature (Lond) 203:257, 1964
16. Weber MJ, Demoss JA: The inhibition by chloramphenicol of nascent protein formation in *E coli*. Proc Natl Acad Sci (Wash) 55:1224, 1966

17. Monroe RE, Maden BEH, Traut RR: The mechanism of peptide bond formation in protein synthesis, Genetic Elements—Projections and Functions. Edited by D Shugar. New York, Academic, 1967
18. Cundliffe E, McQuillen K: Bacterial protein synthesis: the effects of antibiotic. J Mol Biol 30:137, 1967
19. Folette JH, Shugarman PM, Reynolds J, et al: The effect of chloramphenicol and other antibiotics on leukocyte respiration. Blood 11:234, 1956
20. Erslev AJ, Iossifides IA: In vitro action of chloramphenicol and chloramphenicol analogues on the metabolism of human immature red blood cells. Acta Haematol (Basel) 28:1, 1962
21. Yunis AA, Harrington WJ: Patterns of inhibition by chloramphenicol of nucleic acid synthesis in human bone marrow and leukemic cells. J Lab Clin Med 56:831, 1960
22. Zelkowitz L, Arimura GK, Yunis AA: Chloramphenicol and protein synthesis in mammalian cells. J Lab Clin Med 71:596, 1968
23. Ambrose CT, Coons AH: Studies on antibody production. VIII. The inhibitory effect of chloramphenicol on the synthesis of antibody in tissue culture. J Exp Med 117:1075, 1963
24. Daniel TM, Suhrland LG, Weisberger AS: Suppression of the anamnestic response to tetanus toxoid in man by chloramphenicol. N Engl J Med 273: 367, 1965
25. Hartman BK, Pettengill OS, Sorenson GD: Chloramphenicol: effects on mouse myeloma cells in tissue culture. Science 165:297, 1969
26. Rendi R: The effect of chloramphenicol on the incorporation of labeled amino acids into proteins by isolated subcellular fractions from rat liver. Exp Cell Res 18:187, 1959
27. Roodyn DB, Reis PJ, Work TS: Protein synthesis in mitochondria. Biochem J 80:9, 1961
28. Truman DES, Korner A: Initial stages in the incorporation of amino acids into protein in rat liver mitochondria. Biochem J 85:154, 1962
29. Kroon AM: Protein synthesis in heart mitochondria. II. A comparison of mitochondria from liver and heart with special reference to the role of oxidative phosphorylation. Biochim Biophys Acta (Amst) 91:145, 1964
30. Garren LD, Crocco MR: Amino acid incorporation by mitochondria of the adrenal cortex: the effect of chloramphenicol. Biochem Biophys Res Commun 26:722, 1967
31. Martelo OJ, Manyan DR, Smith US, et al: Chloramphenicol and bone marrow mitochondria. J Lab Clin Med 74:927, 1969
32. Yunis AA, Smith US, Restrepo A: Reversible bone marrow suppression from chloramphenicol. Arch Intern Med 126:272, 1970
33. Smith U, Smith DS, Yunis AA: Chloramphenicol-related changes in mitochondria ultrastructure. J Cell Sci 7:501, 1970
34. Manyan DR, Yunis AA: The effect of chloramphenicol treatment on ferrochelatase activity in dogs. Biochem Biophys Res Commun 41:926, 1970
35. Manyan DR, Arimura GK, Yunis AA: Chloramphenicol-induced erythroid suppression and bone marrow ferrochelatase activity in dogs. J Lab Clin Med 79: 137, 1972a
36. Wheeldon LW, Lehninger AL: Energy linked synthesis and decay of membrane proteins in isolated rat liver mitochondria. Biochemistry 5:3533, 1966
37. Neupert W, Brdiczka D, Bucher T: Incorporation of amino acids into the outer and inner membrane of isolated rat liver mitochondria. Biochem Biophys Res Commun 27:488, 1967

38. Beattie DS, Basford RE, Koritz SB: The inner membrane as the site of the in vitro incorporation of L-^{14}C leucine into mitochondrial protein. Biochemistry 6:3099, 1967
39. Jones MS, Jones OTG: The structural organization of haem synthesis in rat liver mitochondria. Biochem J 113:507, 1969
40. McKay R, Druyan R, Getz GS et al: Intramitochondrial localization of δ-aminolevulinate synthetase and ferrochelatase in rat liver. Biochem J 114: 455, 1969
41. Firkin FC: Mitochondrial lesions in reversible erythropoietic depression due to chloramphenicol. J Clin Invest 51:2085, 1972
42. Yunis AA, Arimura GK: Biochemical predisposition to chloramphenicol induced bone marrow aplasia. Clin Res 11:201, 1963

John D. Hines
and Dale H. Cowan

12
Anemia in Alcoholism

The ingestion of excessive amounts of alcohol is associated with the development of a wide variety of hematologic abnormalities, including vacuolated marrow precursor cells,[1] iron deficiency after gastrointestinal hemorrhage,[2] megaloblastic anemia secondary to folate deficiency,[3–5] reversible sideroblastic anemia,[5] chronic hemolysis associated with cirrhosis,[2] granulocytopenia,[6] depressed granulocyte mobilization,[6,7] and thrombocytopenia.[8–13] In rare instances acute hemolytic anemia occurs in association with hyperlipidemia.[14]

Jandl[15] in 1955 suggested that excessive alcohol ingestion could exert a direct suppressive effect on bone marrow function. This, coupled with chronic hemolysis accompanying Laennec's cirrhosis, could lead to an uncompensated chronic anemia. Sullivan and Herbert[3,4] emphasized the increased frequency of megaloblastic anemia secondary to folate deficiency in alcoholics and showed conclusively that excess alcohol ingestion per se was hemosuppressive ostensibly through its effect on cellular utilization of folate. This effect could be overcome with pharmacologic amounts of folic or folinic acid. Other predisposing factors leading to folate deficiency in chronic alcoholics include: poor dietary intake, altered absorption, and defective hepative storage. Hines,[5] in 1969, found a high incidence of marrow sideroblastic abnormalities (increased iron stores and ring sideroblasts) in alcoholic patients admitted for acute withdrawal symptoms. (Figure 1). These marrow abnormalities reversed rapidly when alcohol intake ceased and a normal diet was instituted, findings confirmed by other investigators.[16,17] Grasso and Hines[18] demonstrated that the iron in these abnormal sideroblasts was located principally in the mitochondria, suggesting a defect in heme biosynthesis. The incidence of various hematologic abnormalities in alcoholics was determined by Eichner and Hillman.[16] Anemia (hematocrit below 38%) was present in 40 of 65 unselected chronic alcoholic patients admitted to the hospital. Megaloblastic anemia secondary to folate deficiency occurred in 40% of patients, and sideroblastic marrow abnormalities were present in 30%. The remaining anemic patients had iron deficiency, inflammation (hypoproliferative), or "resolving megaloblastic anemia."

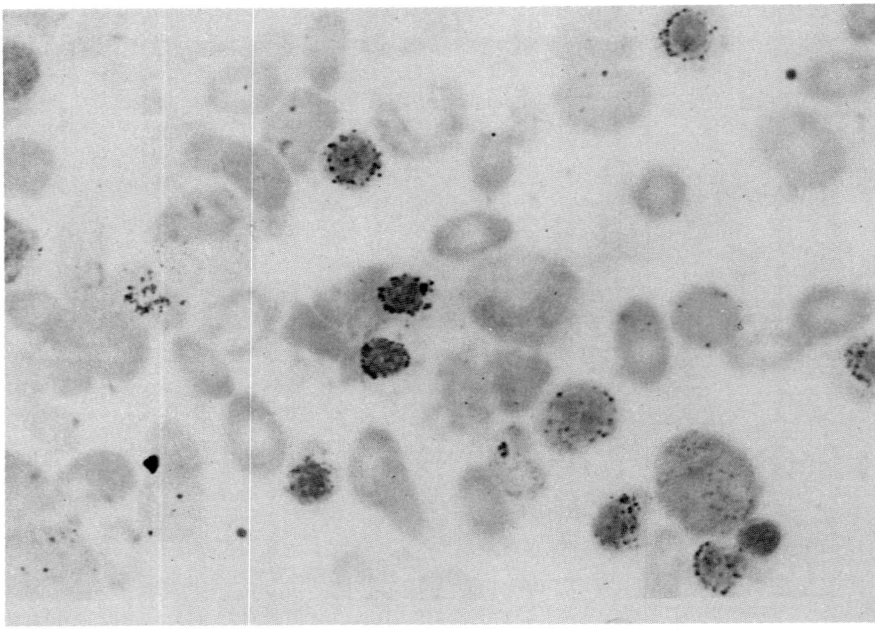

Fig. 1. Erythroblasts containing massive amounts of iron; ring sideroblasts in a bone marrow specimen from an alcoholic patient.

The current study reviews our experience in delineating hematologic abnormalities involving red cell production in 70 unselected acute and chronic alcoholics (55 male, 15 female) admitted to Cleveland Metropolitan General Hospital for acute alcohol withdrawal symptoms. Additionally, data will be presented which bears on the pathogenesis of alcohol-induced sideroblastic marrow abnormalities commonly observed in such patients.

MATERIALS AND METHODS

Seventy patients admitted to the hospital for acute alcoholic withdrawal symptoms were investigated (55 male, 15 female). The minimum period of excessive alcohol ingestion was 3 years, and most gave a nutritionally suboptimal dietary history prior to admission. Venipuncture and bone marrow aspiration were obtained in nearly all patients within 12 hours of admission, and the only medications administered prior to these studies were thiamine and paraldehyde (60 patients). Eleven patients (all male) were selected for subsequent investigation in the metabolic ward and were administered graded amounts of 86 proof whiskey, while on a normal or supplemented diet. Informed signed consent was obtained from every patient and each was monitored carefully both clinically and biochemically. None of these 11 patients had clinical or biochemical evidence of liver, renal, neurologic, or cardiovascular disease.

Routine hematologic studies were performed according to standard methods.[19] Serum folate estimations were performed by the aseptic addition method using *Lactobacillus casei*.[20] Serum vitamin B_{12} assays were performed using the *Euglena gracilis*,[21] and erythrocyte folate was determined using the *Lactobacillus casei* assay.[22] Serum and erythrocyte pyridoxal phosphate (PLP) levels were determined by the method of Hines and Love.[23] Biochemical assessment of hepatic function, and renal function including electrolytes, were determined by standard methods. Serum magnesium levels were determined by atomic absorption spectrometry. Erythrocyte and hepatic pyridoxal phosphokinase estimations were performed as previously described.[24] Serum iron and total iron binding capacity was performed according to the method of Schade.[25] Bone marrow specimens were stained with Wright's stain and for iron using the Prussian blue method. Marrow iron stores were graded from 0–6+.

METABOLIC STUDIES

Eleven patients with a history of chronic alcohol abuse but without clinical or biochemical evidence of hepatic, renal, or neurologic disease were investigated on the Metabolic Ward of Cleveland Metropolitan General Hospital. All studies performed were in accord with the Helsinki Declaration, with informed signed consent obtained in each. All patients were withdrawn from alcohol on a standard hospital diet for 4 weeks. All hematologic parameters were normal except for 2 subjects in whom a persisting subnormal serum folate was observed without any other detectable abnormality. At the start of administration of alcohol (86 proof bar whiskey), all patients exhibited normal serum B_{12}, serum and erythrocyte PLP, erythrocyte folate, and serum iron levels. Erythrocyte pyridoxal phosphokinase levels were normal in each subject. Five of the 11 patients were placed on a folate-deficient diet[24] during the initial phase of the investigation. All 11 patients were administered alcohol, between 900 and 1200 ml per day (average 1000 ml). Six of the 11 patients were fed a standard hospital diet and received 1000 μg of pterolyl glutamic acid (PGA) parenterally per day. Three of these 6 patients were maintained on a daily oral multivitamin preparation containing ascorbic acid 50 mg, pyridoxine 1.0 mg, riboflavin 2.0 mg, and thiamine 2.0 mg. Alcohol was isocalorically substituted for carbohydrate in all diet regimens.

RESULTS

Seventy adult patients (55 male, 15 female) admitted to the hospital principally for acute alcohol withdrawal symptoms were investigated. Clinical and/or biochemical evidence of hepatic disease were present in 75% of patients (hepatomegaly 60%, splenomegaly 35%). Hypomagnesemia and/or hypokalemia occurred in 65% of patients. Other medical complications were not uncommon, including acute delerium tremens, gastrointestinal hemorrhage, pancreatitis, hepatic encephalopathy, and bronchopneumonia. Six patient fatalities were recorded.

HEMATOLOGIC STUDIES

Most of the hematologic findings are summarized in Table 1. Anemia, as defined as a hematocrit below 40% (male) or 37% (female), occurred in 48% of patients (median of three successive determinations). Abnormalities of peripheral blood smear and bone marrow morphology were detected in 70% of patients. A significant degree of macrocytosis (ovalomacrocytes) was observed in 25 patients (5 nonanemic) and megaloblastic marrow alterations were detected in 24 patients (4 nonanemic). Twenty patients had dimorphic erythrocyte populations on peripheral smear, and all 20 exhibited marrow sideroblastic alteration with between 9% and 65% ring sideroblasts. Ten of these 20 marrow specimens exhibited some degree of megaloblastic change in the erythyroid series confined largely to the polychromatophilic erythroblast series. Sixty-five of the 70 bone marrow specimens revealed some degree of myeloid cytoplasmic vacuolization. Serum folate levels were subnormal in 61 patients, but subnormal erythrocyte levels were present in only 30. Serum PLP values were subnormal in 55 patients, whereas low erythrocyte levels were detected in only 33. Serum iron, expressed as per cent saturation of TIBC, was elevated in 43 patients and was slightly but not significantly higher in the sideroblastic group. Bone marrow iron stores were increased in the megaloblastic and sideroblastic groups (43 patients). Other types of anemia documented in 5 patients were: iron deficiency in 3 and inflammation and infection in 2. None of the 70 patients exhibited a subnormal serum B_{12} level.

The differences between those patients with megaloblastic anemia and those with sideroblastic marrow alteration with or without megaloblastic-like changes were: (a) significantly lower serum and erythrocyte folate levels in the megaloblastic group (Student's t test $p < 0.01$), and (b) significantly lower serum and erythrocyte PLP levels in patients with sideroblastic marrow alteration. No definite correlation relative to the amount of alcohol consumption or dietary habits could be established.

Minimal to severe degrees of thrombocytopenia were observed in 75% of patients (platelet count range 16,000–98,000 per cubic millimeter). In all thrombocytopenic patients the platelet count returned to a minimum value of 150,000 per cubic millimeter within 12 days, irrespective of therapy. There was

Table 1

							Iron	
	No. of Patients	Hct (%)	Serum Folate (ng/ml)	RBC Folate (ng/ml)	Serum PLP (ng/ml)	RBC PLP (ng/ml)	Serum (% Sat.)	Marrow
Normal		39–50	4–18	160–650	30–60	180–700	30–65	1+
Megaloblastic	20	28.5	2.0	119	28.2	195	88	3–4+
Sideroblastic*	23	27	3.8	144	14	110	92	4–6+
Other	5	32	3.7	185	32.5	220	26	0–2+
Nonanemic	22	42	3.9	245	33	280	45	1–2+

* Sideroblastic and/or megaloblastic

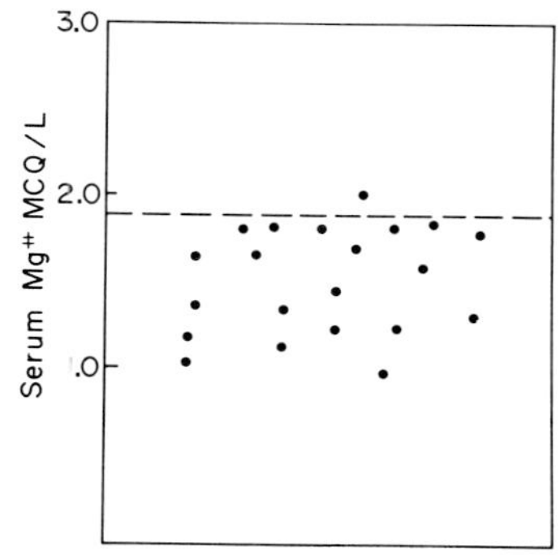

Fig. 2. Serum magnesium levels in 21 alcoholic patients with sideroblastic marrow alterations on hospital admission; the hatched line indicates the lower limit of normal.

no significant difference in the incidence of thrombocytopenia in the sideroblastic and megaloblastic patient groups.

Serial bone marrow aspiration was obtained in 15 of the 23 sideroblastic patients. The earliest disappearance of ring sideroblasts was 3 days and the latest was 12 days after hospital admission. Ten of these patients received PGA 100–300μg per day, orally, and no correlation could be established between this therapy and the time of disappearance of ring sideroblasts. None of the 23 patients received pyridoxine or PLP therapy. Serum magnesium levels (Figure 2) were subnormal in 20 of 21 patients with sideroblastic marrow alterations compared to 20 of the 47 remaining patients. This observation is similar to previous data obtained in alcohol-associated marrow sideroblastic abnormalities in this laboratory.

Figure 3 illustrates the serum PLP levels in 17 age-matched normal control subjects with 16 randomly selected chronic alcoholic patients admitted to the hospital for withdrawal symptoms. There is a significantly lower serum PLP in the alcoholics. Figure 4 illustrates whole blood PLP values in the same patients and controls. The hematocrits had been corrected to 50% in all subjects. There is a significantly lower whole blood value in alcoholic patients. Figure 5 illustrates serum PLP values in a selected group of alcoholic patients with and without marrow sideroblastic abnormalities. The lowest recorded values occurred only in the sideroblastic group.

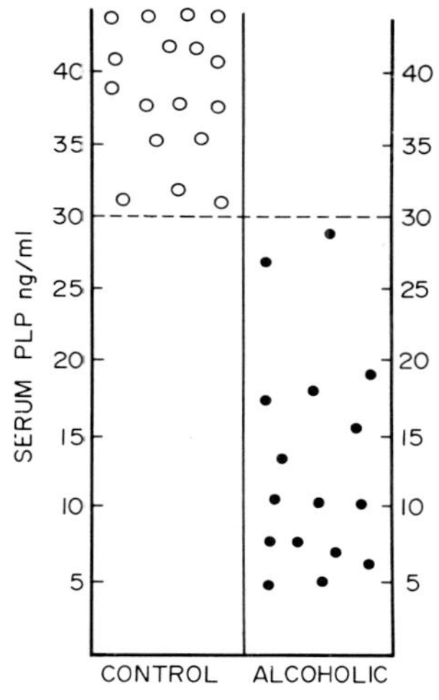

Fig. 3. Serum pyridoxal phosphate levels (PLP) in age-matched normal control subjects compared to alcoholic subjects. Hatched line indicates lower limit of normal.

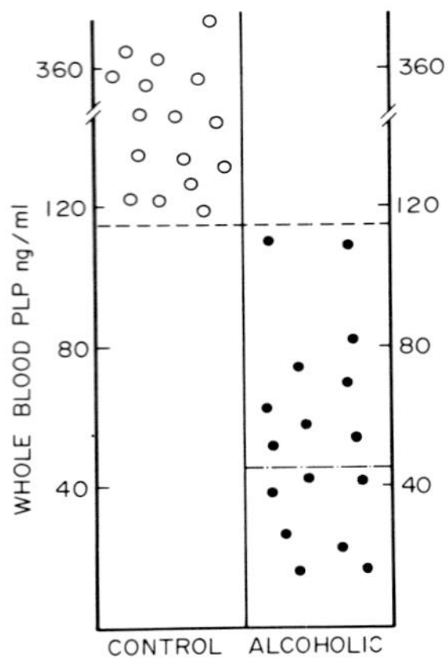

Fig. 4. Whole blood PLP levels in age-matched normal controls compared to alcoholic subjects; upper hatched line is the lower limit of normal; lower hatched line indicates (below) patients with sideroblastic marrow, upper group is nonsideroblastic.

METABOLIC STUDIES

As previously indicated, the 11 volunteer subjects were hematologically normal except for 2 who had subnormal serum folate levels without other hematologic abnormality. Eight patients were given the folate-deficient diet without supplementation in association with approximately 1000 ml of 86 proof bar whiskey per day for 8 days. Figure 6 depicts the serum folate data in these patients. A dramatic fall in serum folate occurred in each patient, and in 7 of 8 patients these lebels decreased to subnormal values without a significant change in red cell folate levels (not illustrated). These findings are similar to those described by Eichner and Hillman.[16] No inhibitor to *Lactobacillus casei* could be detected in serum from any of these patients. A similar decrease in serum PLP levels was observed in these 8 patients (not illustrated). By day 8 of alcohol administration, the initially normal serum PLP levels had decreased to subnormal values in 7 of 8 patients. No serum inhibitor to the enzymatic PLP assay system could be detected within this period of time.

Five of the 11 study subjects were maintained on the folate-deficient diet in association with alcohol administration. Serum folate levels remaining subnormal throughout the observation period (4 to 9 weeks). Erythrocyte folate values became subnormal within 5 to 6 weeks of alcohol administration (120 and 135 ng per milliliter, respectively). Megaloblastic marrow alteration occurred

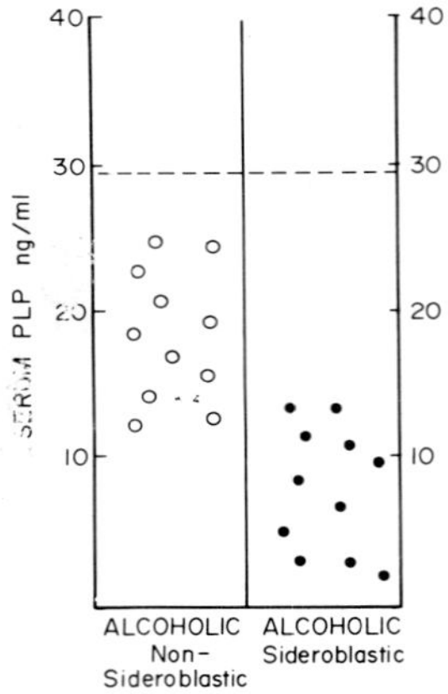

Fig. 5. Comparison of serum PLP levels in sideroblastic and nonsideroblastic patients.

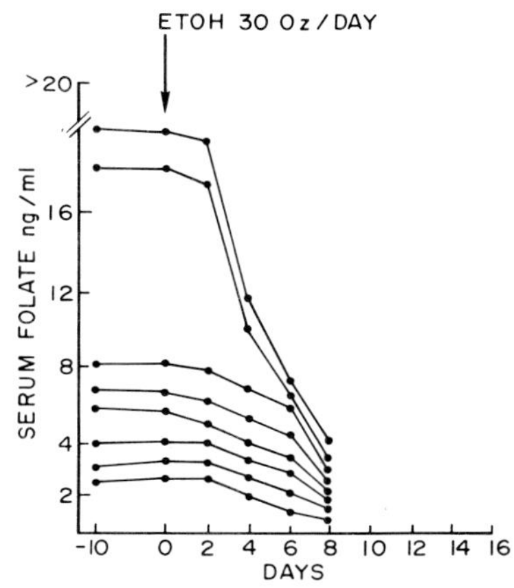

Fig. 6. Serum folate levels in 8 alcoholic volunteer subjects before and after the administration of 30 ounces of alcohol on the Metabolic Unit.

in all 5 subjects within 2 to 3 weeks of alcohol administration. A mild degree of anemia occurred in 3 of 5 subjects (Hct 37%–39%). Marrow ring sideroblastic alterations evolved in 3 of 5 subjects ranging from 22% to 69% in number. Per cent saturation of serum iron levels increased progressively in all subjects, ranging from 80% to 100% saturation.

Intramuscular PGA, 1000 μg per day, was administered to 3 of these 5 subjects. The marrow megaloblastic features reverted to normal maturation, but the ring sideroblasts persisted unchanged. No significant change in per cent saturation of serum iron occurred nor was there any associated elevation in reticulocyte count. After 10 days of the PGA regimen, two separate "pulse" doses of pyridoxine were administered intravenously 6 days apart in a dose of 20 mg. Five days after the last dose, the marrow ring sideroblast abnormality was unaltered in the 2 subjects. No change in reticulocyte count or serum iron was detected up to 7 days postpyridoxine therapy. Ten days subsequent to the last pyridoxine injection, a therapeutic regimen of pyridoxal phosphate was instituted, consisting of 10 mg of PLP intramuscularly every 6 hours. After 6 days of the PLP regimen, each patient exhibited a dramatic fall in serum iron (per cent saturation) to between 30% and 45%, a reticulocyte response between 4.2% and 5.8%, and complete disappearance of marrow ring sideroblasts. These findings support previous studies in this laboratory indicating an alcohol-induced marrow sideroblastic abnormality secondary to some derangement in the erythroid marrow utilization of pyridoxine leading to defective heme biosynthesis, which can be overcome with parenteral administration of the coenzyme form of the vitamin.

When a dose of 20 mg of pyridoxine is administered intravenously to normal individuals, a predictable rise in serum PLP occurs within 4 hours. Figure 7 illustrates the results in normal individuals as compared to an alcoholic volunteer ingesting a standard hospital diet with isocaloric substitution of alcohol (1000 ml per day) for carbohydrate. These data indicate a severe impairment of oxidation and phosphorylation of pyridoxine to PLP during alcohol administration and illustrate the return towards normal of this in vivo assay system after 3 weeks of alcohol withdrawal.

The remaining 6 subjects received one of two regimens. Three were placed

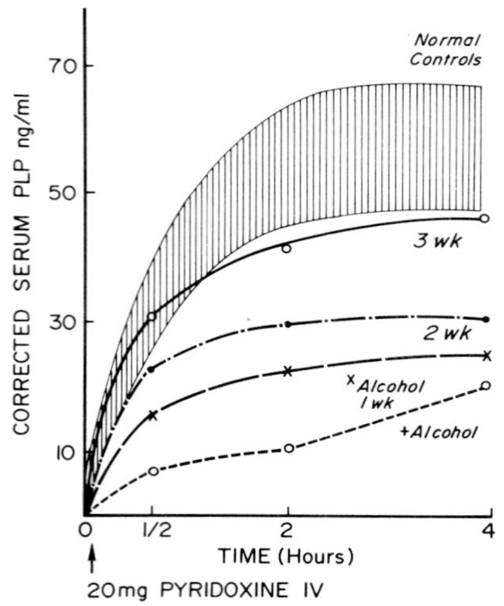

Fig. 7. In vivo intravenous pyridoxine load, 20 mg; results are the corrected increase in serum PLP levels in normal controls (hatched area) compared to an alcoholic subject ingesting 1000 ml of alcohol per day, during ingestion and after withdrawal, for 3 weeks.

on the normal hospital diet and alcohol with the addition of PGA 1000 μg per day, and 3 received the same regimen with the addition of the multivitamin preparation. Two of the 3 former patients developed marrow ring sideroblast alterations by the fourth week along with hyperferremia without anemia or megaloblastic marrow changes. Serum PLP levels decreased to subnormal levels in each of these 3 patients by 2 weeks of alcohol administration and erythrocyte levels decreased to subnormal levels in all 3 by 4 weeks of alcohol administration. The last 3 subjects were administered the multivitamin preparation in addition to alcohol and PGA 1000 μg per day. Only 1 of the 3 developed the marrow ring sideroblast abnormality (fifth week), and the per cent ring forms never exceeds 15. Marrow vacuolization was observed in all 6 subjects along with variable degrees of hyperferremia. Serum PLP levels decreased to subnormal in the 3 subjects ingesting multivitamins, but erythrocyte values decreased to a subnormal range in only the single patient exhibiting the ring sideroblast alteration. Of the 6 subjects receiving PGA supplementation only the 3 with sideroblastic marrow alteration showed an increase in plasma iron turnover (PIT) ranging from a two- to fourfold increase and diminished erythrocyte incorporation of the radioiron label. These results indicate that erythroid mitochondrial iron overload occurs in some well-nourished chronic alcoholic subjects during excessive alcohol ingestion despite the ingestion of a nutritionally replete diet and multivitamin supplementation.

These results suggested a defect in heme biosynthesis possibly related to defective conversion of dietary pyridoxine to its coenzyme PLP. Estimation of erythrocyte pyridoxal phosphokinase was performed in 10 of 11 of these alcoholic volunteer subjects before, during, and after alcohol ingestion. Figure 8 depicts the mean net increases in erythrocyte hemolysate PLP generation in 10 normal controls and in the 10 alcoholic subjects before and during their alcohol ingestion. By 9 weeks, erythrocyte pyridoxal phosphokinase activity had markedly decreased, compared to controls. In order to test whether or not some factor in the plasma of these subjects was inhibitory to this phosphokinase system, plasma from 3 of the alcoholic subjects was mixed in equal volumes with ery-

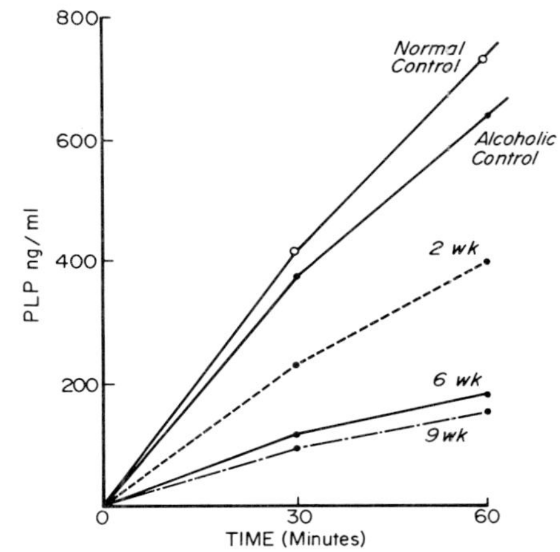

Fig. 8. Erythrocyte pyridoxal phosphokinase levels in 10 normal control subjects compared to 10 alcoholic subjects before (control) and during 9 weeks of alcohol ingestion.

throcyte hemolysate and preincubated 30 minutes at 37° C. Subsequently, the erythrocyte phosphokinase was estimated in the usual fashion. Figure 9 illustrates the results of incubation of plasma from 1 such patient. The sample was incubated with hemolysate at varying times before and during alcohol ingestion. The plasma obtained during the third week of ingestion showed a marked inhibitory effect on the patient's erythrocyte phosphokinase activity. These erythrocytes possessed normal enzyme activity when incubated with plasma obtained before alcohol ingestion. Figure 9 illustrates a similar experiment em-

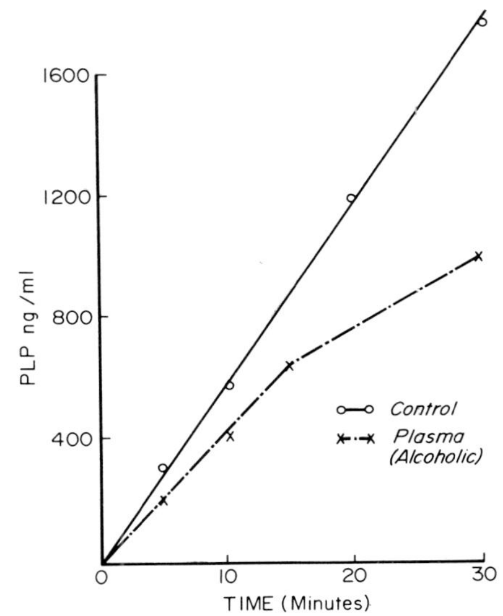

Fig. 9. Estimation of hepatic (rat liver) pyridoxal phosphokinase levels preincubated with normal plasma (control) and plasma obtained from an alcoholic subject during alcohol ingestion.

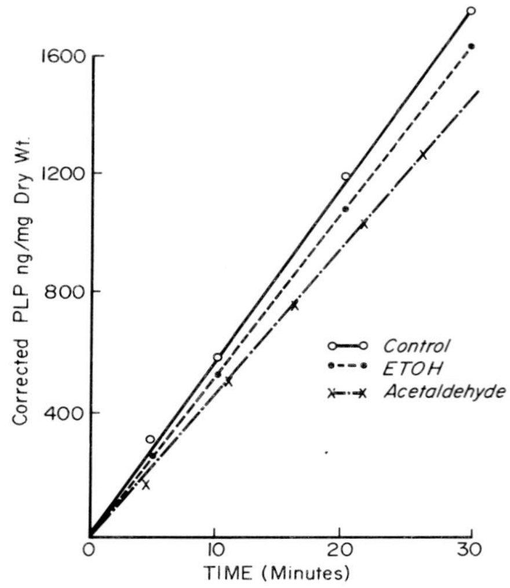

Fig. 10. Estimation of hepatic (rat liver) pyridoxal phosphokinase preincubated with "physiologic" amounts of ethyl alcohol, acetaldehyde as compared to normal control; no significant differences are observed in enzyme activity.

ploying rat liver, with preincubation of normal plasma and plasma obtained from an alcoholic subject at 3 weeks. There is a similar inhibitory effect on enzyme activity. Figure 10 illustrates an experiment designed to test whether rat liver phosphokinase would be affected by preincubation with alcohol (ethyl alcohol 250 mg%) or with acetaldehyde. No significant inhibition was observed.

Recent studies show that the inhibiting material is nondialyzable, and on sephadex gel G 200 filtration appears to be found (or contained) in protein (or polypeptide) fractions less than 5000 MW. The precise structural identity of this material awaits further characterization.

COMMENT

The results of these and other investigations have shown that chronic alcoholic patients will frequently develop certain hematologic abnormalities when administered excessive amounts of alcohol, both with a normal and folate-deficient diet. Supplementation with pharmacologic amounts of PGA and multivitamins will not affect the development of cytoplasmic vacuolization, elevation of serum iron, and sideroblastic marrow alterations in some subjects (with or without anemia).

Alcohol-induced vacuoles in early erythroid and myeloid forms are probably the most commonly detected marrow abnormality.[1,26] Sullivan and Herbert[3,4] conclusively demonstrated that 15 ounces of alcohol daily could prevent or abort a reticulocyte response in 3 alcoholic subjects ingesting a folate-deficient diet when these patients were administered physiologic doses of PGA. This hemosuppressive effect of alcohol on folate utilization could be overcome with pharmacologic amounts of folic or folinic acid. Reticulocytosis and a decrease in serum iron could be elicited in these patients with physiologic amounts of PGA when alcohol was discontinued. Lindenbaum and Lieber [27] recently reported metabolic findings in 9 well-nourished alcoholic volunteers who were maintained on an excellent diet with generous mineral and vitamin supplementation and alcohol administration. The hematologic abnormalities were: vacuolization of erythroid-myeloid cells, slight rise in serum iron, and modest thrombocytopenia in 4. These abnormalities reverted to normal when alcohol intake ceased.

Finding significant numbers of ring sideroblasts in marrows of acute and chronic alcoholics prompted study of vitamin B_6 metabolism in such patients. Hines and Cowan[24] reported studies on three well-nourished alcoholic volunteers housed on a metabolic ward. Each was given a low folate diet plus 900–1000 ml of 86 proof bar whiskey, daily, for 8 to 12 weeks. The dietary pyridoxine was estimated to be twice normal. All 3 subjects became anemic, with megaloblastic marrows, and 2 developed sideroblastic changes associated with hyperferremia. Serum levels of PLP decreased in all subjects, as did serum folate levels. The in vivo estimation of phosphorylation of pyridoxine to pyridoxal phosphate was impaired during alcohol ingestion but returned to normal after several weeks of alcohol withdrawal. Treatment with pyridoxal phosphate but not pyridoxine or PGA was associated with modest reticulocyte elevation and disappearance of ring sideroblasts. This suggested that alcohol caused sideroblastic marrow alteration by interfering with the conversion of pyridoxine to PLP.

The present results in the 70 patients closely agree with those of Eichner and Hillman[16] with respect to the incidence of megaloblastic and sideroblastic abnormalities in unselected severe alcoholic patients. In studies of 65 alcoholic patients consecutively admitted to the hospital these authors found that 75% had disorders of red cell production. The most frequent finding was megaloblastic marrow changes due to folate deficiency (40%) or sideroblastic marrow alteration (30%). Eichner and Hillman also studied the evolution of anemia in selected volunteer alcoholics on a metabolic ward and concluded that the first stage is that of negative vitamin balance, which begins as alcohol is ingested and food intake is decreased. During this period, there is a sharp reduction in serum folate, more pronounced when subjects are on low folate diets. No associated abnormalities in erythropoiesis accompany this stage. The second stage, which may occur as early as 7 days after alcohol ingestion and a poor diet, is megaloblastic change in the marrow. This is seen earliest in patients ingesting a low folate diet plus alcohol, compared to low folate diet alone.[28] The third stage observed by these workers in some patients was the development of marrow sideroblastic conversion probably related to abnormal vitamin B_6 metabolism (or deficiency).

The metabolic results reported here show that alcohol administration, in the range of a fifth of bar whiskey per day, with a normal diet will, in some patients, produce megaloblastic and sideroblastic marrow alterations, vacuolization, and hyperferremia. The addition of pharmacologic amounts of PGA daily will not alter the sideroblastic conversion, nor will the addition of multivitamins and PGA. The presumed reason for this is the demonstrated defective in vivo conversion of pyridoxine to PLP in these subjects. A circulating inhibitor to the erythrocyte enzyme pyridoxal phosphokinase is described in some alcoholic patients during alcohol ingestion. The precise structure and characteristics of this material require further investigation.

REFERENCES

1. McCurdy PR, Pierce LE, Rath CE: Abnormal bone-marrow morphology in acute alcoholism. N Engl J Med 266:505, 1962
2. Jandl JH: Hematologic changes in chronic liver disease. Am J Gastroenterol 30:46, 1958
3. Sullivan LW, Herbert V: Suppression of hematopoiesis by ethanol. J Clin Invest 43:2048, 1964
4. Sullivan LW, Herbert V: Mechanism of hematosuppression by ethanol. Am J Clin Nutr 14:238, 1964
5. Hines JD: Reversible megaloblastic and sideroblastic marrow abnormalities in alcoholic patients. Br J Haematol 16:87, 1969
6. Brayton RG, Stokes PE, Schwartz MS, et al: Effect of alcohol and various diseases on leukocyte mobilization, phagocytosis and intracellular bacterial killing. N Engl J Med 282:123, 1970
7. Crowley JP, Abramson N: Effect of ethanol on complement-mediated chemotaxis. Clin Res 19:415, 1971
8. Lindenbaum J, Hargrove RL: Thrombocytopenia in alcoholics. Ann Intern Med 68:526, 1968
9. Post RM, Desforges JF: Thrombocytopenia and alcoholism. Ann Intern Med 68:1230, 1968
10. *Idem*: Thrombocytopenic effect of ethanol infusion. Blood 31:344, 1968
11. Ryback R, Desforges J: Alcoholic thrombocytopenia in three inpatient drinking alcoholics. Arch Intern Med 125:475, 1970
12. Sullivan LW, Liu YK, Talarico L, et al: Alcohol-induced thrombocytopenia in man. J Clin Invest 47:95a, 1968
13. Cowan DH, Hines JD: Thrombocytopenia of severe alcoholism. Ann Intern Med 74:37, 1971
14. Kessel L: Acute transient hyperlipemia due to hepatopancreatic damage in chronic alcoholics (Zieve's syndrome). Am J Med 32:747, 1962
15. Jandl JH: The anemia of liver disease: Observations on its mechanism. J Clin Invest 34:390, 1955
16. Eichner ER, Hillman RS: The evolution of anemia in alcoholic patients. Am J Med 50:218, 1971
17. Eichner ER, Buchanan B, Smith JW, et al: Variations in the hematologic and medical status of alcoholics. Am J Med Sci 263:35, 1972
18. Grasso J, Hines JD: A comparative electron microscopic study of refractory and alcoholic sideroblastic anemias. Br J Haematol 17:35, 1969
19. A Syllabus of Laboratory Examinations in Clinical Diagnosis. Edited by LB Page, PJ Culver. Cambridge, Harvard University Press, 1960
20. Herbert V: Aseptic addition method for Lactobacillus casei assay of folate activity in human serum. J Clin Pathol 19:12–16, 1966
21. Anderson BB: Investigations into the Euglena method for the assay of vitamin B12 in serum. J Clin Pathol 17:14–26, 1964
22. Hoffbrand AV, Newcombe BFA, Mollin DL: Method of assay of red cell

folate activity in the value of the assay as a test for folate deficiency. J Clin Pathol 19:17–28, 1966
23. Hines JD, Love DS: Determination of serum and blood pyridoxal phosphate concentrations with purified rabbit skeletal muscle phosphorylase b. J Lab Clin Med 73:343, 1969
24. Hines JD, Cowan DH: Studies on the pathogenesis of alcohol-induced sideroblastic bone marrow abnormalities. N Engl J Med 283:441, 1970
25. Schade AL, Oyama J, Reinhart RW, et al: Bound iron and unsaturated iron-binding capacity of serum: rapid and reliable quantitative determination. Proc Soc Exp Biol Med 87:443, 1954
26. Jarrold T, Will JJ, Davies AR, et al: Bone marrow-erythroid morphology in alcoholic patients. Am J Clin Nutr 20:716, 1967
27. Lindenbaum J, Lieber CS: Hematologic effects of alcohol in man in the absence of nutritional deficiency. N Engl J Med 281:333, 1969
28. Eichner ER, Pierce HI, Hillman RS: Folate balance in dietary-induced megaloblastic anemia. N Engl J Med 284:933, 1971

R. L. Gordon*
and S. B. Kahn†

13
Hematologic Effects of Anticonvulsant Drugs

Since the introduction of diphenylhydantoin (Dilantin ® by Merritt) in 1938 for the treatment of seizure disorders,[1] complications of this therapy have become apparent and include neurologic, dermatologic, and gastrointestinal side effects.[2–4] However, the hematologic complications were not noted in the literature until 1952 when Mannheimer published a report of two cases of megaloblastic anemia arising as a complication of therapy with hydantoin-related drugs.[5]

It is now recognized that megaloblastic anemia is the most common hematologic complication of anticonvulsant therapy; but other side effects include leukopenia, thrombocytopenia, pancytopenia, red cell aplasia, polycythemia, immunohemolytic anemia, and a pseudolymphoma like syndrome (Table 1).[6]

Megaloblastic anemia may occur with any of the anticonvulsants (diphenylhydantoin, primidone, phenobarbital) either used singly or in combination. Diphenylhydantoin alone, or combined with phenobarbital has been the prime offender.[7–9] The incidence of megaloblastic anemia in patients on continuous diphenylhydantoin therapy (average duration 6 years) is 0.15% to 0.75%.[10,11] Megaloblastic anemia has appeared from 1 month to 21 years after continuous diphenylhydantoin therapy with 200–300 mg per day.[12,13] While this disease is most common in adults, megaloblastic anemia due to drug therapy has been seen in children.[14] The incidence of macrocytosis in nonanemic patients on anticonvulsants varies from 11% to 53% while greater than 30% of these same patients who demonstrate no peripheral macrocytosis have megaloblastic changes in the bone marrow.[15–17]

The etiology of the megaloblastic picture is folic acid deficiency, and over 50% of patients on long-term anticonvulsant therapy demonstrate low serum and red cell folate levels.[18] The serum folate depression does not correlate with the degree of macrocytosis or with the dosage or duration of drug use.[19,20] How-

* Supported in part by a grant from the American Cancer Society.
† Supported by funds from Clinical Cancer Training Grant CA 08034, National Cancer Institute, National Institutes of Health.

Table 1
Hematologic Disorders Associated With Anticonvulsant Therapy

1.	Megaloblastic anemia
2.	Leukopenia
3.	Thrombocytopenia
4.	Pancytopenia (aplastic anemia)
5.	Red cell aplasia
6.	Polycythemia
7.	Immunohemolytic anemia
8.	Pseudolymphoma

ever, a direct relationship exists between the degree of macrocytosis and the dose of anticonvulsant drug.[21] These hematologic changes can be readily corrected with folic acid treatment. Interestingly enough, this therapy is associated with a fall in serum B_{12} levels in over 50% of patients.[22,23] The cause and significance of this is unknown, especially since B_{12} levels normally rise when folate deficiency is treated.[24]

The mechanism whereby folate metabolism is disturbed by anticonvulsant therapy remains to be clearly defined. A list of hypotheses are presented in Table 2.

Benn and her associates proposed that alkalinization of the jejunum, the optimal site of folic acid absorption,[25] by diphenylhydantoin caused malabsorption of the monoglutamate form of folic acid.[26] This was not confirmed by Doe, et al who gave a folate-deficient epileptic on long-term diphenylhydantoin therapy 100 mg of this drug as a suspension, after which they could demonstrate no rise in the resting intraluminal pH of 6.5 after a 45-minute period.[27]

It has been suggested by Hoffbrand and Rosenberg that anticonvulsants inhibit intestinal conjugases, which act to reduce the poorly absorbed polyglutamates (that account for 75% of dietary folate) to the more readily absorbed monoglutamate form.[28,29] Against this is the fact that the study was not per-

Table 2
Proposed Mechanism of Altered Folate Metabolism During Anticonvulsant Therapy

1.	Alkalinization of jejunal contents leading to malabsorption
2.	Inhibition of intestinal conjugase
3.	Direct effect on jejunal cells leading to malabsorption
4.	Displacement of folate from plasma proteins
5.	Interference of cellular uptake of folate
6.	Increased metabolic requirement for folate

formed at the normal intraluminal pH of the jejunum. In addition, a report by Baugh refutes their claim of in vitro intestinal conjugase inhibition by diphenylhydantoin. These workers found no evidence of inhibition of conjugase extracted from the brain, liver, or intestine.[30] Data from our laboratory confirms Baugh's work. Perhaps the discrepancy in results lies in the fact that at the pH maximum for liver or intestinal conjugase, diphenylhydantoin is not soluble.[31]

Impairment of intestinal conjugase should have no effect on the absorption of monoglutamates, which are present in sufficient quantity in all diets to satisfy daily requirements.[32] Recently, Gerson and his associates demonstrated that diphenylhydantoin inhibits the absorption of monoglutamate folate at the intestinal mucosa. The degree of inhibition is minimal, but this amount of malabsorption could be sufficient to impair normal folate nutrition.[34]

Another theory states that diphenylhydantoin displaces folate from its plasma protein carrier,[18] but this does not explain the reduction of tissue folate also found.[24] There is no evidence for interference of cellular uptake of folate either in in vitro or in vivo testing.[32] Growth of the organism, *L Casei*, used in the microbiologic assay, is also not inhibited by diphenylhydantoin.[18]

These first five mechanisms do not fully explain the altered folate metabolism induced by the anticonvulsants. However, a newer theory has been recently proposed—that is, increased metabolic requirement for folate.

The anticonvulsant drugs are potent enzyme inducers, stimulating enzyme activity in the endoplasmic reticulum of the liver. For example: phenobarbital is used to reduce the level of indirect bilirubin in the treatment of congenital and neonatal jaundice[35,36] by induction of the enzyme bilirubin glucuronyl transferases.[37,38]

Maxwell and his co-workers have postulated that the reduction of serum and red cell folate in patients on chronic anticonvulsant therapy was the result of an increased metabolic requirement for folate by the liver.[39] These workers noted that folate is a cofactor for certain hydroxylations by hepatic microsomal enzymes. One such example is presented in Figure 1.

A glycerol ether, in the presence of oxygen and tetrahydrofolate (PTH_4), is hydroxylated (reaction 2). This product then forms glycerol and an aldehyde (reaction 2), which is then oxidized to an acid (reaction 4). At the same time, dihydrofolate is generated and then reduced to the tetrahydro form by the enzyme dihydrofolic acid reductase. If the anticonvulsants induce enzyme 1, folate turnover increases and folate is diverted from marrow and blood stores

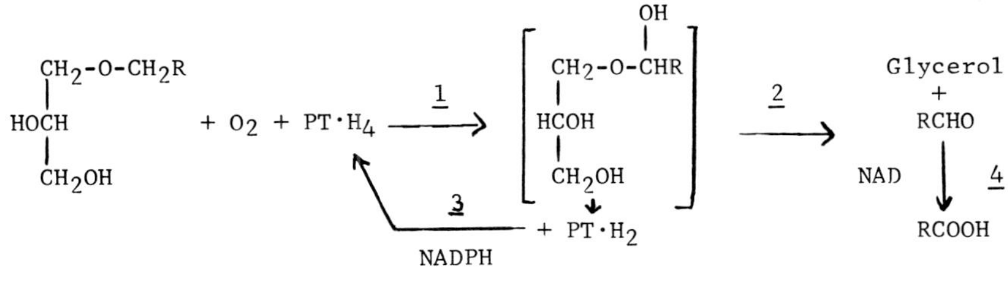

Fig. 1. Postulated reaction scheme for the oxidation of glyceryl ethers (after Tietz, et al[40].)

for use in the liver. It should be noted, that many steroids in the body are hydroxylated by the same enzyme system, and a requirement for folate in these reactions has also been shown.[40,42]

Measurement of urinary D-glucaric acid, a product of glucuronic acid metabolism in the liver, is an easy way to assess hepatic enzyme induction by anticonvulsants. Hunter has shown that patients taking a single anticonvulsant drug excreted a mean of 75 more μ moles per day of D-glucaric acid than those taking none.[42]

Maxwell has demonstrated a linear relationship between increased D-glucaric acid excretion and reduction of serum and red cell folate.[39]

The chronic administration of any drug capable of inducing activity of microsomal drug-metabolizing enzyme may result in an increased demand for folate. Since body stores are limited, and the dietary intake of folate is usually sufficient only for daily requirements, depletion of folate cofactor may occur.[43]

Over a decade ago, it was noted that the administration of folate to diphenylhydantoin treated folate-deficient epileptics might increase their seizure frequency. Diphenylhydantoin is converted in the body to an inactive hydroxylated metabolite, *p*-hydroxyphenytoin. According to the schema in Figure 1, diphenylhydantoin actually induces its own conversion and utilizes tetrahydrofolate to do so. Folate-deficient patients on anticonvulsants thus limit the conversion of diphenylhydantoin and prolong the effective half-life of the drug. If this block is removed by adding supplemental dietary folic acid, a rapid increase in the rate of drug metabolism may ensue, causing a fall in the blood level and possibly loss of seizure control,[39] a phenomenon that has been observed clinically.[44]

Further work will be necessary before this most attractive theory can be confirmed. However, the data suggest that a small degree of drug-induced folate malabsorption, along with an increased metabolic requirement for folate, may account for the mechanism of anticonvulsant-induced megaloblastic anemia.

Leukopenia, induced by anticonvulsants, an uncommon finding, is believed to be a hypersensitivity reaction to the anticonvulsant drug(s), although folate deficiency may also play a role. The occurrence rate is about 2%, and most of the patients have white counts between 3000–4000 per cubic millimeter.[45,46] Thrombocytopenia without megaloblastic anemia is rare and also may be the result of a hypersensitivity reaction.[45] A case of diphenylhydantoin induced, reversible erythroid aplasia has been reported, the mechanism of which remains obscure.[47] A serious complication is the development of pancytopenia with marrow aplasia. This is more commonly associated with mesantoin therapy and less commonly with diphenylhydantoin. The mortality rate is around 75% and deaths occur most often during the first 30 to 60 days of therapy.[48] There have been several case reports of polycythemia after anticonvulsant-induced megaloblastic anemia has been treated with folic acid, after which polycythemia disappeared when folic acid was withdrawn.[49,50] Immunohemolytic anemia is another reported complication of anticonvulsant therapy.[51]

Some patients on anticonvulsant therapy may exhibit an unusual type of hypersensitivity reaction that clinically resembles malignant lymphoma. This is characterized by significant adenopathy (most frequently involving the cervical nodes), fever, dermatitis, eosinophilia, and hepatosplenomegaly.[52] The association of this syndrome complex with diphenylhydantoin was first reported in 1940 by Cooper and Burrows.[53] Their patient developed a severe maculopapular eruption, fever, and posterior cervical adenopothy 1 week after being placed on diphenylhydantoin therapy. These symptoms disappeared when the drug was discontinued and reappeared when the drug was readministered.

The clinical picture of pseudolymphoma may begin as soon as 1 week or up to 24 months after therapy is started; but generally, most patients develop symptoms within a few weeks to months.[52] Pathologic examination of involved lymph glands may show a picture almost indistinguishable from that of a malignant lymphoma. Distinguishing features, however, are lack of architectural obliteration and cellular invasion of blood vessels and capsule in cases of pseudolymphoma.[54]

Regression of adenopathy will occur within 1 to 2 weeks after the offending drug(s) are discontinued, and this finding is the best differential diagnostic test.[55] There are reports in the literature of malignant lymphoma developing from 1 to 12 years after anticonvulsant therapy has been started. In each case, the adenopathy did not regress after the medication was discontinued, and pathologic examination revealed them to be clearly "malignant." The question to be answered is whether or not anticonvulsant drugs are carcinogenic, in certain susceptible hosts, rather than allergenic.[54]

In summary, the hematologic side effects of anticonvulsant drug therapy covers the spectrum from megaloblastic anemia to pseudolymphoma. Although the incidence of any of these hematologic side effects is small, in view of the frequency and chronicity of drug use these toxic effects are important limiting features of anticonvulsant drug therapy.

REFERENCES

1. Merritt H, Putnam TJ: Sodium diphenylhydantoinate in the treatment of convulsive disorders. JAMA 111:1068, 1938
2. *Idem*: Sodium diphenylhydantoinate in treatment of convulsive seizures. Toxic symptoms and their prevention. Arch Neurol Psychiatry 42:1053, 1939
3. Kimball OP: The treatment of epilepsy with sodium diphenylhydantoinate. JAMA 112:1244, 1939
4. Drill's Pharmacology in Medicine. Third Edition. Edited by JRD Palma. New York, McGraw-Hill, p 236
5. Mannheimer R, Pakesch F, Reimir EF, et al: The hematologic complications of epilepsy therapy with hydantoin drugs. Med Klin 47:1397, 1952
6. Sparberg M: Diagnostically confusing complications of diphenylhydantoin therapy. Ann Intern Med 59:914, 1963
7. Newman MJO, Sumner DW: Megaloblastic anemia following the use of primidone. Blood 12:183, 1957
8. Hawkins CF, Meynell MJ: Megaloblastic anemia during anticonvulsant therapy. Lancet 2:846, 1957
9. Calvert RJ, Hurworth E, Macbean AL: Megaloblastic anemia from methophenobarbital. Blood 13:894, 1958
10. Benians RC, Hunter RH: Megaloblastic anemia occurring during treatment of epilepsy with phenytoin sodium, primidone, and phenobarbital. J Ment Sci 103:606, 1957

11. Flexner JM, Hartman RC: Megaloblastic anemia associated with anticonvulsant drugs. Am J Med 28:386, 1960
12. Sherwin AL, Wart RH, Cooper BA: Megaloblastic anemia associated with phenobarbital therapy. Can Med Assoc J 82:365, 1960
13. Macintosh PC, Hutchinson JL: Megaloblastic anemia due to anticonvulsant therapy. Report of a case responding to vitamin B_{12}. Can Med Assoc J 82:368, 1960
14. Kahn SB, Baker L, Lischmer H, et al: Megaloblastic anemia following phenobarbital and primidone therapy. Pediatrics, 1963
15. Reynolds EH, Preece J, Chanarin I: Folic acid and anticonvulsants. Lancet 1:1264, 1969
16. Child JA, Khattak BZ, Knowles JP: Macrocytosis in patients on anticonvulsant drugs. Br J Haematol 16:451, 1969
17. Reynolds EH, Milner G, Matthews DM, et al: Anticonvulsant therapy, megaloblastic haemopoiesis, and folic acid metabolism. QJ Med 35:521, 1966
18. Klipstein FA: Subnormal serum folate and macrocytosis associated with anticonvulsant therapy. Blood 23, 1964
19. Dahlke MB, Mertens-Roesler E: Malabsorption of folic acid due to diphenylhydantoin. Blood 30:341, 1967
20. Child JA, Khattak BZ, Knowles JP: Folic acid deficiency and the megaloblastic anemias. Br J Haematol 16:451, 1969
21. Eastman RD, Jancar J: Macrocytosis associated with anticonvulsant therapy. Epilepsia 11:275, 1970
22. Hunter R, Barnes J, Matthew DM: Effect of folic acid supplement on serum B_{12} levels in patients on anticonvulsants. Lancet 11:666, 1969
23. Reynolds EL, Wrighton RJ, Johnson AL, et al: Inter-relations of folic acid and vitamin B_{12} in drug treated epileptic patients. Epilepsia 12:165, 1971
24. Chanarin I: The megaloblastic anemias. Oxford, Blackwell, 1969
25. Chanarin I, Anderson BB, Mollin DL: The absorption of folic acid. Br J Haematol 4:156, 1958
26. Benn A, Swan C, Cook WT, et al: Effect of intraluminal pH on the absorption of pteroylmonoglutamin acid. Br Med J 1:148, 1971
27. Doe WF, Hoffbrand AV, Reed PI, et al: Jejunal ph and folic acid. Br Med J 1:669, 1971
28. Hoffbrand AV, Nechels TF: Mechanism of folate deficiency in patients receiving phenytoin. Lancet 2:528, 1968
29. Rosenberg IH, Streiff RR, Godwin HA, et al: Impairment of intestinal deconjugation of dietary folate. Lancet 2:530, 1968
30. Baugh CM, Krumbaugh CL: Effects of phenytoin on folic acid conjugases in man. Lancet 2:519, 1969
31. Gordon RL, Kahn SB, Brodsky I: Hematologic effects of anticonvulsant therapy. Unpublished data
32. Hurdle ADF, Barton D, Searles IH: A method for measuring folate in food and its application to a hospital diet. Am J Clin Nutr 21:1202, 1968
33. Corcino JJ, Waxman S, Herbert V: Uptake of tritiated folates by human bone marrow cells in vitro. Br J Haematol 20:503, 1971
34. Gerson CD, Hepner GW, Brown N, et al: Inhibition by diphenylhydantoin of folic acid absorption in man. Gastroenterology 63:246, 1972
35. Arias IM: Chronic nonhemolytic unconjugated hyperbilirubinemia with glucuronyl transferase deficiency. Am J Med 47:395, 1969
36. Black M, Sherlock S: Treatment of Gilbert's Syndrome with phenobarbitone. Lancet 1:1359, 1970

37. Werk EE, MacGee J, Sholeton LJ: Effect of diphenylhydantoin on cortisol metabolism in man. J Clin Invest 43:1824, 1969
38. Thompson RPH, Eddleston ALWF, Williams R: Low plasma bilirubin in epileptics on phenobarbitone. Lancet 1:21, 1969
39. Maxwell JD, Hunt J, Stewart DA, et al: Folate deficiency after anticonvulsant drugs: an effect of hepatic enzyme induction? Br Med J 1:297, 1972
40. Tietz A, Lindberg M, Kennedy EP: A new pteridine requiring enzyme system for the oxidation of glycerol ethers. J Biol Chem 239:4081, 1964
41. Hagermann DD: Pteridine cofactors in enzymatic hydroxylations of steroids. Fed Proc 23:480, 1964
42. Hunter J, Maxwell JD, Williams R: Urinary D-glucaric acid excretion as a test for hepatic enzyme induction in man. Lancet 2:47, 1971
43. Baylis EM, Crowly JM, Preece JM, et al: Influence of folic acid on blood phenytoin levels. Lancet 1:62, 1971
44. Reynolds EH: Mental effects of anticonvulsants and folic acid metabolism. Brain 91:197, 1968
45. Sparberg M: Diagnostically confusing complications of diphenylhydantoin therapy. Ann Intern Med 59:914, 1963
46. Kurtzke JF: Leukopenia with diphenylhydantoin. J Nerv Ment Dis 132:339, 1961
47. Brittingham TE, Lutcher CL, Murphy DL: Reversible erythroid aplasia induced by Dilantin. Arch Intern Med 113:764, 1964
48. Robins M: Aplastic anemia secondary to anticonvulsants. Am J Dis Child 104:614, 1962
49. Grønbak P, Larsen JV: Polycythemia vera following treatment of megaloblastic anemia with folic acid. Acta Med Scand 174:781, 1963
50. Amir J, Elian M, DeVries A: Polycythemia following folic acid and vitamin B_{12} treatment of anticonvulsant induced megaloblastic anemia. Israel J Med Sci 6:49, 1970
51. Snapper I, Marks D, Schwartz L, et al: Hemolytic anemia secondary to mesantoin. Ann Intern Med 39:619, 1953
52. Saltztein SI, Ackerman LV: Lymphadenopathy induced by anticonvulsant drugs and mimicking clinically and pathologically malignant lymphoma. Cancer 12:164, 1959
53. Coope R, Burrows RGR: Treatment of epilepsy with sodium diphenylhydantoinate. Lancet 1:490, 1940
54. Hyman GH, Sommer SC: The development of Hodgkin's disease and lymphoma during anticonvulsant therapy. Blood 28:416, 1966
55. Clinicopathologic Conference: Lymphoma or drug reaction occurring hydantoin therapy for epilepsy. Am J Med 32:286, 1962

Albert F. LoBuglio
and Gerald W. King

14

α-Methyldopa and Red Blood Cells

In 1966, Carstairs reported positive red cell antiglobulin reactions in patients receiving α-methyldopa (Aldomet), an antihypertensive drug.[1] This observation led to a flurry of publications describing both clinical and laboratory studies of this unusual immunologic phenomena. This review will attempt to summarize what is known regarding the characteristics of the clinical picture, the immunologic reaction, and the potential mechanism of this adverse drug reaction.

CLINICAL PICTURE

Incidence

Reports regarding the incidence of a positive red cell antiglobulin reaction (direct Coombs test) have ranged from 0%[2] to 28%[3] of patients receiving this drug. However, the incidence in most studies ranged from 10% to 20%, and when the reports were combined, an overall incidence of 15% (214 positive reactions in 1395 patients) was found. In contrast, among 358 hypertensive patients who did not receive α-methyldopa (AMD), there was no instance of a positive antiglobulin reaction.[4] In addition, Hunter[3] noted that if patients were studied serially over several years of therapy with AMD, the overall incidence was 26%, with some patients becoming positive only after several years of treatment. Thus, this effect appears to be one of the most common adverse reactions seen with any drug in common use. Some studies have suggested that this drug reaction might occur less frequently in negroes,[2,5] orientals,[6] and indians.[2]

Effect of Dosage and Duration of Therapy

Carstairs[1] noted a relationship between the incidence of positive Coombs tests and dosage: $<$ 1 g per day, 11%; 1–2 g per day, 19% $>$ 2 g per day, 36%. Other investigators have not noted as striking an effect with dosage. In the four largest series in which dosage was studied, the incidence of positive Coombs tests was 16% at less than 1 g per day and 21% at greater than 1 g per day.[1,3,7,8] It is rare for a patient to develop a positive test during the first 3 months of therapy, and most Coombs tests become positive between the third and twelfth month. In general, if a positive Coombs test occurs, it persists for as long as the patient receives AMD. However, when therapy is discontinued, the antiglobulin reaction will become negative within periods ranging from a few months to over a year, depending on the amount of antibody initially present.[9]

Hemolytic Anemia

Fortunately, the vast majority of patients receiving AMD and in whom positive Coombs tests occur do not develop anemia or evidence of increased red cell destruction. The true incidence of hemolysis is difficult to determine, but it is probably between 0.01%–0.1% of patients receiving the drug and is not dose-dependent.[10] The severity of hemolysis can vary, and clinical and laboratory findings are identical to those of patients with idiopathic autoimmune hemolytic anemia. These findings include reticulocytosis, spherocytosis, shortened red cell survival, positive Coombs test, and splenomegaly. α-Methyldopa has produced more cases of hemolysis than all other drugs known to produce immune hemolysis.[4] It has been suggested that this drug may be the etiology in about 10% of all patients presenting with Coombs positive hemolytic anemia.[11] Most patients with hemolysis improve readily when the drug is discontinued.[10] However, in severe cases, corticosteroids can accelerate improvement in the blood picture but need not be administered for longer than a week or 2.[10,12] Although hemolysis stops readily, it often requires 6 to 18 months before the Coombs test gradually becomes negative. Reinstituting AMD does not cause an accelerated onset of Coombs positivity or hemolysis.[9]

IMMUNOLOGIC REACTION

Antiglobulin Reaction

Most patients who develop this immune reaction have weakly-to-moderately positive direct and negative indirect Coombs tests.[1] If enzyme-treated red cells are used to increase the sensitivity of the indirect test, almost all patients have positive reactions.[1,12] Patients with hemolysis usually have strongly positive direct and indirect Coombs tests, with high titers of antibody, using enzyme-treated red cells.[10] The positive antiglobulin reaction has repeatedly been demonstrated to be due to the presence of IgG globulin on the red cell surface without the presence of complement.[1,12] The only exception to this observation was the study of Perry[5] who noted several patients with complement-coated cells. However, a large number of these patients were receiving hydralazine (Apresoline), which may have been responsible for this finding. The serum of patients with Coombs positive red cells did not have drug-dependent antibody activity, i.e., the sera reacted with a panel of normal or enzyme-treated red cells whether or not AMD was added to the system.[10,12] Thus, the usual method for incriminating a drug in the etiology of immune hemolysis was not present.

Red Cell Eluates

Eluates from red cells of patients on AMD and who had positive antiglobulin reactions contained IgG globulin, which had the ability to react with red cells of normal individuals without the addition of AMD in vitro.[10,12] In addition, these eluates could react with autologous red cells studied after AMD therapy ceased at a time when the direct Coombs test was negative. Thus, the IgG globulin on the red cell surface was an antibody directed against antigens on both homologous and autologous red cells, and, therefore, fits the definition of an "autoantibody." The studies of Bakemeier and Leddy[13] demonstrated that the autoantibody in one patient was clearly polyclonal in that it contained both κ and λ light chains and three heavy chain subclasses of IgG globulin ($IgG_{1,2,\text{ and }3}$).

Antibody Specificity

A number of studies, using both sera and red cell eluates, have demonstrated that these antibodies have specificity for known red cell antigens in the Rh system (anti-e, anti-c, and so forth) as well as to a basic portion of the Rh locus, as demonstrated by lack of reaction with Rh_{null} red cells.[10,12,13] These serologic findings are identical to those found in "idiopathic" autoimmune hemolytic anemia.

Related Autoimmune Reactions

Patients receiving AMD have an increased incidence of antinuclear antibody (10% to 15%), which does not correlate with the presence of positive Coombs tests.[3,9] These patients did not have clinical symptoms or physical findings suggestive of an active "collagen" disease. A small number of patients have had positive LE cell phenomena while receiving AMD.[3] Sherman[14] reported three instances of immune hemolytic anemia in elderly women receiving AMD, 2 of whom also had positive LE cell preparations and rheumatoid factor assays. These immune reactions also appear reversible after therapy ceases.

Drugs Producing Similar Immune Reactions

Recent studies of patients receiving L-dopa in the treatment of Parkinsonism have noted a similar clinical occurrence of positive Coombs tests due to an antibody with the same characteristics as that seen with AMD therapy.[15,16] This drug is almost identical in structure to AMD, suggesting that the dihydroxphenylalanine nucleus is instrumental in producing this immune reaction. There is also some evidence that chronic therapy with mefenamic acid (Ponstan) may rarely produce the same clinical picture.[17]

MECHANISM AMD AUTOIMMUNITY

The observation that administration of AMD can reproducibly result in a high incidence of autoantibody synthesis has led to renewed interest in the role of extrinsic or environmental causes of autoimmune phenomena. The mechanism of this drug effect on the immune system is unknown. A lucid and entertaining exchange of letters in the *New England Journal of Medicine* illustrated best the two most debated mechanisms of this reaction.[11,18] If AMD adversely affected the patient's immune system, tolerance to "self" antigens (Rh locus) may be interrupted, with the subsequent production of antibodies directed against autologous red cells. Alternatively, AMD may react with or modify red cell antigens, resulting in the production of antibodies by the patient's normal immune system directed at these "neoantigens." This explanation would require that these antibodies are able to cross-react with the normal unmodified Rh locus. Vyas[19] has demonstrated in vitro that AMD has the ability to polymerize into melanin-like pigments which have the ability to bind to the red cell surface and even nonspecifically attach immunoglobulins to the red cell surface. It is difficult to construct experimental techniques to discriminate between these two mechanisms of AMD autoimmunity. However, the mechanism involved has application to the whole field of autoimmunity and will require continued investigation in the future. It is frightening to realize that AMD was used clinically for several years before its role in autoimmunity was recognized, despite the high incidence of this adverse reaction. If other chemicals or infectious agents produce this effect in less than 1.0% of patients, it will require more sophisticated methods of identification.

CLINICAL SIGNIFICANCE

A large number of hypertensive patients with AMD-induced Coombs positive red cells have been followed for periods of up to 3 to 5 years.[4] Theoretically, this chronic autoimmune state may lead to serious "collagen" diseases or even neoplasia of the lymphoid system. However, this has not been observed to date. If a patient develops a positive antiglobulin reaction without hemolysis while on AMD, indications for this therapy should be reviewed. Therapy should probably be changed if a reasonable alternative exists. However, in many instances of moderate-to-severe hypertension, AMD is part of the optimal regimen; then the patient should be followed carefully for hemolytic anemia, collagen disease, and lymphoma.

The patient who develops Coombs positive hemolytic anemia can usually be treated simply by discontinuing AMD therapy. If the anemia is severe, corticosteroids will hasten recovery and need not be maintained over a long period of time. In addition, drug-induced immune hemolysis should be considered in all cases of Coombs positive hemolytic anemia. Table 1 compares the char-

Table 1
Characteristics of Drug-Induced Immune Hemolysis

		Coombs Test			Serum Antibody In Vitro			
Mechanism	Hemolysis	Direct	Indirect	Antibody Type	Drug Dependent	Reaction	Antibody in Eluate	Drugs
Hapten Type Complement Fixing	INT	± (complement)	−	IgM	Yes	Agglutination/lysis	No	Phenacetin Dipyrone Orinase
Hapten Type Noncomplement Fixing	EXT	+ (IgG)	−	IgG	Yes	Coombs reaction	Yes (Drug-dependent)	Penicillin
Autoimmune	EXT	+ (IgG)	+	IgG	No	Coombs reaction	Yes	Methyldopa L-Dopa Mefenamic acid
Nonspecific Protein Attachment	None	+ (IgG)	−	None	None	None	None	Keflin
Idiopathic Autoimmune Hemolytic Anemia	EXT	+ (IgG)	+	IgG	No	Coombs reaction	Yes	

INT Intravascular
EXT Extravascular

acteristics of various types of drug-induced hemolytic anemias and idiopathic "autoimmune" hemolytic anemia. As outlined, there are no discernible differences between AMD and idiopathic autoimmune hemolytic anemia. Thus, a history of AMD ingestion is prerequisite for this disorder, and clinical improvement after AMD therapy is discontinued confirms this diagnosis.

SUMMARY

The chronic administration of α-methyldopa, an antihypertensive medication, results in the development of red cell autoantibodies in 15% of patients. Fortunately, the incidence of anemia in these patients with autoantibodies is only about 1%, but this does represent the most frequent form of drug-induced immune hemolytic anemia. These red cell antibodies are IgG immunoglobulins and have a structure and antigenic specificity similar to those of the autoantibodies in idiopathic autoimmune hemolytic anemia. Discontinuing therapy with α-methyldopa results in rapid improvement of anemia with the gradual disappearance of autoantibody production. The mechanism of this drug-induced autoimmune syndrome is unknown, but it may serve as a model to unravel the mechanisms involved in various autoimmune diseases.

REFERENCES

1. Carstairs KC, Breckenridge A, Dollery CT, et al: Incidence of a positive Coombs test in patients on α methyldopa. Lancet 2:113, 1966
2. Seedat YK, Vawda EI: The Coombs test and methyldopa. Lancet 1:427, 1968
3. Hunter E, Raik E, Gordon S: Incidence of positive Coombs test, LE cells and antinuclear factor in patients on alpha-methyldopa therapy. Med J Aust 2:810, 1971
4. Worlledge SM: Immune drug-induced hemolytic anemias. Semin Hematol 6:181, 1969
5. Perry HM, Chaplin H, Carmody S, et al: Immunologic findings in patients receiving methyldopa: a prospective study. J Lab Clin Med 78:905, 1971
6. Burns-Cox CJ: Negative Coombs tests in Chinese on methyldopa. Lancet 2:673, 1970
7. Louis WJ, Doyle AE, Jerums G: Methyldopa and haemolytic anemia. Med J Aust 2:104, 1967
8. Hodge JV, Casey TP: Methyldopa and the direct antiglobulin test. NZ Med J 68:240, 1968
9. Breckenridge A, Dollery CT, Worlledge SM, et al: Positive direct Coombs tests and antinuclear factor in patients treated with methyldopa. Lancet 2:1265, 1967
10. Worlledge SM, Carstairs KC, Dacie JV: Autoimmune hemolytic anemia associated with α methyldopa therapy. Lancet 2:135, 1966
11. Jandl JH, LoBuglio AF: Alpha-methyldopa red cell antibody: cross-reaction or forbidden clones? N Engl J Med 276:1382, 1967
12. LoBuglio AF, Jandl JH: The nature of the alpha-methyldopa red cell antibody. N Engl J Med 276:658, 1967
13. Bakemeier RF, Leddy JP: Erythrocytes autoantibody associated with alpha-methyldopa: heterogeneity of structure and specificity. Blood 32:1, 1968

14. Sherman JD, Love DE, Harrington JF: Anemia, positive lupus, and rheumatoid factors with methyldopa. Arch Intern Med 120:321, 1967
15. Joseph C: Occurrence of positive Coombs test in patients treated with levodopa. N Engl J Med 286:1401, 1972
16. LoBuglio AF, Masouredis SP, Pisciotta AV, et al: Immunoglobulin coating of red cells following L-dopa therapy. Fed Proc 28:315, 1969
17. Scott GL, Myles AB, Bacon PA: Autoimmune haemolytic anemia and mefenamic acid therapy. Br Med J 3:534, 1968
18. Dameshek W: Alpha-methyldopa red-cell antibody: cross-reaction or forbidden clones? N Engl J Med 276:1382, 1967
19. Vyas GN, Sassetti RJ, Petz LD, et al: Experimental study of aldomet-induced positive antiglobulin reaction. Br J Haematol 16:137, 1969

PART III

Drug Effects on Leukocytes

Frederick Stohlman, Jr.
and Peter Quesenberry

15
The Kinetics of Myelopoiesis and Their Relationship to Drug-induced Neutropenia

In considering drug-induced changes in the production of neutrophils, it seems appropriate to first review current concepts of the regulation of myelopoiesis. It should be remembered, however, that this field is in a developmental stage and that we are presenting a working model which, in many respects, will undoubtedly need to be modified as new information develops.

MODEL OF MYELOPOIESIS

It is abundantly clear that the differentiated myeloid compartment is not self-sustaining but rather is derived from a precursor pool of cells which share a common cell of origin with erythroid and megakaryocytic lines of cells and, perhaps, also the lymphoid cells (Figure 1). Between the pluripotent cell (CFU) and the identifiable myeloid elements of bone marrow, there is reason to suspect that there is an intermediate precursor compartment committed to differentiation along a single cell line. Evidence for such a committed compartment, in the case of the erythroid series, is clear and has been recently reviewed.[1] Evidence for a similar committed myeloid stem cell (CFC) rests on evaluation of changes in *concentrations* of CFC after a variety of experimental maneuvers.

The CFU maybe assayed in mice by transplanting bone marrow or spleen into heavily irradiated recipients, as described by Till and McCulloch,[2] and the CFC by growth in soft agar, as described by Bradley and Metcalf.[3] It has been reported that after the administration of agents selectively lethal for cells in DNA synthesis, (hydroxyurea or ^{3}H-thymidine) 0%–15% of the CFU will be killed but that a greater proportion of CFC are lethally damaged 25%–50%, suggesting that the cells monitored by these two techniques have different

Supported in part by Grants from the National Heart and Lung Institute (HL 5600 and 7542) and the General Research Support Grant National Institute of Health (FR 5587).

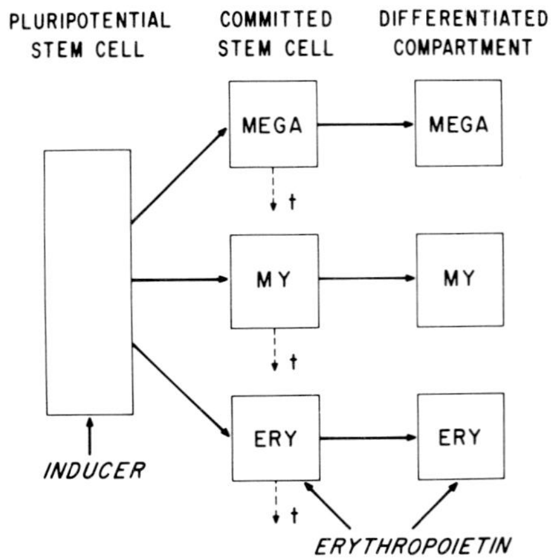

Fig. 1. A schematic model of hematopoiesis. MEG–megakaryocytic, MY–myelocytic, ERY–erythropoietic. **Dashed line** and **cross** indicate cell death (Reprinted from Stohlman F Jr, by permission from Appleton-Century-Crofts.[36]).

cell cycle characteristics.[4,5] This, in turn, suggests separate identities for the two. After intense erythroid stimulation, the CFU will migrate from bone marrow to the spleen,[6] where perhaps the microenvironment is more favorable for erythroid growth. There is parallel migration of the CFC from bone marrow to spleen.[7] Further, in liquid suspension cultures the presence of colony stimulating factor (CSF) (*vide infra*) favors maintenance of both CFC and CFU conventrations.[8] These latter data, taken together, might be interpreted as indicating a common identity for CFC and CFU; they migrate together and both are affected by CSF. If this is the case, then the experiments with cycle-specific agents might be explained as reflecting functionally identical cells in different stages of cell cycle, i.e., G_0 compared with active cycle, rather than a truly separate and more differentiated cell in the case of CFC.

When triggered, the pluripotent stem cell enters its cycle and undergoes a series of division which "magnifies" the size of the compartment; at some point in time, given the appropriate stimulus, cells within this compartment become committed to myelopoiesis. This latter cell is responsible for growth in soft agar and serves as the immediate precursor for myeloblasts. There is some experimental information to suggest that both long range[9] (hormonal) and short range[6,10,11] (cell interaction) regulation is responsible for maintaining the pluripotent compartment size. As yet there is not enough substantive information to warrant a detailed consideration of these interrelationships in a presentation of this sort.

Differentiation of the CFC is thought to be under humoral control, but the nature of the stimulus is still unproven. It is clear, from studies in neutropenic animals, that the numbers of CFC[12] and the size of the myeloblast-promyelocyte (MPC) compartment[13] are related to the concentration of peripheral neutrophils. For example: if one shields the hind limb of a mouse and then gives varying doses of irradiation to the remainder of the animal, a dose-dependent neutropenia will result. The response of the myeloid compartment in the unirradiated, shielded limb has shown to be directly related to the degree of peripheral neutro-

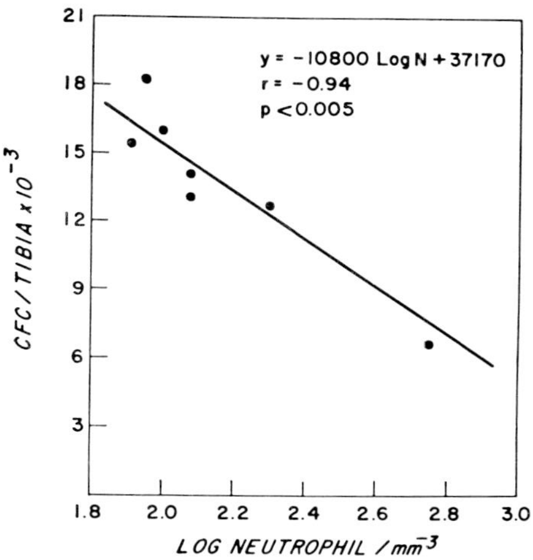

Fig. 2. The relationship between the size of the CFC compartment and the blood neutrophil count in ILS mice for days 2–8 postirradiation. CFC are the average of mean values for composite results of at least three experiments per point. Correlation coefficient r and the regression line are calculated from these values and are significant when $p < 0.005$. (Reprinted from Rickard, et al, by permission from Blood[12]).

penia. On the fifth postirradiation day, the concentration of cells in both the CFC and MPC is a linear function of the log of the peripheral neutrophil count (Figures 2 and 3). From this we have concluded that the feedback control of myelopoiesis is governed by the concentration of peripheral neutrophils or a function thereof. Further evidence for this relationship was provided by studies in which bone marrow was implanted into millipore chambers, which were then

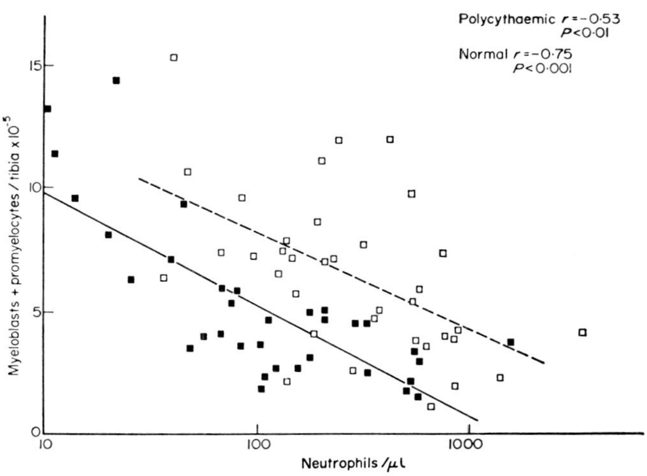

Fig. 3. Correlation of myeloblast-promyelocyte compartment with the logarithm of the neutrophil count in both normal and polycythaemic animals on day 4 after various doses of irradiation. (Reprinted from Morley, et al, by permission from Br J Haematol[37]).

inserted intraperitoneally into host animals, some of which had been rendered neutropenic by pretreatment with cyclophosphamide and others, serving as controls, were injected with saline.[9] Release of cells from the chamber does not occur, as is the case with intact marrow. We observed that the rate of myelopoiesis was greater in chambers implanted in neutropenic animals. Further a dose-dependent relationship was seen.

The above observations present cogent evidence for a long-range humoral control of myelopoiesis. It is tempting, therefore, to suggest that a hormone, analogous to erythropoietin, is responsible for regulating white cell production. However, proof for a granulopoietin would require the demonstration of a sustained increase in myelopoiesis after the putative protein has been injected. As yet, no such rigorous proof has been provided, and we must rely on indirect relationships. The evaluation of these relationships, however, is complicated by the nature of myelopoiesis within the differentiated compartment. In several critical areas this is quite distinct from that seen in the erythroid compartment. First, there is no histochemical marker, such as the reticulocyte, nor unique protein, such as hemoglobin, which may be labeled to identify the newly released granulocytes. The best approximation is with ^{3}H-Tdr labels, but because of the short intravascular life span of the granulocyte, this does not lend itself to quantitative studies of regulation. Second, there is a large intramedullary pool of granulocytes which can be released promptly in response to a variety of stimuli. Thus, granulocytosis, rather than reflecting increased production, may reflect only the release of cells from the storage pool. Finally, and perhaps of less importance in evaluating granulocyte production is the relationship of marginal and circulating pools of granulocytes. Under normal circumstances these are in equilibrium, but this balance may be shifted in either direction by physiologic or pathologic processes. Thus, to evaluate the regulation of myelopoiesis at the present time, it is necessary to resort to in vitro techniques, e.g., the soft agar, or the closed in vivo millipore chamber system.

HUMORAL REGULATION

Gordon and his associates[14] demonstrated that when endotoxin was given a protein was released into the plasma, which, when transferred to normal animals, produced a leukocytosis thought to result from the release of granulocytes from the storage pool. This was subsequently confirmed by Boggs, et al.[15] The relationship of this factor to granulocyte production, however, is unknown. It is possible, for example, that this protein has two effects, one of which is to initiate CFC differentiation into myeloblasts, the other to release mature granulocytes from the storage pool. This seems unlikely to us. A second possibility would be that the discharge of granulocytes from the storage compartment initiates an intramedullary feedback circuit which induces differentiation. However, in view of the increased myelopoiesis observed in chambers implanted into neutropenic animals, it seems more likely that a long-range regulation is responsible for granulocyte differentiation and that an intramedullary loop, responding to the depletion of the storage compartment, is an unlikely primary control mechanism.

A more likely candidate for the regulation of myelopoiesis is the colony stimulating factor or CSF. As noted before, myelocytic colonies may be grown from bone marrow explants in soft agar (or methyl cellulose), providing an appropriate stimulus is present. This stimulus—CSF—may be provided by medium conditioned by a variety of tissues and may also be found in the serum of some species of normal mice and in human urine. It is a glycoprotein which may be present as a polymer; molecular weights varying from 15,000 to 60,000 have been ascribed to it. Human bone marrow may also be grown in agar. Initially, this was accomplished by using an underlayer containing buffy coat cells from normal blood.[16] More recently it has been recognized that both peripheral blood cells from normal human beings and human bone marrow will give rise to colony formation in soft agar without a feeder layer, provided the concentration of cells is sufficiently great. This type of autostimulation is not seen with normal cells of murine origin.

There is also present in serum an inhibitor of colony formation. This is thought to be a lipoprotein of relatively high molecular weight.[17] Because of this high molecular weight, its activity is greatly diminished when one uses a double layer technique and places the serum in the underlayer. With this technique, CSF will diffuse readily into the overlayer, but the inhibitor, being of larger molecular weight, will diffuse poorly. The inhibitor may be removed by a variety of other techniques, such as column separation, ether extraction, and so forth. It is noteworthy that in a number of reports of changes in CSF under experimental or clinical conditions, little attention has been paid to this inhibitor. Evaluation of inhibitor levels, however, is essential, for apparent changes in CSF concentrations may reflect only changes in inhibitor. The physiologic role of the inhibitor, if any, is unknown. We think that it is probably a nonspecific effect and that its importance is only in the assay.

It has been suggested that CSF is produced by the granulocyte.[18] The evidence cited in favor of this hypothesis is that granulocytes are the most common cell in the buffy coat used for feeder layers that provide the stimulus for growth of human bone marrow in culture. Additional evidence might be the prompt rise in CSF when immune neutropenia is induced. However, this could also be explained by the release of endogenous pyrogen. If the granulocyte were the source of CSF, it would mean that granulopoiesis was controlled by a positive feedback. In consequence, increasing amounts of CSF would be produced as the white count rose, thus producing an ever greater granulocytic response. It would not, however, provide for a response to neutropenia. It seems to us more likely that CSF production relates to a function of the neutrophil rather than being produced by the granulocyte. It is not unreasonable to suggest that the cell of origin is ubiquitous, since CSF may be obtained by conditioning media with a variety of tissues and the body must provide for a granulocytic response to local infection. The macrophage-monocyte system and collagen-vascular system might be considered candidates. Pertinent to this consideration are observations of Moore[19] and of Chervenick[20] who independently demonstrated that after physical separation of monocytes from granulocytes, the monocyte fraction supported the growth of colonies in vitro but the granulocyte fraction did not. We have also found that in implanted millipore chambers the addition of large numbers of granulocytes will impede cell growth.[21]

Perhaps this inhibition reflects the release of lysozymal enzymes after the death of mature granulocytes which have an inhibitory effect on growth under the existing cultural conditions. It may, however, reflect a more specific effect and raises anew the question of whether the intramedullary storage pool might play a role in regulating granulopoiesis, in this case exerting a "braking" effect. It should be noted, however, that under the conditions which apply in experiments using millipore chambers, granulocytes are undergoing breakdown and cell death in situ, whereas under normal circumstances there is not a firm estimate as to the extent of ineffective myelopoiesis, if it occurs.

Under normal conditions CSF may be seen in the serum or urine but only in low concentrations. Frequently, it is not detectable. The latter is true in some species of mice. In irradiated animals, as neutropenia develops increased con-concentrations of CSF are observed in serum[22] and concurrently, as shown in Figure 4, there is an increase in CFC and then the myeloblast-promyelocyte compartment (of the hind-leg shielded animal). The sequence of changes suggest a physiologic role for CSF. In some experiments with whole body irradiated mice, after the initial increase in serum CSF activity on day 5–10, its activity declined in the presence of continued neutropenia. The early peak of CSF and myeloid activity coincide with the abortive recovery of granulopoiesis. This early peak and fall is reminiscent of that seen in serum concentration of

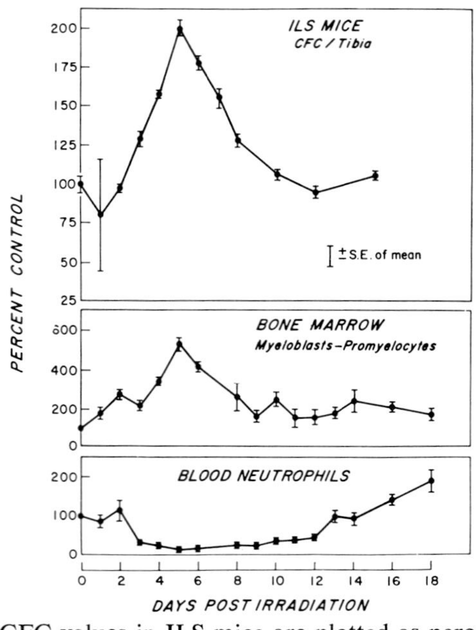

Fig. 4. CFC values in ILS mice are plotted as percent control for days 1–15 postirradiation. Absolute values for the MPC compartment and the blood neutrophil count are similarly plotted as per cent control. Values for CFC/tibia in ILS mice are calculated by compiling the results from at least three experiments per point (Day 5, 13 experiments). The average of mean values so obtained is expressed as per cent of control values obtained from normal mice. Vertical bars represent the standard error. (Reprinted from Rickard, et al, by permission from Blood[12]).

erythropoietin after exposure to altitude. The inability to detect CSF elevations, in some experiments, at later intervals, e.g., 10–15 days after irradiation when neutropenia is marked, may relate to the insensitivity of the methods used or, alternatively, to the development of tolerance to the CSF-elevating effect of host endotoxin (*vide infra*).

The initial rise in CSF is temporally correlated not only with the onset of granulocytic recovery but it also coincides with the bacteremia and endotoxemia resulting from intestinal injury associated with irradiation. It was of interest, therefore, to consider the role of endotoxin in the generation of CSF. We noted that germ-free irradiated animals did not develop elevated serum CSF levels.[23] However, when endotoxin was given to normal animals or animals rendered severely neutropenic by irradiation, there was a prompt and striking increase in serum CSF (Figure 5).[24] Thus, generation of CSF apparently is related more to neutrophil function, i.e., bactericidal, than directly to neutrophil levels. On the basis of these observations, one might suggest that, normally, granulocytopoiesis is in part controlled by intermittent bacteremia and endotoxemia.

There are a number of problems yet to be resolved before the final chapter can be written on the role of CSF and endotoxin in myelopoiesis. Chief among these are that tolerance develops to endotoxin, and this is true for the production of CSF.[25] Further, myelopoiesis develops in germ-free animals. In part, this may be accounted for by endotoxins in the diet. Tissue break down and resultant "endogenous stimulation" may also play a role. The latter mechanism would also provide an explanation for the rapid increase in CSF when antineutrophil serum is given.

CLINICAL APPLICATIONS

One might classify drugs which potentially can produce neutropenia into perhaps four separate categories. These would be those that affect: (a) pluripotent stem cells, (b) the committed stem cell or CFC, (c) differentiated cells, (d) microenvironment. Unfortunately, in man we are restricted in our evalua-

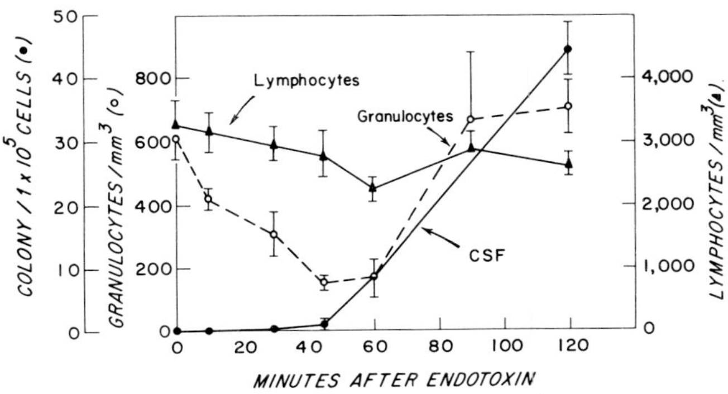

Fig. 5. Changes in serum CSF. Granulocytes and lymphocytes shown as a function of time after intraperitoneal injection of 5ug of endotoxin (each point represents the mean ± SE of 10–12 mice). (Reprinted from Quesenberry, et al, by permission from N Engl J Med[24]).

tion by several considerations which do not apply to experimental animals. The pluripotent stem cell can be assayed only after transplantation into heavily irradiated syngeneic recipients. Accordingly, we cannot assay CFU in man except perhaps in the unusual situation in which transplantation of bone marrow is being carried out as a therapeutic maneuver. This clearly does not permit one to evaluate CFU under most clinical circumstances. The CFC may be measured in soft agar, but there are limitations in man which do not apply in animals. In man, the CFC can be evaluated only in terms of cell concentration, i.e., CFC per 10^6 nucleated cells. In the mouse, it is possible to measure total numbers of CFC in a given organ, e.g., the tibia or whole body. This clearly is a more meaningful value. If, as might be expected in some hypoplastic marrows, there is a proportional reduction in differentiated cellular elements, then a change in the concentration of CFC per 10^6 cells would not be anticipated. Conversely, a decrease in the number of differentiated elements without a change in absolute CFC would produce an increase in CFC per 10^6 cells, and so forth. However, within these constraints, one may get some insight into the response of committed myeloid compartment in various clinical settings. The relationship of microenvironment to growth of bone marrow cells is still poorly understood. It is clear from studies in irradiated animals,[26] as well as those in which the marrow has been removed mechanically,[27] that the stromal structure is of major significance in hemopoiesis. Further, it has been shown that the hemopoietic inductive microenvironment will affect differentiation along the erythroid or myeloid line.[28] Physiologic evaluation of the microenvironment is not possible at the present time, but it is to be anticipated that assay systems will be developed and in the not too distant future.

There are clearly a number of agents which affect the pluripotent stem cell. Perhaps the most commonly used agents are those employed in the chemotherapy of malignant disease. These drugs produce a dose-dependent effect on cells in active cycle. In the bone marrow, the initial effect is confined to the differentiated and committed stem cells, which normally are in active cycle. Hence, relatively few pluripotent stem cells, the bulk of which are in G_0, would be affected by the first dose of drug. When no further drug is given, the initial damage to the committed and differentiated compartments is repaired by two mechanisms: (a) increased replication of the remaining cells within the committed compartment and (b) increased influx from the pluripotent into the committed compartment. The latter will lead to a temporary decline in pluripotent stem cells. In some experimental studies this late fall in CFU has been interpreted as indicating an effect of the chemotherapeutic agent on the pluripotent cell itself. It should be emphasized, however, that these agents affect primarily cells in active cycle and not those which are resting or in G_0. However, after the initial administration of chemotherapeutic agent, the CFU will enter cycle to restore compartment size, which would be reduced due to the aforementioned efflux of CFU from the compartment to repair committed and differentiated compartments. In consequence, subsequent doses of drug will have a direct effect on the pluripotent stem cell compartment.

The effect of these agents will be dose related and hence the degree of marrow damage will vary. In the case of the neutrophil, this can lead to rather interesting changes in white cell production. When damage to the stem cell compartment is moderate, granulocyte production will be curtailed and, as a result, the size of the storage compartment will be reduced significantly. Normally, granulocyte production has an inherent tendency to oscillate because of feedback regulation, but oscillatory changes in peripheral neutrophil concentration are not observed because the storage compartment tends to dampen these oscillations.[29] The reduction in size of the storage compartment after chemotherapy removes this dampening effect and thus permits oscillations of granulocyte concentrations in the peripheral blood, i.e., a cyclic neutropenia. With higher doses of drug and further suppression of granulocyte production, a noncyclic neutropenia would be expected to develop for the bone marrow would be driven at maximum capacity. We have shown this to be the case experimentally, and a representative study is presented in Figure 6.[30] A cycling type of neutropenia has been observed after treatment of malignant disease with cytotoxic agents. These considerations are important in the use of those chemotherapeutic agents which suppress bone marrow function. The peripheral white count is commonly measured as a guide to drug toxicity. Since cycling may develop, care must be taken to be certain that one is not sampling the nadir or apogee of a cycle, for if this is done the effect of drug therapy on bone marrow function will be improperly evaluated.[30]

Chloramphenicol may produce selective aplasia of differentiated elements, most commonly erythroid, but this is a dose-related phenomenon and usually is transient. The more ominous generalized aplastic anemia is, fortunately, rare, and as awareness of this possible complication has become more generally appreciated and alternative antibiotics have become available, the use of chloramphenicol has diminished. Accordingly, the frequency of chloramphenicol-induced aplasia has decreased, and cases have not been available for clinical studies of

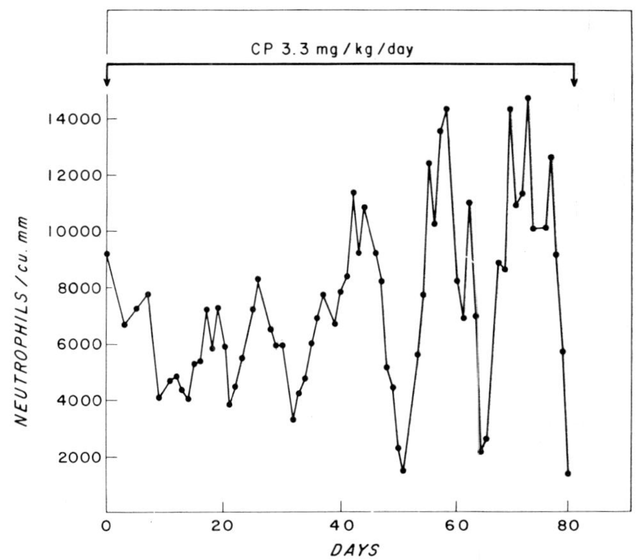

Fig. 6. Serial neutrophil counts during cyclophosphamide (CP) administration. (Reprinted from Morley, et al, by permission from N Engl J Med[30]).

the effect of chloramphenicol-induced aplasia on CFC and CSF. It is likely that in this disease the CFU compartment is primarily affected, for all three differentiated cell lines are involved, but it is entirely possible that damage to the stroma plays a significant role by altering the necessary environment for hemopoiesis. In some instances, the onset of aplasia may occur several weeks after chloramphenicol has been discontinued. This time sequence is most compatible with the thesis that stromal changes play an important role. It is similar to the time sequence observed in permanent aplasia after high doses of radiation. Under these experimental conditions the aplasia has been shown to be due to changes in stroma and environment.[26]

Drugs that affect only the committed myeloid compartment would be expected to result in a selective neutropenia, which would be associated with a depletion of the differentiated myeloid compartment of the marrow. The neutropenia associated with agents such as propylthiouracil (PTU), tapazole, phenylbutazone, and phenothiazine derivatives would be cases in point. We have had the opportunity to study a patient with moderately severe neutropenia associated with PTU. The patient had hyperthyroidism and had been doing well on PTU for a period of several months when she developed pharyngitis for which she called her physician. He found her to be neutropenic, and we were consulted. Her bone marrow had a selective granulocytic aplasia. Evaluation of the bone marrow at that time revealed a normal concentration of CFC. We were unable to sequentially measure the CFC, for this would have required multiple bone marrow aspirations. Sequential measurement of CSF was possible and showed a slight increase at day 4 just prior to the recovery of granulopoiesis (Figure 7). This rise in activity was not associated with overt infection. Shadduck[31] studied a similar case with a more severe neutropenia and prior to recovery noted a rise in CSF of somewhat greater proportions than in our case. In these studies, the sequential changes in CSF suggest, but do not prove, a central role for CSF in the regulation of granulopoiesis. The mechanism of PTU-induced neutropenia is not settled. McIntyre, et al[32] have suggested that it has an immunologic basis, and, using a test which depends on phagocytic function, they provided data to support this thesis. If this is the case, then the antibody must affect not only peripheral cells but also differentiated precursors, for the myeloid compartment may be totally aplastic. This is an unusual feature, since most types of immune cytopenias are not associated with this degree of aplasia of precursor elements. The rather prompt recovery of myelopoiesis after the drug is discontinued, however, might be viewed as offering further indirect evidence for an immune mechanism.

Immune neutropenias have been difficult to evaluate, for the tests of autoantibody and drug antibodies directed at the neutrophil do not have the precision seen with erythrocyte autoantibodies. The effect of white cell antibodies on leukocyte kinetics, however, is well established from experimental studies.[33] Thus, one would anticipate a rapid fall in peripheral granulocyte count, followed by the increased generation of CSF. Initially, there would be a decrease in CFC due to efflux into the differentiated compartment. This would be compensated for by a return of the CFC compartment to normal, either through increased generation or turnover within the compartment and/or influx from the pluripotent

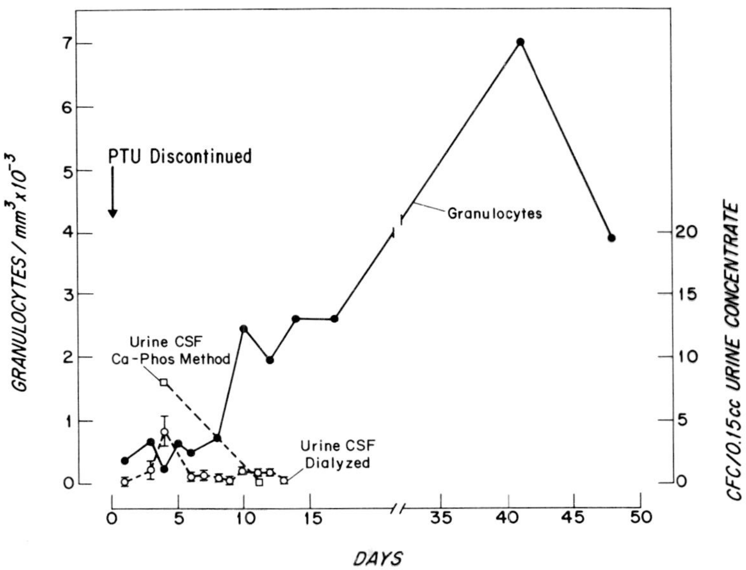

Fig. 7. Sequential changes in granulocytes and colony-stimulating factor (CSF) after discontinuation of propylthiouracil (PTU) in a patient with drug-induced neutropenia. Inhibitors were removed by dialysis against H_2O or by calcium phosphate gel absorption (the latter method being more effective). The activity of the CSF is measured as the numbers of colonies produced when 0.15 ml of concentrated urine was used to stimulate murine bone marrow in soft agar.

compartments. One can only speculate on the duration of CSF elevation. In mice, after a single injection of antineutrophil serum, it peaks within 2–8 hours and returns toward normal much as in the endotoxin treated animals (Figure 5). The continued presence of antibody in an autoimmune neutropenia might modify this response. Drug-associated immune neutropenias would be expected to behave much like the animal model, once the drug is removed.

In the case of phenothiazines, Pisciotta[34] has demonstrated interference with DNA replication, and one might suggest a similar mechanism for phenylbutazone. This type of disorder, then, represents an effect of the drug on cell proliferation itself. Presumably, the immediate precursor cells as well as the more differentiated cells are affected. The reason, however, that myeloid elements appear to be selectively affected, in many cases, is obscure. To date, we have not had the opportunity, nor have others, to evaluate myelopoiesis, in the present context, in patients with neutropenia of this type. It is to be anticipated that such studies will be done when the opportunity presents, and these should provide further insight into the mechanism of drug toxicity in this interesting group of patients.

It should be noted that any drug that affects nuclear replications may produce a transformation in the stem cell compartment which could theoretically lead to a variety of change in hemopoiesis, ranging from selective aplasia through paroxysmal nocturnal hemoglobinuria to leukemia. It was well documented that irradiation and radioactive compounds, such as ^{32}P, induce leukemia. As more experience is gained with the use of cytotoxic drugs in the chemotherapy of malignancy, it becomes clear that these drugs are also potentially leukemogenic. In our clinic, we have seen two instances of acute leukemia in patients with polycythemia vera treated with busulfan and in one treated for Hodgkins disease with the combination program, MOPP. We are aware of cases from other clinics in association with busulfan, chlorambucil, and phenylalaine mustard. Leukemia has been reported in 3 patients receiving chloramphenicol,[35] and we have seen one in which phenylbutazone appeared to be the offending agent.

It would be beyond the scope of this presentation to catalog all drugs that affect myelopoiesis. We have, however, attempted to present the spectrum of effects which might be seen in the clinical practice of medicine and to illustrate some of these. As is evident from this presentation, too little information is currently available on the application of some of the newer concepts of myelopoiesis to clinical problems, particularly those of drug-induced neutropenia. However, severe drug neutropenia, other than those cases associated with cytotoxic therapy, is relatively uncommon.

REFERENCES

1. Stohlman F Jr, Miller M: Erythropoietic cellular proliferation. Physiol Pharmacol (In press)
2. Till JE, McCulloch EA: A direct measurement of the radiation sensitivity of normal mouse bone marrow cells. Radiat Res 14:213–221, 1969
3. Bradley TR, Metcalf D: The growth of mouse bone marrow cells in vitro. Aust J Exp Biol Med Sci 44:287–299, 1966
4. Iscove NN, Till JE, McCulloch EA: The proliferative status of mouse granulopoietic progenitor cells. Proc Soc Exp Biol Med 134:33–36, 1970
5. Rickard KA, Shadduck RK, Howard DE, Stohlman F Jr: A differential effect of hydroxyurea on hemopoietic stem cell colonies in vitro. Proc Soc Exp Biol Med 134:152–156, 1970
6. Rencricca N, Rizzoli V, Howard D, Stohlman F Jr: Stem cell migration and proliferation during severe anemia. Blood 36:764–775, 1970
7. Rickard KA, Rencricca NJ, Shadduck RK, Manetta FC, Howard DE, Garrity M, Stohlman F Jr: Myeloid stem cell kinetics during erythropoietic stress. Br J Haematol 20:537–547, 1971
8. Rickard KA, Morley A, Howard D, Garrity M, Stohlman F Jr: Stem cell stimulatory properties in vitro of an agar colony stimulating factor. Proc Soc Exp Biol Med 136:608–611, 1971
9. Tyler W, Niskanen E, Stohlman F Jr, Keene J, Howard D: Effect of neutropenia on myeloid growth and the stem cell in an in vivo culture system. Blood 40:634, 1972
10. Goodman JW, Grubbs CG: The relationship of the thymus to erythropoiesis, Hematopoietic Cellular Proliferation. Edited by F Stohlman, Jr. New York, Grune & Stratton, 1970, pp 27–35
11. McCulloch EA, Till JE: Cellular interactions in the control of hemopoiesis.[10] pp 15–25
12. Rickard KA, Morley A, Howard D, Stohlman F Jr: The in vitro colony-forming cell and the response to neutropenia. Blood 37:6–13, 1971
13. Morley AA, Stohlman F Jr: Studies on the regulation of granulopoiesis I. The response to neutropenia. Blood 35:312–321, 1970

14. Gordon AS, Handler ES, Siegel CD, Dornfest BS, Lobie J: Plasma factors influencing leukocyte release in rats. Ann NY Acad Sci 113:766–779, 1964
15. Boggs DR, Chervenick PA, Marsh JC, Cartwright GE, Wintrobe MM: Neutrophil releasing activity of dogs injected with endotoxin. J Lab Clin Med 72:177–185, 1968
16. Robinson WA, Pike BL: Colony growth of human bone marrow cells in vitro.[10] pp 249–259
17. Chan SH, Metcalf D, Stanley ER: Stimulation and inhibition by normal human serum of colony formation in vitro by bone marrow cells. Br J Haematol 20: 329–341, 1971.
18. Robinson WA, Mangalik A: Regulation of granulopoiesis: Positive feedback. Lancet 2:742–744, 1972
19. Moore MAS, Williams N: Physical separation of colony-stimulating cells from in vitro colony forming cells in hemopoietic tissue. J Cell Physiol 80:195–206, 1972
20. Chervenick PA, Lobuglio AF: Human blood monocytes: Stimulators of granulocyte and mononuclear colony formation in vitro. Science 178:164–166, 1972
21. Niskanen E, Symann M, Tyler W, Howard D, Stohlman F Jr: Evidence of negative feedback regulation of granulopoiesis by mature granulocytes. Unpublished data
22. Morley AA, Rickard KA, Howard D, Stohlman F Jr: Studies on the Regulation of Granulopoiesis. Blood 37:14–20, 1971
23. Morley A, Quesenberry P, Stohlman F Jr: Wilson R: Serum colony stimulating factor levels in irradiated germfree and conventional CFW mice. Proc Soc Exp Biol Med 140:478–480, 1972
24. Quesenberry P, Morley A, Stohlman F Jr, Rickard K, Howard D, Smith M: Effect of endotoxin on granulopoiesis and colony-stimulating factor. N Engl J Med 286:227–231, 1972
25. Quesenberry P, Halperin J, Ryan M, Stohlman F Jr: The role of endotoxin in colony-stimulating factor (CSF) elevations seen after irradiation. Presented at the American Society of Hematology Fifteenth Annual Meeting, December 3–6, 1972
26. Knopse WH, Blom J, Crosby WH: Regeneration of locally irradiated bone marrow. Blood 28:398–415, 1966
27. Patt HA, Maloney MA: Reconstitution of bone marrow in a depleted medullary cavity.[10] pp 56–66
28. Trention JJ: Influence of hematopoietic organ stroma on stem cell differentiation, Regulation of Hematopoiesis. Edited by AS Gordon. New York, Appleton-Century-Crofts, 1970, pp 159–184
29. Morley A, King-Smith EA, Stohlman F Jr: The oscillatory nature of hemopoiesis.[10] pp 3–14
30. Morley AA, Stohlman F Jr: Cyclophosphamide-induced cyclical neutropenia. N Engl J Med 282:643–646, 1970
31. Shadduck RK: Personal communication
32. McIntyre PA, Leleli YR, Hodkinson BA, Wagner HN Jr: Evidence for antileukocyte antibodies as a mechanism for drug-induced agranulocytosis. Trans Assoc Am Physicians 134:217–228, 1971
33. Shadduck RK, Nagabhushanam: Granulocyte colony stimulating factor I response to acute granulocytopenia. Blood 38:559–568, 1971
34. Pisciotta AV: The effect of chlorpromazine of peripheral leukocytes, in drugs and hematologic reactions. Edited by NV Dimitrov, and JH Nodine. New York, Grune & Stratton.

35. Brauer MJ, Dameshek W: Hypoplastic anemia and myeloblastic leukemia following chloramphenicol therapy. N Engl J Med 277:1003–1005, 1967
36. Stohlman F Jr: Kinetics of erythropoiesis.[28] pp 317–326
37. Morley A, Howard D, Bennett B, Stohlman F Jr: Studies on the regulation of granulopoiesis II. Relationship to other differentiation pathways. Br J Haematol 19: 523–532, 1970

N. Raphael Shulman

16

Drug-induced Antibodies to Blood Cells

In this brief review of drug-induced antibodies, an attempt will be made to point out the practical clinical implications of information derived from laboratory and theoretical analyses of drug antibody reactions. Table 1 lists drugs that have been proved to induce antibodies that attach to blood cells. As shown in Table 2, the antibodies induced by these drugs have been detected by techniques of classical immunology as well as by certain indirect techniques that reflect cellular injury by immunologic reactions. White cells are missing from Table 1; the only drug suspected of inducing acute agranulocytosis by an apparent immunologic mechanism is aminopyrine. Aminopyrine agranulocytosis appears to be immunologic on the basis of the immediate decrease in circulating cells observed when test doses are given,[1] but there is no in vitro test for antibody that can be reproduced in a consistent manner. A number of other drugs not listed in Table 1 have been implicated clinically as possible inducers of antibodies that cause thrombocytopenia, e.g., digitoxin, hydrochlorothiazide, and acetaminophen, but as yet the participation of these drugs in immunologic reactions has not been generally confirmed.

Some questions that come immediately to mind concerning drug antibodies are (1) what the basis is for cellular specificity of antibodies against different drugs or of different antibodies against the same drug, (2) why some easily measured drug antibodies are of relatively little clinical significance whereas others cause catastrophic destruction of blood cells, and (3) what possible reasons exist for a so-called "idiosyncrasy" to a drug. Answers to these questions involve consideration of mechanisms of formation of antibody, of attachment of antibody to cells, and of secondary reactions evoked by antibodies on cell surfaces, as well as of physiologic processes involved in survival, production, and destruction of different cell types.

First, we will consider the nature of formation of drug antibodies in terms of the classical haptene chemistry. In order for a molecule as small as the usual drug to become antigenic, it must combine with some large molecule in a nondissociable manner, usually by covalent bonding, to form an antigenic

Table 1
Drugs That Can Have an Immunologic Effect on Blood Cells

Red Cells	Platelets
Penicillin	Sedormid
(cephalothin)	Quinine
Methyldopa	Quinidine
Quinine	Stibophen
Quinidine	Salicylamide
Stibophen	
Salicylamide	

complex, the so-called haptenic complex described initially by Landsteiner[2] (Fig. 1). The binding of drug (haptene) to a large molecule (carrier), usually a protein, permits the small molecule to gain access to antibody-forming cells. Antibody specificity induced by the antigenic haptene-carrier complex can be directed against the complex itself, the carrier, or the haptene. A theoretical possibility shown in line 1 of Fig. 1 is an antibody with double specificity against the carrier molecule and the haptene, a circumstance which has not yet been demonstrated experimentally. Antibody against carrier alone, as shown in line 2, occurs only when a foreign protein, rather than an autologous protein, is used as carrier. As shown in line 3, antibody induced by haptene characteristically shows specificity for the haptene, whether the haptene is combined with carrier or free. The type of antibody specificity shown in line 4, not yet observed in sensitivities that develop clinically, is directed against the molecular configuration at the site of combination of haptene and carrier.

None of the drugs that induce antibodies clinically are sufficiently active in the native state to combine covalently with body proteins or other macromolecules. Generally, it has been considered, and in the case of penicillin, proved, that a chemically active metabolic product of the drug is responsible for forming covalent bonds with proteins. As shown in Fig. 2, there are many reactive derivatives of penicillin, the major one responsible for sensitization apparently being benzyl penicillenic acid[3] because of its ability to form covalent bonds with protein. Antibodies against this penicillin derivative react with an antigenic configuration shared by native penicillin and various modifications of

Table 2
Tests Helpful in Diagnosis of Drug Antibodies

Red Cells	Platelets
Agglutination	Complement fixation
Antiglobulin	Release phenomena
(gamma and	(factor III, Cr^{51}, serotonin,
nongamma)	nucleotides)
Complement fixation	Aggregation
(hemolysis)	Agglutination
	Inhibition of clot retraction

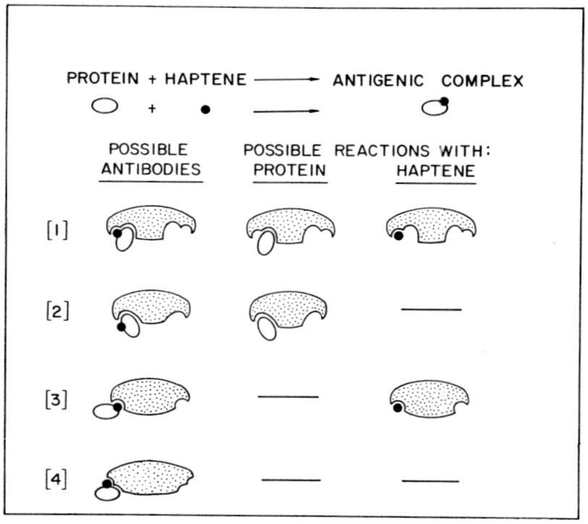

Figure 1

the penicillin molecule. In the case of quinine or quinidine, the sensitizing compound has not been identified, for metabolites that combine firmly with protein have not yet been clearly delineated. It appears, however, that an oxidative product of these drugs is involved in sensitization; although most of the drug antibodies developed clinically are specific either for quinine or quinidine, occasionally an antibody is formed that cross-reacts with both drugs as well as with quininone[4] (Fig. 3). Four of the 20 antibodies that we tested reacted with both quinine and quinidine. These same four antibodies also reacted with quininone, which is an oxidative derivative of both quinine and qunidine at the stereoisomeric site of the molecule. It appears likely that the more usual antibodies against quinine and quinidine are formed against metabolites that are re-

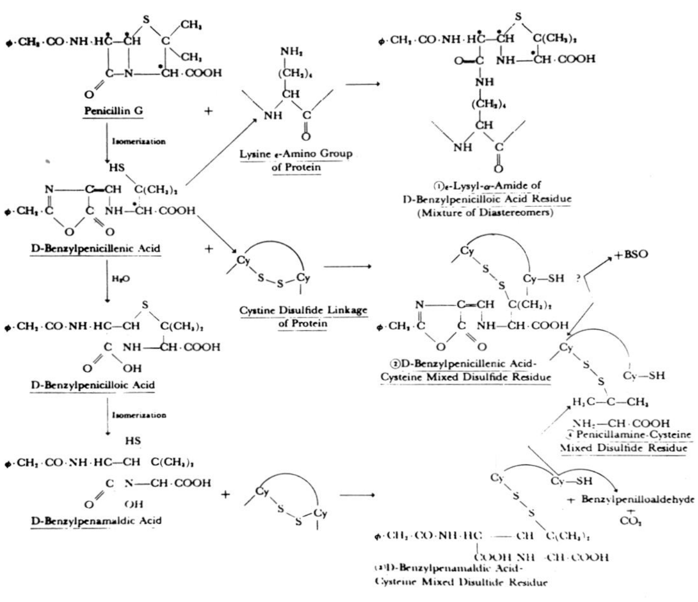

Figure 2

Sensitizing Drug	Reaction With		
	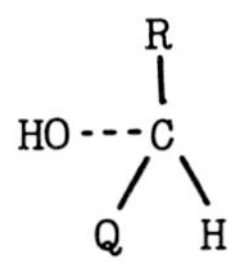 quinine	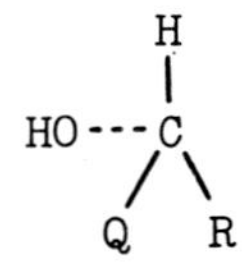 quinidine	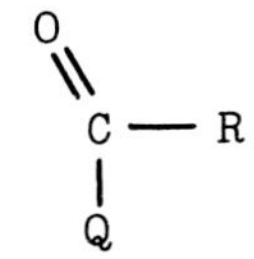 quininone
Quinine - 4	4	2^{*}	2^{*}
Quinidine - 16	$2^{\dagger}$	16	$2^{\dagger}$

Q = quinoline
R = quinuclidine
* † same sera

Figure 3

active with proteins but still retain the stereoisomeric site. The recent report by Eisner and Shahidi[5] on an antibody induced by a metabolic derivative of acetaminophen that reacts with platelets only in the presence of the metabolite, if corroborated, will provide further substantiation of the general principle that the metabolic products of a drug rather than the drug itself are involved in haptenic complex formation that leads to sensitization.

The initial concept of the mechanism of cellular injury by drug antibodies involved the attachment of drug to cell and then attachment of antibody to cell by virtue of its specificity for the drug.[6] However, as shown in Fig. 4, there are several distinct mechanisms documented as the basis for attachment of different drug antibodies to cells. In the case of penicillin (diagrams on the left of Fig. 4), the cells first react with a penicillin derivative to form a firm cell-drug complex,[7] and antipenicillin antibodies then agglutinate the drug-coated cells. When testing for penicillin antibodies in vitro, red cells are incubated with a very high concentration of penicillin that sensitizes the cells because relatively low concentrations of reactive contaminants such as benzyl penicillenic acid (BPO) form covalent bonds with proteins of the red cell membrane. After the cells are sensitized, it is necessary to wash them thoroughly in order to remove free penicillin from the incubation mixture, for, as indicated in the lower left-hand diagram of Fig. 4, free penicillin would combine with the drug antibody and compete with penicillin groups that are attached to red cells, thereby inhibiting attachment of antibody to red cells and preventing agglutination. Thus, free penicillin (haptene) causes so-called haptenic inhibition of the reaction.

With quinine, quinidine, salicylamide, or stibophen sensitization, the mechanism of attachment of antibody to cells, whether to red cells or platelets, is quite different from that of penicillin antibodies, and there is no haptenic inhibition of the reaction. Antibodies reacting with these drugs will not attach to the cell surface unless the drug is present in high concentration in mixture with antibody and cells (the center diagrams of Fig. 4). If cells are exposed to a high concentration of drug and then washed once, the cells will not react with antibody. These drugs, in contrast to penicillin, do not combine directly with cellular membranes in vivo or in vitro. However, all of the drug antibodies studied so far combine directly with drug in a typical haptenic fashion (Fig. 1, line 3). In the case of quinine, quinidine, salicylamide, and stibophen, the first step of the reaction is combination of drug with antibody and then this antigen-antibody complex is adsorbed onto the cell. The secondary reaction in which the cell participates is a relatively nonspecific adsorption reaction that is not dependent primarily on drug specificity, but rather on the unique ability of certain cell membranes to adsorb certain antigen-antibody complexes. The ability of the complex to be adsorbed is determined as much by the nature of the antibody as by the drug. This is clear from the observation that some antibodies against quinine, quinidine, or stibophen attach only to platelets while others attach only to red cells. Some patients' sera have been found to contain two types of quinidine antibody, a 7S globulin that reacted only with platelets and a 19S globulin that reacted with red cells.[8] The membrane properties that predispose to adsorption of immunologic complexes have not been defined biochemically. Note in the center diagrams of Fig. 4 that the high concentrations of free drug do not interfere with antibody attachment to cells; antibody attaches only as an antibody-drug complex, and there is essentially no cell-bound drug with which free drug would compete. Whenever antigen-antibody complexes are adsorbed on cells, there appears to be no haptenic inhibition of antibody attachment.

There is a known third mechanism of drug-induced attachment of gamma globulin to cells (Fig. 4, diagrams on right) recognized in association with α-methyldopa therapy. The term gamma globulin rather than antibody more accurately describes the substance coating red cells after methyldopa therapy, for it is not yet clear whether the gamma globulin has specific combining sites

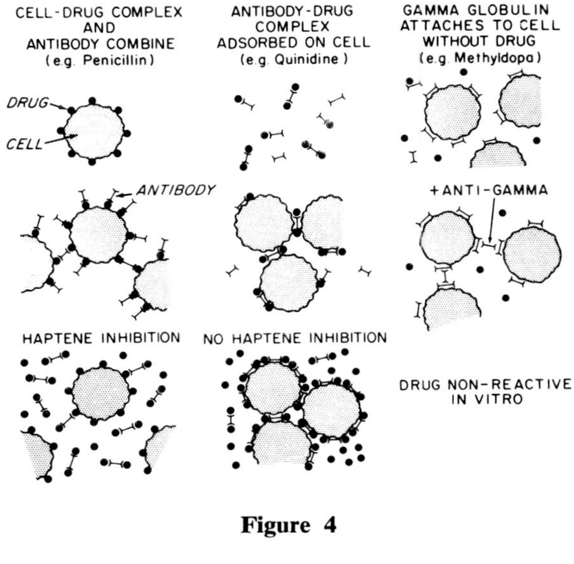

Figure 4

for an antigen in the manner of a true antibody. It is clear, however, that the gamma globulin has *no* specificity for α-methyldopa or its derivatives. The gamma globulin coating induced by methyldopa is detected by the agglutination of affected red cells with antiglobulin serum, i.e., by development of a positive Coomb's test.[9–11] Approximately 20% of patients receiving α-methyldopa develop a positive antiglobulin reaction within 3–6 mo after initiation of therapy. The antiglobulin reaction is almost always the direct type and regresses slowly after withdrawal of the drug. In those instances in which gamma globulin that attaches to cells can be demonstrated to circulate by an indirect antiglobulin reaction, drug is not required to effect the attachment. Gamma globulin eluates of sensitized cells from individuals receiving methyldopa coat normal red cells in the manner of a panagglutinin rather than showing isoantibody or drug specificity,[11] although some investigators suggest that certain Rh specificities may be involved.[10,12] All of the various observations point to the following mechanism for the α-methyldopa phenomenon: gamma globulin is altered probably by combination with highly reactive polymerized α-methyldopa, which is known to form in vivo, and this altered gamma globulin is adsorbed onto red cells in a manner similar to the adsorption by red cells of gamma globulin denatured by other physical or chemical processes.[13] Since the cells are coated in vivo with gamma globulin, drug is not necessary to complete the antiglobulin reaction in vitro. Addition of the drug itself to normal plasma or plasma from patients treated with α-methyldopa will not induce a positive antiglobulin reaction, apparently because α-methyldopa does not undergo the type of oxidation and polymerization necessary for interaction with protein unless appropriately metabolized in vivo. Thus, α-methyldopa appears to act chemically as a denaturing agent to change gamma globulin in such a way that it is adsorbed onto red cells. It is possible, however, that in rare instances antibodies may develop against gamma globulin denatured by α-methyldopa. This has been demonstrated in animals[11] but has not been documented clinically.

The physiologic effects and clinical manifestations of the different drug antibodies are diverse. Although approximately 20% of individuals receiving penicillin develop antipenicillin antibodies, only rarely has an antipenicillin antibody been implicated as the cause of hemolytic anemia. There are several reasons for this. Plasma levels of reactive penicillin derivatives (e.g., BPO) after therapeutic doses of penicillin usually are not high enough to cause coating of red cells to a degree detectable by agglutination with antipenicillin antibodies. Since plasma proteins react as avidly as cellular proteins with penicillin derivatives, the plasma proteins protect red cells from sensitization by competing for reactive penicillin derivatives. However, this protection sometimes may be overcome by high doses of penicillin used intravenously. Under these circumstances, BPO may coat the red cells in vivo, antipenicillin antibodies attach, and the direct antiglobulin tests become positive. An occasional patient treated with intravenous penicillin may develop hemolytic anemia on the basis of penicillin antibodies, but unless the antibodies have complement fixing properties, which they rarely do, hemolysis is usually insufficient to require discontinuation of therapy. Antipenicillin antibodies have not been well documented as causing thrombocytopenia or leukopenia. Noteworthy is the fact that there is no correlation between the presence or absence of antipenicillin antibodies of the type described and development of other forms of penicillin sensitivity such as anaphalyaxis, serum sickness-like manifestations, or skin reactions. Antibodies against cephalothin appear to have the same significance as those against penicillin.

Antibodies against quinine, quinidine, salicylamide, or stibophen are recognized clinically because they cause severe thrombocytopenia or hemolytic anemia or both. The marked effect of these antibodies on cells is probably related to their ability to lyse cells directly in the circulation by complement-fixing reactions that occur when antibody-drug complexes are adsorbed on the cells. If therapy is stopped, antibody-drug complexes no longer form and those that have already become attached to cells reverse as drug concentration decreases in vivo. Even though plasma antibody persists and the titer may rise, there is no further sensitization of cells as long as there is no circulating drug. If sublytic amounts of complement have become attached to red cells in association with antigen-antibody complexes, these complement components remain on the cells even when antibodies detach. Reversal of drug-antibody complexes by washing or dialysis in vitro or by discontinuation of drug in vivo is depicted schematically in Fig. 5. Complement components fixed by secondary immunologic reactions remain firmly attached to the cells and can be detected by reaction with anti-nongamma globulin, the so-called nongamma Coomb's test.[8] An incomplete sequence of complement components deposited on red cells does not lyse the cells and has only a minor effect on cell survival in vivo, as shown in Fig. 6. Following recovery from stibophen hemolytic anemia, the red cells of the patient in Fig. 6 remained coated with complement components and therefore give a positive anti-*nongamma* Coomb's test. Antiglobulin serum directed against human *gamma* globulin does not react with cells following recovery from drug hemolytic anemia, for antibody detaches soon after drug is stopped. These obser-

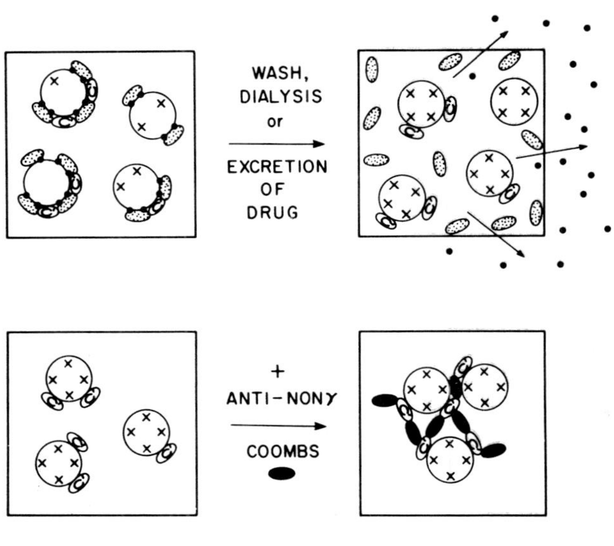

Figure 5

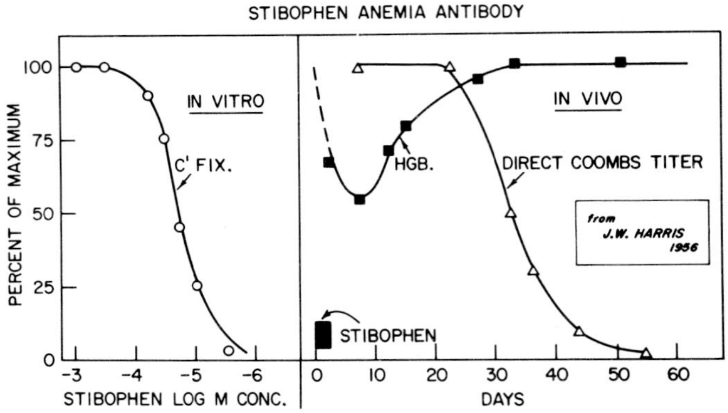

Figure 6

vations have bearing on the types of serologic tests observed clinically in obscure or idiopathic acquired hemolytic anemia. In these patients a drug cannot be implicated and the antigen of sensitization is unknown, but the mechanism by which the cells become coated through adsorption of antigen-antibody complexes and associated complement fixation may be similar to that of drug-hemolytic anemia.

Although the acute clinical manifestations of drug antibodies subside with discontinuation of drugs, measurable antibody levels may remain for weeks or years. At any time prior to disappearance of drug antibodies from the circulation, reinstitution of therapy with a provocative drug will cause immediate recurrence of blood cell destruction. If the titer of antibody has fallen below levels that are capable of inducing clinical manifestations, reinstitution of drug may be followed by the same acute occurrence after a delay of the 3-5 days required for an anamnestic response. The first episode of an antibody-dependent drug reaction never occurs prior to 2 weeks after exposure to the medication, because this period of time is required for development of sufficient antibody during primary sensitization. However, there is no way to predict when initial sensitization may take place; in some cases, the drug has been taken for years before antibodies develop.

Development of antibodies that cause thrombocytopenia or hemolytic anemia is a rare occurrence. In the past it was generally considered that individuals who developed drug antibodies were "hyperallergenic," i.e., more prone to develop other diseases of sensitivity such as asthma or hayfever. Over the years, however, it has become clear that patients with drug antibodies have not developed other allergies more frequently than the general population. The idiosyncrasy, rather than being a vague predisposition to sensitization, appears to be explained best by chance formation of a high affinity antibody. All of the drug-hemolytic anemia or drug purpura antibodies that have been studied have been found to have unusually high association constants.[14] That a high association constant is necessary in order for a drug antibody to have a physiologic effect is apparent from considerations summarized in Table 3. Drugs that are involved in antibody reactions rarely attain concentrations in plasma greater than 10^{-6} M after therapeutic doses, and these drugs are bound nonspecifically by

Table 3

By Equilibrium Dialysis

$$K = \frac{[\text{Pr-Drug}]}{[\text{Pr}][\text{Drug}]} = 3 \times 10^3$$

$$K_1 = \frac{[\text{Ab-Drug}]}{[\text{Ab}][\text{Drug}]} = > 10^6$$

By Antibody Adsorption

$$K_2 = \frac{[\text{Ab-Drug-Cell}]}{[\text{Ab-Drug}][\text{Cell}]} = > 10^7$$

Antibody concentration [Ab] = 10^{-8} to 10^{-7} *M*.
Protein concentration [Pr] = 7×10^{-3} *M*.
Drug concentration [Dr] = 10^{-6}

albumin and nonantibody globulins that are present in plasma at the relatively high concentrations of 10^{-3} *M*. Since specific antibody is present at extremely low concentrations (10^{-7} *M* or less), it must have unusually high affinity for drug in order to compete effectively with albumin and nonantibody globulin, since these proteins bind the various drugs under consideration with an affinity equal to an association constant between 10^3 and 10^4. The association constants of specific drug antibodies that have been studied have been in the range of 10^7 to 10^9.[14] Moreover, the affinity of cells for antibody-drug complexes has been found to be as high as affinity of antibody for drug.[14] Thus, despite marked competition for drug by normal plasma proteins, specific antibodies at extremely low concentrations, by virtue of their high affinity for drug and by virtue of the high affinity of cells for drug-antibody complexes, form antibody-drug-cell complexes that lead to cellular destruction. Theoretically other factors may predispose individuals to sensitization by drugs; for example, genetic variation in drug metabolism could lead to formation of excess or more highly reactive intermediates, or genetic variations in certain macromolecules might facilitate formation of haptenic complexes, but as yet there has been no indication of an inherited or familial tendency to develop drug antibodies.

The affinity of antibodies in a single antiserum sample varies widely, but each antiserum has an average affinity that may be treated as an association constant. The average affinity of antibodies varies in different individuals following a single exposure to antigen and changes from time to time with continued immunization of one individual.[15] The affinity of most antibodies would be equivalent to an association constant of 10^4 to 10^6, with some higher or lower, essentially describing a bell-shaped curve. Antibodies with average or low affinity would not effectively compete for drug in plasma, and hence would not evoke clinical manifestations. Only rare drug antibodies with unusually high affinity would be responsible for clinical manifestations. This implies that many people may develop antibodies against drugs, but that clinical manifestations may occur only in those who by chance develop high affinity antibodies in relatively high titer. Patients who have had drug purpura or drug-hemolytic anemia might not

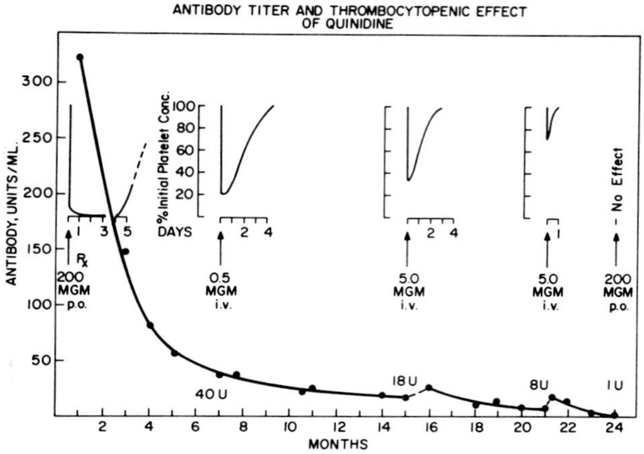

Figure 7

necessarily respond on repeated immunization by forming the same high affinity antibody. That such is the case is evident from observations such as those shown in Fig. 7. The patient shown in this figure was followed for a long period until drug antibody fell below levels detectable by in vitro tests or decrease in platelets when carefully controlled intravenous test doses were used.[16] Repeated doses of the drug that had caused purpura did not result in detectable anamnestic antibody formation. It seems likely that antibody was present after reexposure to drug but in a form not detectable by in vitro tests or in vivo reactions. Although development of a drug complication on one occasion does not invariably preclude the use of the same drug, there is no completely reliable way of determining when an individual may reform an anamnestic high affinity antibody. Reinstitution of therapy with a drug that has caused a serious reaction remains hazardous.

REFERENCES

1. Moeschlin S: Immuno-leucopenie et immuno-agranulocytose. Rev Hemat 8:249, 1953
2. Landsteiner K: The specificity of Serological Reactions. Dover, 1962
3. Levine BB: Studies on the mechanism of the formation of the penicillin antigen. I. Delayed allergic cross-reactions among penicillin G and its degradation products. J Exp Med 112:1131, 1960
4. Shulman NR: Immunologic reactions to drugs. N Engl J Med 287:8, 1972.
5. Eisner EV, Shahidi NT: Immune thrombocytopenia due to a drug metabolite. N Engl J Med 287:8, 1972
6. Ackroyd JF: The pathogenesis of thrombocytopenic purpura due to hypersensitivity to Sedormid. Clin Sci 7:249, 1949
7. Levine BB: Immunochemical mechanisms involved in penicillin hypersensitivity in experimental animals and in human beings. Fed Proc 24, 1965

8. Shulman NR: A mechanism of cell destruction in individuals sensitized by foreign antigens and its implications in auto-immunity. Ann Int Med 3:60, 1966
9. Carstairs KC, Breckenridge A, Dollery CT, Worlledge SM: Incidence of positive direct Coombs test in patients on α-methyldopa. Lancet 2:133–135, 1966
10. LoBuglio AF, Jandl HH: The nature of the alpha-methyldopa red-cell antibody. N Engl J Med 12:276, 1967
11. Vyas GN, Sassetti RJ, Petz LD, Fudenberg HH: Experimental study of aldomet-induced positive antiglobulin reaction. Brit J Haemat 16:137, 1969
12. Worlledge SM, Carstairs KC, Dacie JV: Autoimmune hemolytic anemia associated with methyldopa therapy. Lancet 2:135–139, 1966
13. Grob PJ, Frommel D, Isliker HC, Masouredis SP: Interaction of IgG and its fragments with red cells. Immunology 13:489, 1967
14. Shulman NR: Mechanism of blood cell damage by adsorption of antigen-antibody complexes. Third International Symposium, La Jolla, California, pp 338–352, 1963
15. Kabat EA, Mayer MM: Experimental Immunochemistry. Springfield, Ill. Thomas, 1948
16. Shulman NR: Immunoreactions involving platelets. IV. Studies on the pathogenesis of thrombocytopenia in drug purpura using test doses of quinidine in sensitized individuals; their implications in idiopathic thrombocytopenic purpura. J Exp Med 107:711, 1958

Arthur A. Trowbridge
and James W. Linman

17
Drug-induced Morphologic Changes in Leukocytes

Drugs commonly produce quantitative changes in leukocytes. Many agents have also been shown to bring about a variety of qualitative changes, such as chromosomal abnormalities,[1] blastic transformation of lymphocytes,[2] and decreased leukocyte alkaline phosphatase scores associated with the administration of female sex hormones.[3] These qualitative changes, however, can be demonstrated only in vitro or with special techniques. An extensive review of the literature has confirmed our impression that drug-induced morphologic changes in leukocytes, evident in routine blood or marrow smears stained with Wright's or some other Romanowsky stain, occur infrequently. Furthermore, morphologic changes which have been observed generally lack diagnostic specificity, even though they may be indicative of important pathophysiologic alterations, e.g., impaired DNA synthesis. Types of drug-induced morphologic changes in leukocytes include: (a) proliferative abnormalities—megaloblastic features consequent to impaired metabolism and/or absorption of vitamin B_{12} or folates, and megaloblastoid changes secondary to the administration of cytotoxic drugs, (b) nuclear defects—acquired Pelger-Hüet anomaly and vacuolization, (c) cytoplasmic abnormalities—inclusion bodies (Döhle bodies), vacuolization, and altered granulation, and (d) miscellaneous changes, e.g., atypical lymphocytes.

DISORDERS OF FOLATE OR VITAMIN B_{12} METABOLISM

Although the morphologic changes consequent to drug-induced disorders in folate or vitamin B_{12} metabolism do not reflect a direct effect of such agents on leukocytes, these leukocytic abnormalities are perhaps the most common ones attributable to medicinal agents. A large number of drugs are capable of impairing the absorption and/or utilization of folates and vitamin B_{12}. Irrespective of the mechanism, the ultimate effect is impaired DNA synthesis, defective mitotic activity, and the production of megaloblastic morphology in bone marrow and other proliferating cellular systems.

The megaloblastic morphology of blood cells caused by drugs which interfere with vitamin B_{12} or folate metabolism is identical with that of better known examples of megaloblastosis (e.g., Addisonian pernicious anemia and nutritional folate deficiency). Megaloblastic abnormalities in granulopoiesis are often overshadowed by the more striking changes in erythropoiesis. However, the nuclei of granulocytes and their precursors maturing in the presence of suboptimal vitamin B_{12} or folate activity are also characterized by a fine basichromatin network, accentuated parachromatin, and asynchrony of nuclear and cytoplasmic maturation, with the latter outdistancing the former. Other leukocytic changes include giant metamyelocytes and band neutrophils in the marrow, and large, hypersegmented neutrophils in the marrow and peripheral blood (Figure 1).

Many drugs are capable of inhibiting the utilization and/or absorption of folates.[4,5] Folate analogues, which have chemical structures sufficiently similar to naturally occurring folates to act as metabolic antagonists, provide a classic example of substances interfering with the utilization of folates. By blocking the action of dihydrofolate reductase, methotrexate and related chemotherapeutic compounds prevent the reduction of dihydrofolate to its metabolically active form. Additional substances with similar, but less marked, activity include protozoacidal agents (pyrimethamine and pentamidine isethionate), diuretics (triamterene), and certain drugs with antibiotic activity (trimethoprim).

A variety of other drugs also function as folate inhibitors, although their mode(s) of action is less clear than is the case for folate analogues. Impaired absorption appears to play a role with many of these agents, a mechanism probably coupled with impaired folate utilization. Included in this category are anticonvulsants (diphenylhydantoin, barbiturates, and primidone), oral contraceptives, antituberculous drugs (isoniazid and cycloserine), and alcohol. Even though these agents may act in different ways, the end result is the same, i.e., megaloblastosis identical with that produced by nutritional folate deficiency. Other factors which bear directly on the frequency and severity of these megalo-

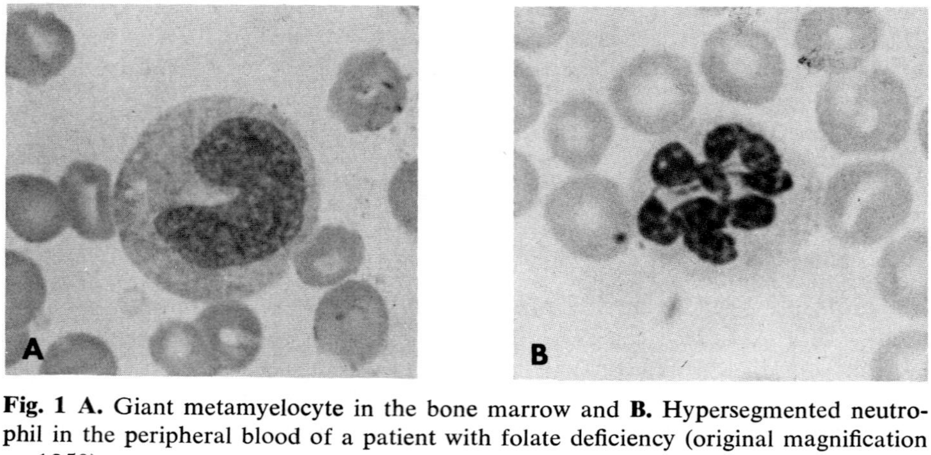

Fig. 1 A. Giant metamyelocyte in the bone marrow and **B.** Hypersegmented neutrophil in the peripheral blood of a patient with folate deficiency (original magnification × 1250).

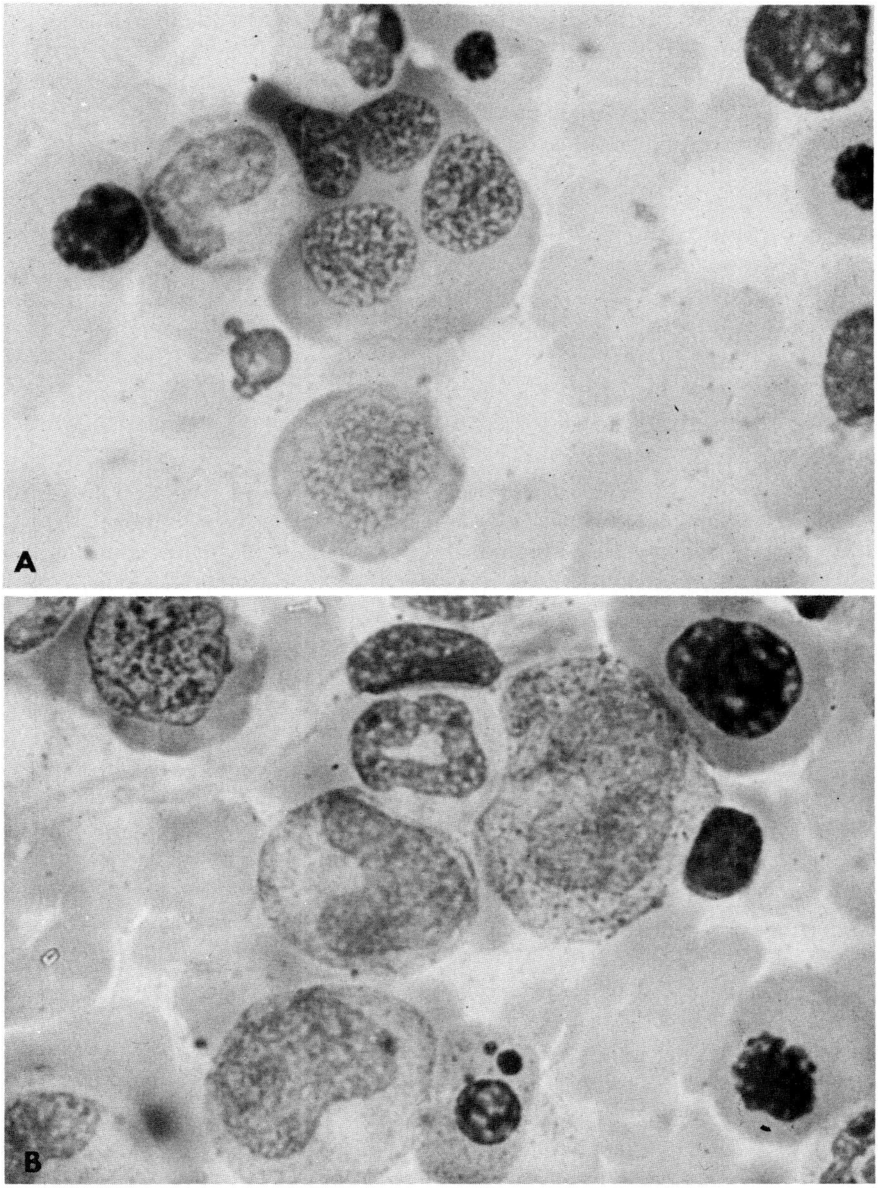

Fig. 2 A. Atypical, megaloblastoid red cell precursor and **B.** Large, abnormal metamyelocytes in a patient treated with cytosine arabinoside (original magnification × 1250).

blastic changes include body folate stores at the onset of treatment and the folate content of the diet.

Several drugs, such as neomycin, colchicine, and *p*-aminosalicylic acid, are known to impair intestinal absorption of vitamin B_{12}.[6] However, relatively abundant body stores and small daily obligatory loss prevent the development of overt megaloblastosis with short-term drug therapy. Vitamin B_{12} analogues, which function as vitamin B_{12} antagonists, have been studied experimentally. These agents may have chemotherapeutic potential and as such would be expected to produce the morphologic changes of vitamin B_{12} deficiency. It can be predicted with reasonable certainty that the list of drugs capable of impairing the absorption and/or utilization of folates and vitamin B_{12} will continue to grow.

CYTOTOXIC DRUGS

Any drug which exerts an oncolytic or cytotoxic effect by affecting cellular proliferation will produce morphologic changes similar to those caused by vitamin B_{12} or folate deficiency. Occasionally, these features are identical with the appearance of megaloblastic blood cell precursors. However, in most instances, there are differences ordinarily discernable at the light microscopic level; the term, megaloblastoid, has often been used to describe these changes. The list of agents that inhibit a cell's proliferative potential is lengthy and varied; it includes antipurines (6-mercaptopurine, thioguanine, and azathioprine); antipyrimidines (5-fluorouracil and cytosine arabinoside); plant alkaloids (vincristine and vinblastin); alkylating agents (nitrogen mustard, cyclophosphamide, busulfan, and chlorambucil); and antibiotics (daunomycin). This list is by no means complete, and any substance capable of impairing DNA synthesis is potentially capable of evoking megaloblastoid morphologic changes.

The morphologic abnormalities caused by cytotoxic drugs are most evident in the erythrocytic compartment (Figure 2). However, granulocytic elements are also affected with the production of giant metamyelocytes and band forms, large hypersegmented neutrophils, nuclear-cytoplasmic asynchrony, and a megaloblastoid nuclear chromatin pattern (Figure 2). Of the more commonly used cytotoxic drugs, cytosine arabinoside produces the most pronounced morphologic changes.

NUCLEAR ABNORMALITIES

The Pelger-Hüet anomaly is characterized by a defect in nuclear segmentation of granulocytes. It is most noticeable in neutrophils, most of which display band, rod-like, or bilobate nuclei with coarsely clumped chromatin (Figure 3). This anomaly is generally indicative of a benign hereditary disorder in which the cells function normally. There are scattered reports of such abnormalities being induced by sulfisoxazole and disappearing when the drug was discontinued.[7,8] In a few instances, similar changes have been causally related to the administration of colchicine.[9] It has also been suggested that there is an increased frequency of these cells in patients with myeloproliferative disorders receiving cytotoxic drugs.[10,11] However, it should be noted that similar changes are demonstrable in certain of these patients before therapy is started.[10–12] The mechanism(s) responsible for a drug-induced Pelger-Hüet-like anomaly is unknown.

Vacuolization of the nuclei and cytoplasm of erythrocytic and granulocytic precursors has been attributed to a variety of substances, including ethanol,[13,14] chloramphenicol,[15] pyrazinoic acid,[14] and daunomycin[16] (Figure 4). The vacu-

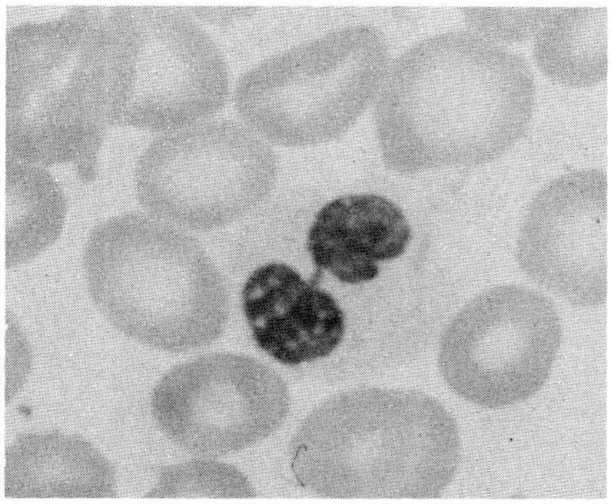

Fig. 3. Pelger-Hüet anomaly (original magnification × 1250).

oles induced by these different agents are morphologically indistinguishable, do not stain with lipid or polysaccharide stains, and appear to lack specificity. The mechanisms responsible for their production are conjectural. Vacuoles are more numerous in the cytoplasm than in the nuclei and more prominent in the erythrocytic series than in granulocytes.

CYTOPLASMIC ABNORMALITIES

Cytoplasmic inclusion bodies that stain pale blue with a Romanowsky stain were first described by Döhle in granulocytes from patients with scarlet fever. Döhle bodies (Figure 5), which may be single or multiple, probably represent

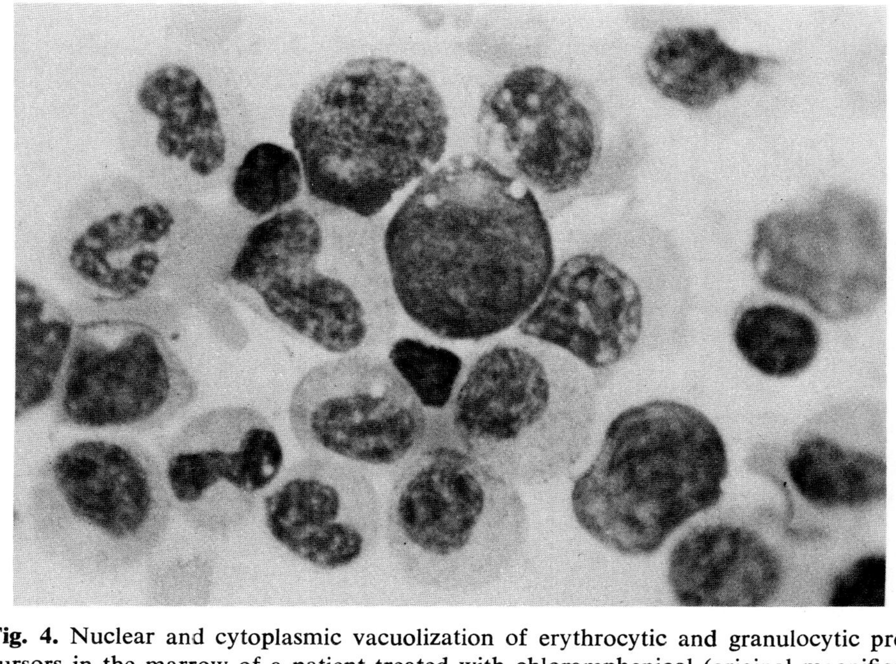

Fig. 4. Nuclear and cytoplasmic vacuolization of erythrocytic and granulocytic precursors in the marrow of a patient treated with chloramphenicol (original magnification × 1250).

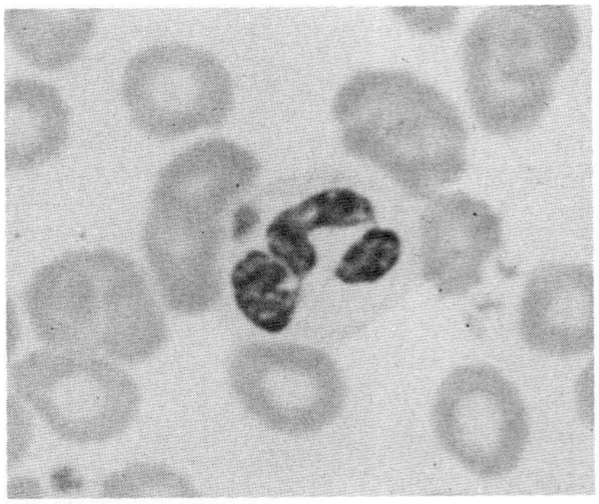

Fig. 5. Döhle body in a neutrophil (original magnification × 1250).

RNA and appear to reflect a nonspecific abnormality in cytoplasmic maturation. They are now known to accompany a wide variety of other disorders, including leukemia, lymphoma, severe burns, tuberculosis, measles, and so forth. They have also been attributed to certain drugs, e.g., cyclophosphamide, nitrogen mustard, busulfan, and chlorambucil.[17] Thus, Döhle bodies are most likely indicative of one or more of several derangements in the metabolism or maturation of granulocytes, and as such they lack specificity. Our experience supports the conclusion that these cytoplasmic inclusion bodies are relatively common findings in a number of diverse conditions.

Abnormal granulation is another cytoplasmic manifestation of altered granulocyte metabolism. Blue-black cytoplasmic granules of variable size (so-called "toxic granulation") are found in the neutrophils and less often in other granulocytes of persons with a variety of "toxic" states (Figure 6). Although such granulation most frequently accompanies acute infections, it also occurs in patients with burns, exposure to heavy metals, and after the ingestion of certain drugs, e.g., cyclophosphamide, *p*-aminosalicylic acid, and chloroquine. These granules, which presumably reflect altered lysosomes, exhibit, on electron microscopy, fine structural abnormalities;[18] however, they appear to be nonspecific and devoid of diagnostic significance.

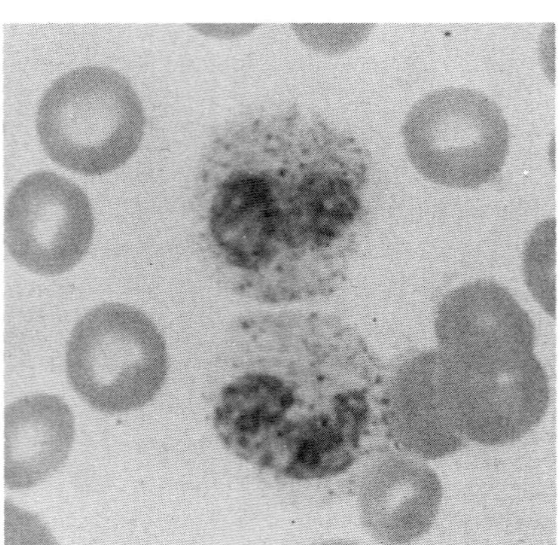

Fig. 6. Toxic granulation of neutrophils (original magnification × 1250).

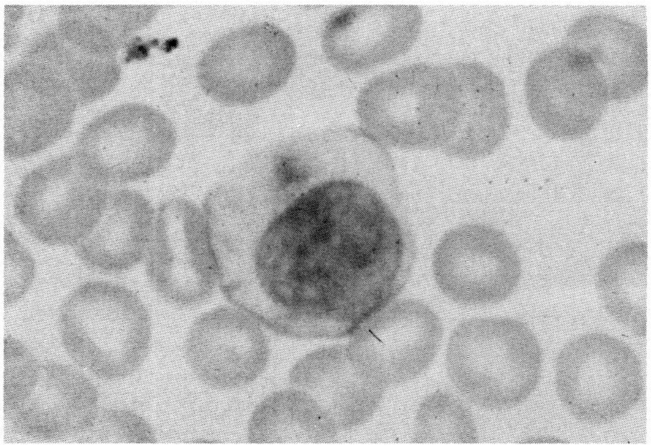

Fig. 7. Atypical lymphocyte (original magnification × 1250).

MISCELLANEOUS CHANGES

Atypical lymphocytes (Figure 7), similar to those demonstrable in a variety of conditions (most notably infectious mononucleosis and cytomegalovirus infection), have been observed rarely in patients who develop hypersensitivity reactions to diphenylhydantoin or *p*-aminosalicylic acid.[19,20] These occurrences are more likely a consequence of an idiosyncratic response on the part of the recipient than a direct or dose-dependent effect of drug on cells.

SUMMARY

Many drugs exert significant changes in the physiology, metabolism, and proliferation of leukocytes and their precursors. However, drug-induced morphologic changes in leukocytes, evident in routine blood and marrow smears, are infrequent and lack specificity. Most common are megaloblastic changes caused by agents that impair the absorption and/or utilization of folates or vitamin B_{12} and the megaloblastoid changes caused by cytotoxic substances that interfere with DNA synthesis and cell division. Certain other nuclear and cytoplasmic findings (acquired Pelger-Hüet anomaly, vacuolization, Döhle bodies, granule abnormalities, and atypical lymphocytes) can be causally related to a number of drugs, but these changes lack specificity; their modes of production and true significance are, for the most part, conjectural.

REFERENCES

1. Shaw M: Human chromosome damage by chemical agents. Annu Rev Med 21:409–432, 1970
2. Chessin LN: Lymphocytes and plasma cells: newer views of their relationships, life cycles and functions, Hematology for Internists. Edited by RI Weed. Boston, Little, Brown 1971, pp 361–378
3. Abul-Fadl Y, Scott RB: Glycogen in human peripheral blood leukocytes. III. Effect of female hormones. Scand J Haematol 6:262–269, 1969

4. Waxman S, Corcino JJ, Herbert V: Drugs, toxins and dietary amino acids affecting vitamin B_{12} or folic acid absorption or utilization. Am J Med 48:599–608, 1970
5. Streiff RR: Disorders of folate metabolism. DM, April 1972, pp 18–22
6. Corcino JJ, Waxman S, Herbert V: Absorption and malabsorption of vitamin B_{12}. Am J Med 48:562–569, 1970
7. Kaplan JM, Barrett O Jr: Reversible pseudo-Pelger anomaly related to sulfisoxazole therapy. N Engl J Med 277:421–422, 1967
8. Brunning RD: Morphologic alterations in nucleated blood and marrow cells in genetic disorders. Hum Pathol 1:99–124, 1970
9. Laszlo J, Rundles RW: Morphology of granulocytes, Hematology. Edited by WJ Williams, E Beutler, AJ Erslev, RW Rundles. New York, McGraw-Hill, 1972, p 566
10. Dorr AD, Moloney WC: Acquired pseudo-Pelger anomaly of granulocytic leukocytes. N Engl J Med 261:742–746, 1959
11. Shanbrom E, Collins Z, Miller S: "Acquired" Pelger-Huët cells in blood dyscrasias. Am J Med Sci 240:732–737, 1960
12. Saarni MI, Linman JW: Myelomonocytic leukemia: disorderly proliferation of all marrow cells. Cancer 27:1221–1230, 1971
13. McCurdy PR, Pierce LE, Rath CE: Abnormal bone-marrow morphology in acute alcoholism. N Engl J Med 266:505–507, 1962
14. Jarrold T, Will JJ, Davies AR, et al: Bone marrow-erythroid morphology in alcoholic patients. Am J Clin Nutr 20:716–722, 1967
15. McCurdy PR: Chloramphenicol bone marrow toxicity. JAMA 176:588–593, 1961
16. Whang-Peng J, Leventhal BG, Adamson JW, et al: The effect of daunomycin on human cells in vivo and in vitro. Cancer 23:113–121, 1969
17. Itoga T, Laszlo J: Döhle bodies and other granulocytic alterations during chemotherapy with cyclophosphamide. Blood 20:668–674, 1962
18. Fedorko M: Effect of chloroquine on morphology of cytoplasmic granules in maturing human leukocytes—an ultrastructural study. J Clin Invest 46:1932–1942, 1967
19. Cannemeyer W, Thompson JR, Lichtenstein MR: Severe para-aminosalicylic acid hypersensitivity. Blood and lymph node studies. Blood 10:62–75, 1955
20. Wood TA, Frenkel EP: The atypical lymphocyte. Am J Med 42:923–936, 1967

Edward S. Henderson

18
The Granulocytopenic Effects of Cancer Chemotherapeutic Agents

The initial use of alkylating agents against lymphoid tumors was prompted by observations of leukocytopenia following exposure to war gases.[1,2] Other drugs, originally designed for therapy of other diseases, such as hypoglycemic agents and antibiotics,[3–5] have also received trials as anticancer agents because of preclinical or clinical observations of untoward myelosuppression. Hence, it is neither surprising that most of the drugs employed in cancer chemotherapy induce some degree of granulocytopenia, nor that in many instances granulocytopenia and infection resulting therefrom is the single factor limiting treatment.

Granulocytopenia is the result of failure of granulocytopoiesis in virtually all such instances, shortened granulocyte survival being uncommon in cancer or in its treatment, even when bone marrow is involved by the malignancy. Granulocytopenia greatly increases susceptibility to infections, particularly those of bacterial and fungal origin, the incidence of which depends upon both the depth and duration of neutrophil depression.[6] Consequently a knowledge of both these parameters is important when evaluating the risk of administering one or another form of chemotherapy.

Both clinical and preclinical evaluations of potentially useful anticancer drugs include some attempt to establish doses and schedules of reasonable tolerability. Earlier in the history of cancer drug development such so called "phase one" clinical toxicology studies were empiric and often superficial. In recent years, considerable sophistication has been incorporated into "phase one" trials, particularly in terms of interrelating animal and clinical dosages and schedules.[7–9] When carefully conducted and reported, these studies provide the best available estimates of absolute and relative toxicities, and the present survey relies heavily on these sources.

Table 1 lists the most widely used, or most promising, of current anticancer drugs, subdividing them according to the risk and severity of granulocytopenia as a side effect. The naturally occurring steroid hormones, of both adrenal and gonadal origin, rarely if ever result in quantitative deficits in granulocyte production. The use of asparaginase, vincristine, and the Japanese antibiotic bleomycin,

Table 1

Granulocytopenic Effects of Anticancer Drugs
(Effects After Therapeutic Doses)

Rarely if ever cause granulocytopenia	
Prednisone	
Androgens and Estrogens	
Asparaginase	
Myelosuppression usually not limiting toxicity	
Vincristine	
Bleomycin	
Myelosuppressive, but other complications equally important	
Procarbazine (CNS,GI), Mitramycin (Liver, DIC)	
Cyclophosphamide (GU), 5-Fluorouracyl (GI)	
Methotrexate (GI), Actinomycin D (GI)	
6-Mercaptopurine (GI)	
Primarily myelosuppressive toxicity	
Cytarabine	Vinblastine
Alkylating agents	Nitrosoureas

although associated with myelosuppression under certain circumstances, is rarely circumscribed by granulocytopenia. For all these compounds, tolerance by the patient almost invariably is determined by other side effects, irrespective of the nature of the underlying disease or the dose and schedule by which the drug is given.

However, most cancer chemotherapeutic agents, as noted earlier, are myelosuppressive. They can be subdivided into drugs whose tolerance depends approximately equally upon myelosuppression and nonhematopoietic toxicities, e.g., procarbazine, cyclophosphamide, methotrexate, and purine antimetabolites, and those in which myelotoxicity (and granulocytopenia) clearly predominated, e.g., cytosine arabinoside, vinblastine, most alkylating agents, and the nitrosoureas.

In reviewing this list, it is of particular interest that antimetabolites and alkylating agents, those classes most frequently synthesized, studied, and explored during the 1950s and early 1960s, are uniformly myelotoxic, while the more recent interest in natural products: plant alkyloids, antibiotics, and enzymes, has brought to light and to medical practice agents for which myelosuppression has been less critical than nonhematopoietic side effects. The introduction of the latter compounds will continue to stimulate investigations of drug combinations and of mechanisms of actions likely to be quite different from those involving interference of DNA synthesis and replication per se.

Table 2 summarizes reported studies of the duration of granulocytopenia after the administration of important anticancer drugs used singly. Taken by class, antimetabolites and vinca alkaloids whose effects are strikingly maximized at particular phases of the cells mitotic cycle, impart the shortest duration of granulocytopenia after single doses or short courses of administration. These drugs have virtually no effect upon cells neither in, nor preparing for, cell division.[44] As a result, single or widely spaced intermittent doses spare a variable but substantial portion of granulocyte progenitors. The most striking example of this type of effect is provided by cytosine arabinoside (Cytarabin, Cytosar ®).

Because its effect is restricted to inhibition of DNA synthesis, and since rapid catabolism renders it inactive in vivo within a matter of minutes, extremely large, single, rapidly administered doses result in little or no observable toxicity.[20] As a corollary, cytosine arabinoside, and to a lesser extent, the other antimetabolites, must be given repetitively or by continuous infusion for maximum antitumor effect. Given by such schedules, these drugs produce strikingly more severe bone marrow suppression.

Alkylating agents and antibiotics, such as actinomycin D and daunorubicin, affect both cell division and the transcriptional events leading ultimately to protein production. The alkylating agents cause cross-linkage between strands of DNA and/or breaks in individual DNA strands. The antibiotics intercalate into DNA copolymers. Both alterations can be permanent or slowly reparable, and thus the effect of a single exposure to such drugs is usually prolonged. These compounds, although most demonstrably active during certain phases of the mitotic cycle, have some activity irrespective of the phase of the mitotic cycle or whether or not the cell is mitotically active or "resting."[44–48] Accordingly, the duration of granulocytopenia after either a single dose or course is characteristically longer than that seen with vinca alkaloids and antimetabolites. For the same reasons the effect of dose schedules is less apparent with the use of semipermanent DNA inhibitors.[8,49]

The most profoundly myelotoxic compounds in frequent clinical use belong to the nitrosourea group. These investigational drugs are clearly effective in the treatment of lymphomas and certain gastrointestinal carcinomas[50,51] and do not show consistent cross-reactivity (or cross-resistance) with alkylating agents.[49,50] The three congeners used clinically, Bis-B-chloroethyl (BCNU), chlorocyclohexyl (CCNU), and methyl chlorocyclohexyl (MCCNU) analogues, have different permissible dosages but nearly identical patterns of toxicity. Cumulative dosage is the major determinant of granulocytopenia, variations in schedule having little influence. At clinically effective doses, the nadir of granulocyte levels occurs 4 to 7 weeks after treatment has been started, and recovery takes an additional 2 to 3 weeks. Predictably, these drugs have been demonstrated to be toxic toward hematopoietic stem cells,[52–54] whether or not they are undergoing cell division. Indeed, recent studies by Sensenbrenner suggest that BCNU is more damaging to latent (Go) progenitors than to rapidly replicating cells.[53] Finally, BCNU, and presumably CCNU and MCCNU as well, can induce prolongation of the time required for cell division[55] and a reduction in the portion of cells in division (i.e., a smaller "growth fraction").[54] These several effects, collectively, provide a rational explanation for the very prolonged depression of granulocytopoiesis observed with these agents.

Extensive studies of the kinetics of myelopoiesis in man have led to conceptual models which have proved consistant with clinically observed events.[56,57] Myelopoiesis can be separated into several functional components (Figure 1): a stem cell compartment with relatively little cell division under normal conditions; a multiplying compartment which includes the mitotically active myeloblasts, promyelocytes, and myeloblasts; and a postmitotic compartment which contains differentiating and maturing metamyelocytes, bands, and polymorphonuclear leukocytes. The average transit time through this latter compartment is estimated to be 10 days. The shortest normal transit time is 72–96 hours[56]

Table 2
Granulocytopenic Effects of Anticancer Drugs[1-3]

Class	Drug	PMN Nadir (days)	Recovery (days)	Modifying Factors	Refs.
Vinca Alkyloids					
	Vincristine	4–5	7	Liver failure	(10,11)
	Vinblastine	5–9	14–21	Liver failure	(12)
		9	15		(13)
		7	14		(14)
Antimetabolites					
	Methotrexate	7	14–21	Renal function	(15)
		7–14	14–21	Schedule	(16)
		4–7	10		(17)
	6 Mercaptopurine	7	14–21	Renal fct	
				Allopurinol	(18)
	6-Thioguanine	7	14–21	Renal fct	(18,19)
	Cytarabine	12–14	22–24	Cytidine kinase	
				Cytidine deaminase	
				Schedule	(20,21)
	5-Fluorouracyl	7–14		Schedule	(22–24)
Antibiotics					
	Actinomycin D	15	25		(25)
		15	22–25		(26)
	Daunorubician	9–13	21–28	Schedule	(27,28)
Miscellaneous					
	Hydroxyurea	7	14–21	Schedule	(29,30)
	Procarbazine	25	35–40	Schedule MAO inhibitors pyridoxin	(31,32)
		36+	50+		(33)

Alkylating Agents				
	Nitrogen mustard	7	28	(34)
		10–15	28	(35)
	Cyclophosphamide	14	25	(36)
		12	24	(37)
		8–12	18	(38,39)
	Melphalan	10–12	—	(7,40)
	Myleran	11–30	24–54	(41)
Nitrosoureas				
	BCNU	26–30	35–49	(42)
	CCNU	40–50	60	(43)
	MCCNU	28–63	82–89	(49–51)

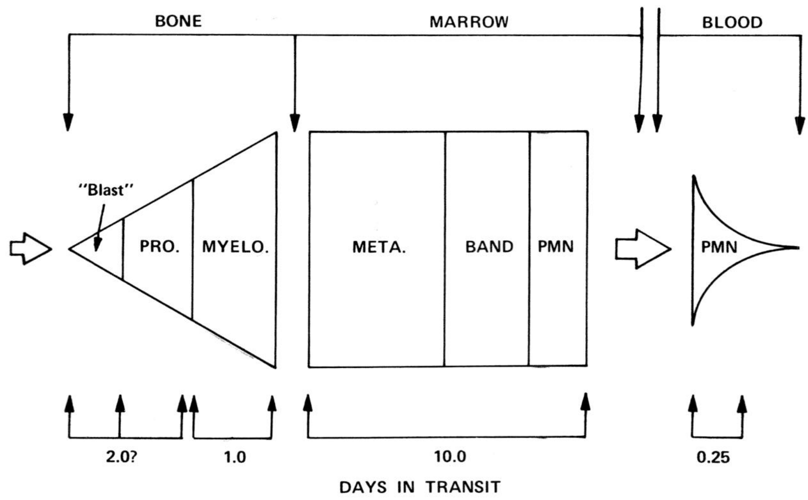

Fig. 1. Schematic representation of granulocytopoiesis in normal man.

which, under the stress of infection, may be reduced to 48 hours. With this system, drugs that exclusively damage cells in division would have no affect on differentiating granulocytes, inflict severe injury to the multiplying population, and, initially at least, would injure pleuripotential stem cells only slightly. Thus, following maximal acute injury by this class of drugs, one would predict a slow fall in peripheral granulocytes to a nadir at about 10 days followed by a return to pretreatment values at day 20 (Figure 2). Recovery would depend upon the

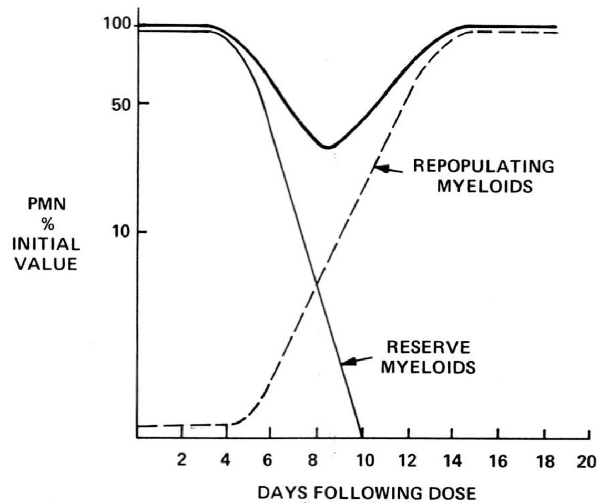

Fig. 2. Schematic representation of the effect on peripheral blood granulocyte levels of a single exposure to a cyclo-active cytotoxic drug. It is assumed that the drug exposure will kill all cells preparing for division, will spare all non-replicating cells, and that pretreatment granulocyte levels and reserves are normal.

time for repopulation of the multiplying cell compartment, estimated at 5–7 days,[39,57] plus an additional time for differentiation, shorter than 10 days in this instance because of the stress of granulocytopenia.

Drugs which injure nondividing as well as dividing cells would cause a delay in the replenishment of all compartments. Depending upon their effect on postmitotic maturing cells, the time to maximum granulocytopenia might be 10 days or less, but the duration of granulocytopenia would, in any case, be extended.

In recent years, techniques have been developed which permit the assessment of drug effects on early hematopoietic progenitors. Such studies have employed in vivo spleen colony assays in mice and rats[44,59] and in vitro myeloid colony formation assays.[60,61] The latter technique has made the investigation of drug effects on human myeloid "stem cells" feasible.[48] Table 3 lists the major antineoplastic drugs in order of increasing duration of granulocytopenia which they produce, and compares this to their documented effects on colony forming units and kinetically determined cell specificities. Compounds cytotoxic within only a portion of the mitotic cycle (phase-specific agents) impart rapidly reversible granulocytopenia (Figure 3). Cycle-specific agents, active throughout cell replication, tend to reduce granulocyte counts as quickly as phase-specific drugs, but recovery is somewhat prolonged. With those few agents which appear to affect cells not preparing to divide, recovery of normal levels of circulating granulocytes is distinctly prolonged, in some cases up to 8 weeks.

There is evidence from studies of mouse bone marrows that BCNU and myleran cause more pronounced damage to hematopoietic stem cells then to

Table 3

Kinetic Class, Effects on Stem Cells, and
Duration of Granulocytopenia of Anticancer Drugs

Kinetic Class	Drug	Extent of Injury to CFU*	Granulocytopenia Nadir (days)	Granulocytopenia Recovery (days)
Phase Specific	Vinca alkyloids	Fraction of dividing cells (48,49)	4–9	7–21
	Hydroxyurea	" " (48)	7	14–21
	Methotrexate	" " (44,49)	7–14	14–21
	Cytarabine	" " (55,62)	12–14	22–24
Cycle Specific	Actinomycin	All dividing CFU (47)	15	25
	Daunorubicin	" (46)	9–13	21–28
	Cyclophosphamide	" (44,45,54)	8–14	18–25
Nonspecific	Nitrogen mustard	All CFU (44,49) (more effective in division)	7–15	28
	Myleran	Nondividing	11–30	24–54
	BCNU	CFU (49,54,55)	26–30	35–49
	CCNU	—	40–50	60

* Colony Forming Units.

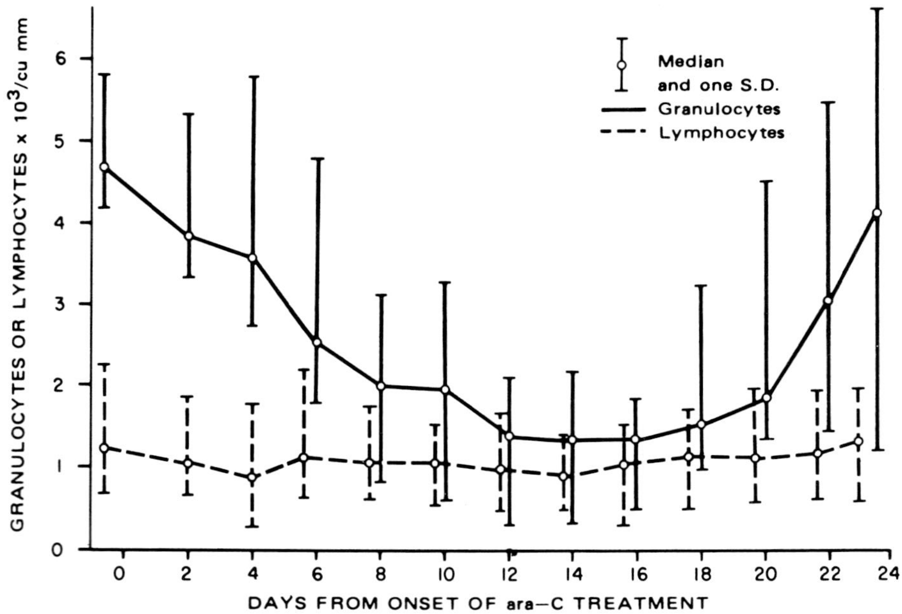

Fig. 3. Effect of cytosine arabinoside on peripheral blood leukocyte levels, (Reproduced by permission from Frei, et al.[20])

their more rapidly multiplying progeny.[53,62] In this regard, it is interesting to note the striking delay in maximal granulocyte depression characteristic of those particular drugs (Figure 4). Although these correlations of observed toxicities and progenitor assays are crude, they demonstrate that the careful evaluation of clinical events (such as granulocytopenia) coupled with an understanding of basic physiology (e.g., bone marrow function), provides an often undervalued insight into important basic drug actions.

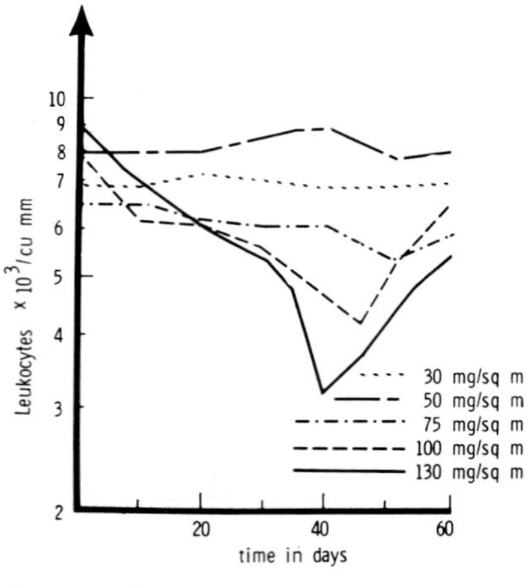

Fig. 4. Effect of chlorocyclohexylnitrosourea (CCNU) on peripheral blood granulocyte levels. (Reproduced by permission from Hansen, et al.[43])

MEASURES TO PREVENT AND/OR AMELIORATE GRANULOCYTOPENIA AND ITS CONSEQUENCES

The major consequence of granulocytopenia is to increase the risk of initiating or aggravating infection. In cancer chemotherapy any measure that will reduce the duration or depth of granulocytopenia without compromising antineoplastic activity should increase the likelihood of a favorable response. Clinical trials to delineate optimum doses and schedules of drug administration, and to evaluate the feasibility and efficacy of drug combinations, represent attempts in this direction. Perhaps the most successful of these trials, has led to the use of methotrexate by a high-dose intermittent schedule,[63,64] the combinations of methotrexate with its antidote citrovorum factor,[65,66] and the combination of cytosine arabinoside with 6-thioguanine[67–69] in the treatment of acute leukemia. In each instance, despite either a modest increase or actually a reduction of myelotoxicity, augmented doses of active drugs have been tolerated, and improved therapeusis has been achieved.

Unfortunately, in most instances greater antitumor effects have been complicated by increased myelotoxicity, and, under these circumstances, ancillary measures must be employed to prevent and ameliorate drug-related infections. Major approaches to this end have been granulocyte replacement and patient insolation. Granulocyte replacement has generally been accomplished by repetitive transfusions of granulocyte-rich fractions of normal blood or blood obtained from patients with chronic myelocytic leukemia (CML).[70–73] Such granulocyte replacement therapy has been successful, together with appropriate antibiotics, in reducing mortality from bacterial septicemias,[73] but it is time consuming and fraught with the problem of securing proper donors and avoiding alloimmunization.

Granulocytes are separated with difficulty from normal blood. Furthermore, the daily requirement of noninfected individuals is approximately 1×10^{11} PMNs,[74] or the equivalent of the number of PMNs in 6–8 blood volumes of the average adult donor. Pooled buffy coats from 50–100 units of fresh whole blood can provide adequate numbers of functional granulocytes,[75] but, in addition to the impractical logistics to this technique, there is inherently an unacceptable risk of red cell incompatability, alloimmunization to histocompatability antigens, and transmission of hepatitis virus. Adequate numbers of granulocytes can be obtained from donors with chronic myelocytic leukemia provided their peripheral granulocyte levels have not been reduced by therapy.[70–72] Although repeated leukophereses of such patients may provide prolonged relief of symptoms and improved red cell and platelet production,[76,77] it is uncommon that CML patients are left untreated and still more rare that they prove compatible donors for multiply transfused granulocytopenic recipients. The most nearly ideal donor is a normal individual, preferably compatible in terms of red and white cell antigens, against whom the recipient has no preformed leukocyte directed antibodies.[73,78] Repetitive granulocyte transfusions of adequate cell count can reverse the downhill course of established life-threatening infections[73] and, given throughout a period of granulocytopenia, should forestall serious infectious complications. Currently, two effective cell-separating devices, the IBM-NCI continuous flow centrifuge[72,73,79] and the leukocyte-filtration unit,[73,80] permit daily collection of therapeutically sufficient numbers of granulocytes from a single donor. The prophylactic utility of this approach is under investigation.

An alternate mechanism for providing granulocytes would involve the transplantation of bone marrow stem cells after myelotoxic chemotherapy. Such grafts are feasible using stored autologous, identical twin donors. The rarity of identical twin donors and the high risk of severe graft-versus-host disease, when autologous marrow is employed, makes these sources of stem cells generally unacceptable. Buckner and co-workers[38] transfused autologous bone marrow stored at −180°C to patients receiving high dose cyclophosphamide. A control group received the same drug doses without attempted bone marrow transplantation. As shown in Figure 5, there was no significant difference in the case of recovery of granulocytopoiesis in the two groups. Thus, at present the use of marrow grafts seems less valuable than granulocyte transfusions in ameliorating drug-induced granulocytopoiesis.

The efficacy of isolation and bacterial decontamination measures is also undergoing active evaluation.[81–84] The key to success in such protocols appears to be the combination of strict isolation, air decontamination by high efficiency filtration, and a reduction of epidermal and gastrointestinal microflora through topical antiseptic and peroral nonabsorbable antibiotics. In patients with short-term, reversible granulocytopenia, results have been encouraging in that both the incidence of infection and mortality from infection have been dramatically diminished.[81,82,84] Whether these procedures will permit a significant augmentation of therapeutic benefit through augmented dosing has yet to be determined.

In conclusion, granulocytopenia is an all too frequent complication of antineoplastic therapy. The depth and duration of granulocyte levels is important

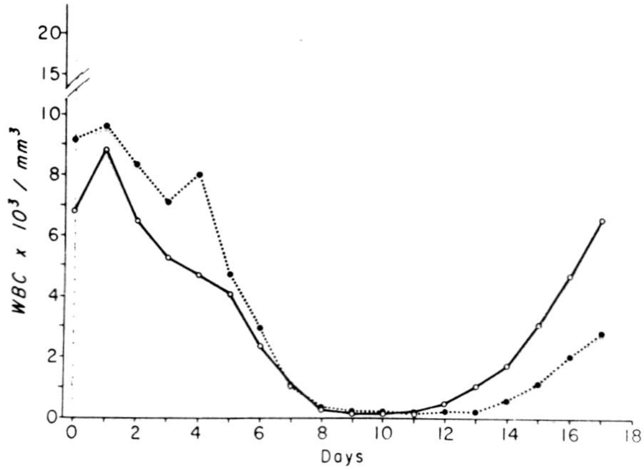

Fig. 5. Granulocytopenia after high dose cyclophosphamide therapy, with and without the subsequent transplantation of autologous bone marrow. (Reproduced by permission from Buckner, et al.[38])

to the pharmacologist and cell biologist in providing clues to the sites of action of the drug employed. It is also vital that the physician (and the patients under his care) understand how to minimize this complication through proper dose scheduling and/or appropriate combinations of drugs, and that he and his medical institution have facilities adequate to minimize or correct the consequences of granulocytopenia. Until therapies are developed which enjoy a degree of specificity sufficient to eradicate tumor cells while sparing normal hematopoiesis from injury, granulocyte depression will remain the major concern of the chemotherapist.

REFERENCES

1. Krumbhaar EB, Krumbhaar HD: The blood and bone marrow in yellow gas poisoning. J Med Res 40:497, 1919
2. Lynch V, Smith HW, Marshall EK: On dichloroethylsulfide (mustard gas). I. The systemic effects and mechanism of action. J Pharmacol Exp Ther 12:265, 1918
3. Johnson IS: The vinca alkaloids: A new class of oncolytic agents. Cancer Res 23:1390, 1963
4. Domagk G: Uber eine neue, gegen tuberkelbazillen in vitro wirksame verbindungsklasse. Naturwissenschaften 33:315, 1946
5. Freedlander BL, French FA: Carcinostatic action of polycarbonyl compounds and their derivatives. II. Glyoxal Bis (Guanylhydrazone) and derivatives. Cancer Res 18:360, 1958
6. Bodey GP, Buckley M, Sathe YS, et al: Quantitative relationships between circulating leukocytes and infection in patients with acute leukemia. Ann Intern Med 64:328, 1966
7. Freireich EJ, Gehan EA, Rall DP, et al: Quantitative comparison of toxicity of anticancer agents in mouse, rat, hampster, dog. Cancer Chemother Rep 50:219, 1966
8. Skipper HE, Schabel FM Jr, Mellett LB, et al: Implications of biochemical, cytokinetic, pharmacologic, and toxocologic relationships in the design of optimal therapeutic schedules. Cancer Chemother Rep 54 (Part 1):431, 1970
9. Goldin A, Sandberg JS, Henderson ES, et al: The chemotherapy of human and animal acute leukemia. Cancer Chemother Rep 55:308, 1971
10. Carbone P, Bono V, Frei E III, et al: Clinical studies with vincristine. Blood 21:640, 1963
11. Karon MR, Freireich EJ, Frei E III: A preliminary report on vincristine sulfate—a new active agent for the treatment of acute leukemia. Pediatrics 30: 791, 1966
12. Warwick O, Darte J, Brown T: Some biological effects of vincaleukoblastine, an alkaloid in *Vinca rosea* Linn in patients with disease. Cancer Res 20:1032, 1960
13. Hertz R, Lipsett M, Moy R: Effect of vincaleukoblastine on metastatic choriocarcinoma and related trophoblastic tumors in women. Cancer Res 21:1050, 1960
14. Vaitkevicius V, Talley R, Tucker JL Jr, et al: Cytological and clinical observations during vincaleukoblastine therapy of disseminated cancer. Cancer 15: 294, 1962

15. Berlin NI, Rall D, Mead JAR, et al: Folic acid antagonists. Ann Intern Med 59:931, 1963
16. Gottlieb JA, Serpick AA: Prolonged intravenous methotrexate therapy in the treatment of acute leukemia and solid tumors. Cancer Res 30:2132, 1970
17. Hertz R, Bergenstal DM, Lipsett MD, et al: Chemotherapy of choriocarcinoma and related trophoblastic tumors in women. JAMA 168:845, 1958
18. Burchenal JH, Murphy ML, Ellison RR, et al: Clinical evaluation of a new antimetabolite, 6-mercaptopurine in the treatment of leukemia and allied diseases. Blood 8:965, 1953
19. LePage GA, Whitecar JP Jr: Pharmacology of 6-thioguanine in man. Cancer Res 31:1627, 1971
20. Frei E III, Bickers JN, Hewlett JS, et al: Dose schedule and antitumor studies of arabinosyl cytosine (NSC 63878). Cancer Res 29:1325, 1969
21. Steuart CD, Burke PJ, Owens AH Jr: Correlation of ara-C metabolism and clinical response in acute leukemia. Proc Am Assoc Cancer Res 12:89, 1971
22. Moertel CG, Reitemeir RJ, Hahn RG: Fluorinated pyrimidine therapy of advanced gastrointestinal cancer. Gastroenterology 46:371, 1964
23. Gold GL, Hall TC, Shnider BI, et al: A clinical study of 5-fluorouracyl. Cancer Res 19:935, 1959
24. Sullivan RD, Young CN, Miller E, et al: The clinical effects of the continuous administration of fluorinated pyrimidines (5-fluorouracil and 5-fluoro-2′-deoxyuridine) Cancer Chemother Rep 8:77, 1960
25. Moore GE, DiPaolo JA, Kondo T: The chemotherapeutic effects and complications of actinomycin D in patients with advanced cancer. Cancer 11:1204, 1958
26. Watke AL, Badillo J, Koike A, et al: Clinical studies of actinomycin D. Ann NY Acad Sci 89:445, 1960
27. Serpick AA, Henderson ES: Observations on the toxicity and clinical trials with daunomycin. Pathol Biol 15:909, 1967
28. Huffman DH, Bachur NR: Daunorubicin metabolism by human hematological components. Cancer Res 32:600, 1972
29. Fishbein WN, Carbone PP, Freireich EJ, et al: Clinical trials of hydroxyurea in patients with cancer and leukemia. Clin Pharmacol Ther 5:574, 1964
30. Thurman WG, Bloedow C, Howe CD, et al: A phase 1 study of hydroxyurea. Cancer Chemother Rep 29:103, 1963
31. DeVita VT, Serpick A, Carbone PP: Preliminary clinical studies with ibenzmethizine. Clin Pharmacol Ther 7:542, 1966
32. Brunner KW, Young CW: A methylhydrazine derivative in Hodgkins disease and other malignant neoplasms. Ann Intern Med 63:69, 1965
33. Stolinsky DC, Solomon J, Pugh RP, et al: Clinical experience with procarbazine in Hodgkins disease, reticulum cell sarcoma, and lymphosarcoma. Cancer 26: 984, 1970
34. Kretchmar AL, Andrews GA, Sitterson BW: Attempted bone-marrow autografts after large doses of nitrogen mustard. N Engl J Med 268:427, 1963
35. Clifford P, Clift RA, Duff JK: Nitrogenmustard therapy combined with autologous marrow infusion. Lancet 1:687, 1961
36. Coggins PR, Ravdin RG, Disman SH: Clinical evaluation of a new alkylating agent: Cytoxan (cyclophosphamide). Cancer 13:1254, 1960
37. Gottlieb JA, Mendelson D, Serpick AA: An evaluation of large intermittent intravenous doses of cyclophosphamide (NSC 26271) in the treatment of metastatic malignant melanoma. Cancer Chemother Rep 54:365, 1970
38. Buckner CD, Rudolph RH, Fefer A, et al: High dose cyclophosphamide therapy for malignant disease. Cancer 29:357, 1972

39. Bergsagel DE, Robertson GL, Hasselback R: Effect of cyclophosphamide on advanced lung cancer and hematological toxicity of large intermittent infusion doses. Can Med Assoc J 98:531, 1968
40. Burns BC Jr, Rutledge F, Gallager HS: Phenylalanine mustard in the palliative treatment of carcinoma of the ovary. Obstet Gynecol 22:30, 1963
41. Sullivan RD: Myleran therapy in bronchogenic carcinoma. Ann NY Acad Sci 68:1038, 1958
42. DeVita VT, Carbone PP, Owens AH Jr, et al: Clinical trials with 1, 3-Bis(2-chloroethyl)-1-nitrosourea, NSC-409962. Cancer Res 25:1876, 1965
43. Hansen HH, Selawry OS, Muggia FM, et al: Clinical studies with 1-(2-choro-ethyl)-3-cyclohexyl-1-nitrosourea(NSC 79037) Cancer Res 31:223, 1971
44. Bruce WR, Meeker BE, Valeriote FA: Comparison of the sensitivity of normal hematopoietic and transplanted lymphoma colony-forming cells to chemotherapeutic agents administered in vivo. J Natl Cancer Inst 37:233, 1966
45. Van Putten LM, Lelieveld P: Factors determining cell killing by chemotherapeutic agents in vivo. II. Melphalan, chlorambucil and nitrogen mustard. Eur J Cancer 7:11, 1971
46. Razek A, Valeriote F, Vietti T: Survival of hematopoietic and leukemia colony-forming cells in vivo following the administration of daunorubicin or adriamycin. Cancer Res 32:1496, 1972
47. Smith WW, Carter SK, Wilson SM, et al: Joint lethal effects of actinomycin D and radiation in mice. Cancer Res 30:51, 1970
48. Ash R, Chaffey JT, Hellman S: The effect of nitrogen mustard on the survival of murine hematopoietic stem cells. Cancer Res 32:1695, 1972
49. Brown CB III, Carbone PP: Effects of chemotherapeutic agents on normal bone marrow growth in vitro. Cancer Res 31:185, 1971
50. Livingston RB, Carter SK: Single Agents in Cancer Chemotherapy. New York, Washington, London IFI/Plenum, 1970
51. Lessner HE: BCNU (1,3,bis(B-chloroethyl)-1-nitrosourea effects on advanced Hodgkin's disease and other neoplasia. Cancer 22:451, 1968
52. Moertel CG, Reitmeier RJ, Hahn RG: Therapy of advanced gastrointestinal cancer with 1,3 bis-(2-chloroethyl)-1-nitrosourea (BCNU). Clin Pharmacol Ther 9:652, 1968
53. Schabel FM Jr, Skipper HE, Trader MW, et al: Experimental evaluation of potential anticancer agents. XIX. Sensitivity of nondividing leukemic cell populations to certain classes of drugs in vivo. Cancer Chemother Rep 48:17, 1965
54. Sensenbrenner LL, Owens AH Jr, Zawatsky LS, et al: Comparative effects of selected cytotoxic agents on transplanted hematopoietic cells. Transplantation 14:347, 1972
55. Preisler HD, Henderson ES: Effect of cytosine arabinoside and 1,3-Bis (2-chloroethyl)-1-nitrosurea on hematopoietic precursors in the mouse. J Nat Cancer Inst 47:971, 1971
56. Young RC, DeVita VT: The effect of chemotherapy on the growth characteristics and cellular kinetics of leukemia L1210. Cancer Res 30:1789, 1970
57. Cronkite EP: Kinetics of granulocytopoiesis, Human Tumor Cell Kinetics. Edited by S Perry. Nat Cancer Inst Monogr 30:51, 1969
58. Boggs DR: The kinetics of neutrophilic leukocytes in health and in disease. Semin Hematol 4:359, 1967
59. Till JE, McCulloch EA: A direct measurement of the radiation sensitivity of normal bone marrow cells. Radiat Res 14:213, 1961
60. Bradley TR, Metcalf D: The growth of mouse bone marrow cells in vitro. Aust J Exp Biol Med 44:287, 1966

61. Pluznik DH, Sachs L: The induction of clones of normal mast cells by a substance from conditioned medium. Exp Cell Res 43:553, 1966
62. Wodinsky I, Swiniarski J, Kensler CJ: Spleen colony studies of leukemia L1210. I. Differential sensitivities of normal and leukemic bone marrow colony-forming units to single and divided dose therapy with cytosine arabinoside (NSC 63878). Cancer Chemother Rep 51:423, 1967
63. Dunn CDR, Elson LA: The comparative effect of busulfan ('myleran') on haemopoietic colony forming units in the rat. Cell Tissue Kinet 3:131, 1970
64. Goldin A, Venditti JM, Humphreys SR, et al: Modification of treatments schedules in the management of advanced mouse leukemia with amethnopterin. J Nat Cancer Inst 17:203, 1956
65. Acute Leukemia Group B.: Acute lymphocytic leukemia in children. Maintenance therapy with methotrexate administered intermittently. JAMA 207:923, 1969
66. Goldin A, Venditti JM, Kline I, et al: Eradication of leukemic cells (L1210) by methotrexate and methotrexate plus citrovorum factor. Nature (Lond) 212: 1548, 1966
67. Hryniuk WM, Bertino JR: Treatment of leukemia with large doses of methotrexate and folinic acid. Clinical-Biochemical correlates. J Clin Invest 48:2140, 1969
68. Gee TS, Yu KP, Clarkson BD: Treatment of adult acute leukemia with arabinosyl cytosine and thioguanine. Cancer 23:1019, 1969
69. Carey RW: Comparative study of cytosine arabinoside (CA) therapy alone and combined with thioguanine (TG) mercaptopurine (MP) or daunomycin (DN) in acute myelocytic leukemia (AML). Proc Am Assoc Cancer Res 11:15, 1970
70. Clarkson BD, Dowling MD Jr, Gee TS, et al: Treatment of acute myeloblastic leukemia. Proceedings of the Fifth International Symposium on Comparative Leukemia Research. Padua 1972 (In press)
71. Freireich EJ, Levin RH, Whang J, et al: The function and fate of transfused leukocytes from donors with chronic myelocytic leukemia in leukopenic patients. Ann NY Acad Sci 113:108, 1964
72. Schwarzenberg L, Mathe G, Amiel JL, et al: Study of factors determining the usefulness and complications of leukocyte transfusions. Am J Med 43:206, 1967
73. Buckner CD, Graw RG Jr, Eisel RJ, et al: Leukopheresis by continuous flow centrifugation (CFC) in patients with chronic myelogenous leukemia (CML). Blood 33:353, 1969
74. Graw RG Jr, Herzig GP, Perry S, et al: Normal granulocyte transfusions: Treatment of gram negative bacterial septicemia. N Engl J Med 287:367, 1972
75. Craddock CG Jr: The physiology of granulocytic cells in normal and leukemic states. Am J Med 28:711, 1960
76. Yankee RA, Freireich EJ, Carbone PP, et al: Replacement therapy using normal and chronic myelogenous leukemia leukemic leukocytes. Blood 24:844, 1964
77. Vallejos CS, McCredie KB, Freireich EJ: Improved leukocyte collections with hydroxyethyl starch (HES) from patients with chronic myelocytic leukemia (CML). Clin Res 20:503, 1972
78. Graw RG Jr, and Henderson ES: Unpublished observations.
79. Goldstein I, Eyre H, Terasaki P, et al: Leukocyte transfusions: role of leukocyte alloantibodies in determining transfusion response. Transfusion 11:19, 1971
80. McCredie KB, Freireich EJ: Increased granulocyte collection from normal donors with increased granulocyte recovery following transfusion. Proc Am Assoc Cancer Res 12:58, 1971

81. Djerassi I, Kim J, Suvansri U: Filtration-leukopheresis for separation and transfusion of large amounts of granulocytes from single normal donors. Proc Am Assoc Cancer Res 12:28, 1971
82. Bodey JP, Freireich EJ, Frei E III: Studies of patients in a laminar air flow unit. Cancer 24:972, 1969
83. Levine AS, Siegel SE, Schreiber AD, et al: Protected environments and prophylactic antibiotics: A prospective controlled study of their utility in the therapy of acute leukemia. N Engl J Med 1972 288:477, 1973
84. Yates J, Holland JF: A controlled study of isolation and endogeneous microbial suppression in acute myelocytic leukemia patients. Cancer: 1973 (In press)

Nikolay V. Dimitrov,
James D. Faix,
and Jørgen Ellegaard

19
Leukocytes and Phenylbutazone

Phenylbutazone, a pyrazolon derivative, is a congener of aminopyrine and antipyrine, with similar pharmacologic and toxic effects. It was introduced in 1949 and since then has been widely used as a nonhormonal antiarthritis and anti-inflammatory agent for the treatment of rheumatoid arthritis, acute gout, acute superficial thrombophlebitis, and in the management of certain musculoskeletal disorders. Phenylbutazone is 3, 5-dioxo-1, 2-diphenyl-4-n butylpyrazolidine. Its structural formula is given in Figure 1. Although the basic structure appears to be stable, most of the pharmacologic effects are due to the activity of its metabolites,[1] the most active of which is oxyphenbutazone, a hydroxy analog.

The pharmacologic properties of phenylbutazone are defined by its anti-inflammatory, uricosuric, and analgesic effects. In addition, this drug causes retention of sodium and chloride, reduces iodine uptake by the thyroid gland, competes for the same binding sites of plasma albumin with warfarin, tolbutamide, indomethacin, glucocorticosteroids, and sulfonamides, and could influence the biosynthesis of many cellular substances. Phenylbutazone is rapidly converted to two metabolites, and only traces of unchanged drug are excreted in the urine.[2]

Since it has a variety of pharmacologic properties and is rapidly absorbed but slowly metabolized in man, phenylbutazone, represented by its major metabolic conversion product, oxyphenbutazone, accumulates in the body after chronic administration. Thus, besides its pharmacologic effects, the drug could exercise a variety of toxic effects, depending on dose, duration of therapy, and functional condition of affected organs. Other factors which should be considered are age, body weight, and concurrent potent chemotherapy. One of the most serious complications during phenylbutazone therapy is the toxic effect of the drug on the hematopoietic system.[3,4]

Less attention has been paid to the effect of phenylbutazone on red cells and platelets and much more consideration has been given to the effect of the drug on leukocytes. Reports on the subject provide information ranging from scientific documentation and interpretation to meager information and speculation.

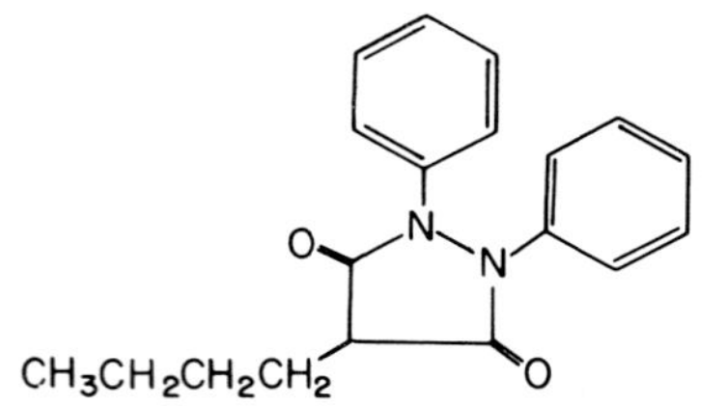

Fig. 1. Structural formula of phenylbutazone (MW 309).

This communication represents a summary of available information in the literature and some data from our own experiments.

PHENYLBUTAZONE AND AGRANULOCYTOSIS

Within the first 5 years after phenylbutazone was introduced, a number of reports appeared attributing a variety of toxic side effects to the drug. In 1955, Mauer[3] presented an extensive review of the available literature. In a series of 3934 patients, 1199 showed toxic reactions of varying degrees of severity. Less common, but more severe, were certain hematologic complications. He found 6 cases of agranulocytosis (0.15%), 32 of leukopenia (0.8%), and 32 of mild-to-moderate thrombocytopenia (0.8%). However, wide discrepancies in the dose of phenylbutazone administered relative to age and duration of therapy make the statistical significance of the reported data dubious. In an effort to provide more detailed information about the toxicity of phenylbutazone, Mauer reviewed case reports for the time between the introduction of the drug and 1955. He collected 49 cases of severe nonfatal reactions, 15 of which were agranulocytosis. Aplastic anemia or thrombocytopenic purpura were not found in this group. Among the 23 deaths, 10 patients had agranulocytosis, 1 had aplastic anemia, and 1 thrombocytopenic purpura. To this, McCarthy and Chalmers[4] added, in 1964, 5 nonlethal cases with agranulocytosis, 6 with aplastic anemia (3 fatal), and 9 with leukemia. The latter authors did not compare hematologic reactions with other complications. This information indicated that the most frequent severe complication during phenylbutazone therapy was agranulocytosis. This complication, in most cases, occurred between 1 to 8 weeks of therapy. Only 2 cases are exceptions from this range, 1 in which therapy was given for 84 days and the other for 450 days. In both cases the patient recovered. The total amount of drug administered ranged from 3.5 to 39.2 g, which suggests that there is no apparent relation between dose and agranulocytosis.

This pattern of agranulocytosis was described in many publications of the late fifties and early sixties that were reviewed by McCarthy and Chalmers.[4] In addition, more information about the influence of age and sex was accumulated. Thus, 76% of the reported cases in adults with agranulocytosis were females and 24% males; ages ranged between 26 and 74. The incidence of toxicity among children and elderly persons was very high. Very few reports of cases with agranulocytosis are available after 1964, because more precautions were taken and probably use of the drug declined somewhat.

The bone marrow picture varies from maturation arrest of the granulocytic series to complete agranulocytosis, with the presence of normal megakaryocytes, lymphocytes, monocytes, and erythroid elements. In advanced cases, a preponderance of monocytes and plasma cells may be found, with a decrease in erythroid precursors and megakaryocytes.

One of the most difficult problems during phenylbutazone therapy, on an outpatient basis, is to provide an effective protective measure against the development of agranulocytosis. It should be emphasized that bone marrow depression continues even after the drug is withdrawn. Under such circumstances, agranulocytosis may appear with dramatic suddenness despite close observation. Thus, weekly blood counts may fail to warn of the impending complication. However, our personal impression is that weekly blood counts will prevent most bone marrow toxicities. As with many other drug reactions, phenylbutazone-induced agranulocytosis should also be considered a result of individual predisposition or sensitivity. Such sensitivity is time related, calling the physician's attention to this complication between the first and eighth week of treatment.

Oxyphenbutazone, the main conversion product of phenylbutazone, shares the same toxic effects.

The clinicians who used phenylbutazone during the last two decades focused their attention primarily on the leukocytes. This not only stimulated clinical investigation but also some laboratory experiments designed to elucidate the effect of phenylbutazone on some physiologic and biochemical properties of polymorphonuclear (PMN) leukocytes. Portions of such studies will be discussed later.

PHENYLBUTAZONE AND LEUKEMIA

The discussion about the relationship between phenylbutazone and leukemia was triggered by case reports revealing leukemia after treatment for arthritis. To date, 38 cases with various types of leukemia after treatment with phenylbutazone have been reported in the available literature (Table 1); 24 are males and 14 females, ranging in age from 29 to 81. Twenty patients were in the 60- to 81-year-old range. The total dose of phenylbutazone before leukemia was diagnosed varied from 1 to 300 g. The duration of therapy ranged from 6 days to 4 years. None of these patients had had bone marrow aspiration prior to therapy or for several weeks before leukemia was diagnosed.

We carefully reviewed all cases reported in the available literature to provide more valuable information about the occurrence of leukemia related to phenylbutazone therapy. However, the situation remains as confusing as it was when the first cases were reported. Good evidence linking phenylbutazone and leukemia is lacking. The picture becomes more blurred when additional information from the literature is considered. For example, several reports indicate an increased incidence of all types of leukemia among patients with rheumatic disease.[5,6] On the other hand, sera from patients with chronic myeloid leukemia have been shown to contain high levels of rheumatoid factor.[7] One should also consider the fact that leukemia, in its early phase, is often associated with joint pain that may simulate arthritis. Such a condition may require treatment with anti-inflammatory drugs until the true cause is discovered. In this case, the drug, by no means, should be considered as leukemogenic. Thus, there is well-documented evidence

Table 1
Malignancy Associated with Phenylbutazone Therapy

Type of Malignancy	No. of Cases Reported	References
Acute lymphoblastic leukemia	6	12,13,26,32,35,36
Acute myelogenous leukemia	13	23,24,29,30,33,36,37,42
Acute monocytic leukemia	1	34
Acute myleo-monocytic leukemia	2	8,31
Acute undifferentiated leukemia	3	27,28,34
Chronic lymphocytic leukemia	1	35
Chronic myelogenous leukemia	6	13,24,25,39
Hodgkin's disease	2	35
Lymphosarcoma	1	12
Reticulum sarcoma	1	12
Polycythemia vera	2	35
Total	38	

supporting an association between leukemia and rheumatic disease. At this point, however, it is fair to say that there is scant evidence that phenylbutazone is one of the leukemogenic agents. On the other hand, we do not ignore the possibility, discussed by Hamer and Gunz,[8] that phenylbutazone-induced bone marrow hypoplasia could be followed by conversion to leukemia after a certain latent period, providing the appropriate genetic background is present. That multiple etiologic factors are involved in leukemia is an old proposition. To add phenylbutazone to these factors on the basis of an isolated case will not avoid the confusion already existing about this drug and the etiology of leukemia. Accumulation of more well-documented cases may shed some insight on this difficult problem.

The possible mechanisms by which phenylbutazone may produce leukemia include interference with intermediary metabolism, stimulation (through bone marrow depression) of a leukopoietic mechanism which may have a genetic flaw, and possible chromosome damage. It has been shown that the drug does cause some chromosome abnormalities in cultured human lymphocytes.[9–11] The hypothesis that bone marrow aplasia plays a role in leukemia is suspect, because phenylbutazone-associated leukemia is not always preceded by an aplastic state.[4,12,13]

PHENYLBUTAZONE AND PHAGOCYTOSIS

Phagocytosis of bacteria and intracellular killing are important functions of polymorphonuclear (PMN) leukocytes. Attempts to identify the exact energetic and metabolic events associated with these functions have shown that phagocytosis is an energy-requiring process, and the energy for actual engulfment probably comes from increased anaerobic glycolysis.[14] Intracellular killing, as it is discussed elsewhere in this Symposium, appears to be related to oxidative events, including increased oxygen consumption, increased flow of glucose through the hexose-monophosphate pathway (HMP), and increased formation of H_2O_2.[14,15]

Phenylbutazone inhibits the engulfment of particles by both guinea pig[16] and human[17] PMN leukocytes. The probable mechanism appears to be inhibition of glycolysis. It inhibits the oxidation of glucose-6-phosphate (G-6-P) by affecting G-6-P dehydrogenase (G-6-PD), the first step in the HMP.[16] This results in increased intracellular G-6-P, which inhibits hexokinase[18] and suppresses glucose intake. However, a mechanical factor involved in the inhibitory mechanism has not been excluded. The possibility that the drug coats the leukocyte or bacterial surface and interferes with the migration ability of the cell should be considered. Such attention appears to be more appropriate after Ward[19] reported that phenylbutazone suppressed chemotaxis.

The inhibition of G-6-PD and also 6-phospho-gluconate dehydrogenase (6-P-GD) results in a decrease in reduced $NADP^+$ cofactor. That phenylbutazone apparently has no significant effect on the reduction of O_2 to H_2O_2 directly indicates that suppression of intracellular killing is due to the drug's effect on G-6-PD and 6-P-GD.[16,17] In addition, it has been shown that phenylbutazone stabilizes the lysosomes,[20] which may further interfere with the killing effect of PMN leukocytes.[16]

It must be noted that these in vitro experiments were performed using drug concentrations far in excess of the blood levels reached with therapeutic doses. We have investigated the effect of phenylbutazone on the glucose metabolism of PMN leukocytes within 8 hours after patients with rheumatoid arthritis or normal volunteers had taken a large dose (Figure 2). The patients had been

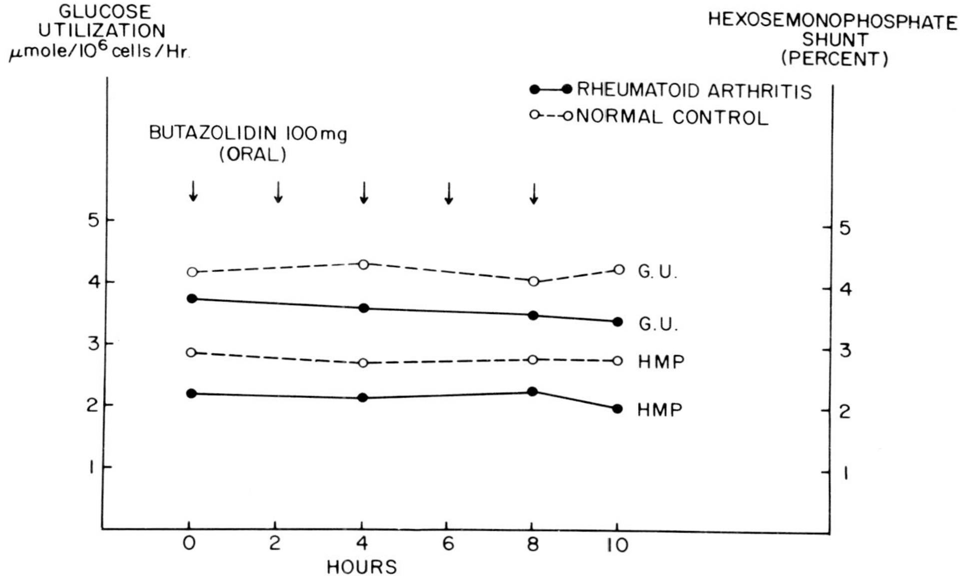

Fig. 2. Effect of phenylbutazone on glucose metabolism of PMN leukocytes. Each group represents the mean of three experiments. Patients with rheumatoid arthritis have been on phenylbutazone (300 mg a day for more than 3 weeks) with no change in peripheral leukocyte count. Leukocyte separation in vitro and determination of glucose utilization (GU) and hexosemonophosphate shunt (HMP) are previously described.[38, 39]

taking phenylbutazone for more than 10 days before the experiment. As is seen in the diagram, lower glucose utilization in patients with rheumatoid arthritis, compared to normal controls, may be a metabolic deficiency. Metabolically abnormal leukocytes in patients with rheumatoid arthritis have been previously described.[21] The usual clinical dose of phenylbutazone should not result in abnormal leukocyte function, as shown in the figure.

PHENYLBUTAZONE AND LYMPHOCYTES

The effect of phenylbutazone on human lymphocytes appears to differ from that on PMN leukocytes, in that in high doses it does not affect oxygen consumption and stimulates the uptake of glucose by human lymphocytes.[22] The reason for this controversial finding is not clear.

Wissmuller has extensively studied the cytogenetic effect of phenylbutazone on cultured human lymphocytes.[9–11] In therapeutic concentrations, the drug prevents cells from starting mitosis and induces a number of chromosomal aberrations. Investigation of this effect with regard to possible interference with the immune response is indicated. If the drug exerts similar cytogenetic effects on leukocytes from the granulocytic series, it may help explain some hematologic toxicities.

We have examined the influence of phenylbutazone on several aspects of lymphocyte metabolism. Some inhibition of RNA and protein synthesis of human lymphocytes, using labeled formate in the presence of phenylbutazone, has been observed (Table 2). Similar experiments performed with bone marrow cultures might offer a better explanation for the effect of phenylbutazone on leukocyte precursors. In these experiments, as in the others with PMN leukocytes, concentrations of the drug exceeded the therapeutic dose in man.

As we mentioned before, it has been shown that phenylbutazone stabilized

Table 2
The Influence of Phenylbutazone upon the In Vitro Synthesis of Serine, RNA, and Protein by Human Lymphocytes

Concentration of Phenylbutazone in Vitro (mg/ml)	^{14}C-Formate Incorporation into		
	Serine	RNA	Protein
0 (Control)	100%	100%	100%
0.1	78±8	69±5	100±11
0.2	101±12	58±4	80±9
0.4	90±13	22±7	8±6
1.0	71±8	9±4	2±2

0.6×10^8 lymphocytes were incubated at 37° C with 10 μCi ^{14}C-formate (specific activity 59 mCi/mM) for 4 hours in a Krebs-Ringer-bicarbonate buffer, pH 7.4, supplemented with 6.7 mM glucose and 1% gelatin. The ^{14}C-incorporation in serine, RNA, and protein in control vials was 1.86×10^6 dpm, 0.79×10^6 and 0.60×10^6 dpm respectively. The results are averages of three incubations and are given as means ± SE.

Table 3
The In Vitro Effect of Phenylbutazone on ATPase Activities of Human Lymphocyte Homogenates

Concentration of Phenylbutazone In Vitro (mg/ml)	Supernatant ATPase (Oligomycin-Sensitive ATPase) μmoles P_i/mg protein/30 min
0	0.36±0.17
0.5	0.37±0.17
1.0	0.31±0.07
10.0	0.13±0.09

Normal human lymphocytes were incubated in vitro with various concentrations of phenylbutazone. After incubation, the cells were homogenized and the ATPase activity of the homogenates determined.[23]

the membrane of some subcellular constituents. ATPase activity participates in a variety of the biochemical reactions taking place in the cell membrane, cytoplasm, and nucleus. We investigated the effect of phenylbutazone on the ATPase activity of human lymphocyte homogenates (Table 3). As in all other experiments, significant inhibition in vitro was achieved only with high concentrations of drug. It is interesting that the supernatant of the homogenate did not show significant inhibition of ATPase activity in the presence of relatively high concentrations of phenylbutazone (1.0 mg/ml). Inhibition occurred only at excessively high concentrations (10 mg/ml). This fraction, obtained after centrifugation of lymphocyte homogenate, is believed to contain mitochondrial ATPase,[23] a finding that may indirectly indicate that phenylbutazone, at therapeutic doses, has no effect on mitochondrial membranes. Further studies are indicated to establish this more clearly.

Whatever the mechanisms involved in the effect of phenylbutazone on PMN leukocytes and lymphocytes, the in vitro experiments cited herein can only lead to suggestion and speculation. When all aspects of the drug are evaluated, conclusions can be more definite. This includes, by all means, dosage, absorption, fate, and excretion of the drug in relation to its toxic effects. Phenylbutazone has a variety of pharmacologic activities. Therefore, its effects on the patient and on isolated organs or systems can be expected to be many and varied. This is especially true of the hematopoietic system where phenylbutazone exerts its most severe toxic effects. In view of the widespread use of this drug, further investigation of its effects on blood cells, both clinically and experimentally, is clearly indicated.

REFERENCES

1. Burns JJ, Yu T'sai-Fan, Dayton PG, et al: Biochemical and pharmacological considerations of phenylbutazone and its analogues. Ann NY Acad Sci 86:253, 1960
2. Woodbury DM: Analgesic-antipyretics, anti-inflammatory agents and inhibitors of uric acid synthesis, The Pharmacological Basis of Therapeutics. Fourth

edition. Edited by LS Goodman, A Gilman. Philadelphia, Saunders, 1970, p 335
3. Mauer EF: Toxic effects of phenylbutazone (Butazolidine). N Engl J Med 253:404, 1955
4. McCarthy DD, Chalmers TM: Hematological complications of phenylbutazone therapy: review of the literature and report of two cases. Can Med Assoc J 90:1061, 1964
5. Abatt JD, Lea AJ: Leukaemogens. Lancet 2:880, 1958
6. Lea AJ: Association between the rheumatic disease and the reticuloses. Ann Rheum Dis 23:480, 1964
7. Innis HD: Latex fixation test in myeloid leukaemia. Lancet 2:947, 1963
8. Hamer JW, Gunz FW: Multiple aetiological factors in a case of acute leukaemia. NZ Med J 71:141, 1970
9. Wissmuller H, Gebhart E: Cytogenetic effects of butazolidine in human leukocytes in vitro. Newsletter Environ Mutagen Soc 3:28, 1970.
10. Wissmuller H: Untersuchungen uber die cytogentische Wirkung von phenylbutazon on menschlicken. Arzneim Forsch 11:1738, 1971
11. Wissmuller H: Zur spezifischen Wirkung von phenylbutazon auf die Mitose menschlicher lymphocyten in vitro. Humangenetik 12:330, 1971
12. Bean RHD: Phenylbutazone and leukemia: a possible association. Br Med J 2:1569, 1960
13. Jensen MK, Roll K: Phenylbutazone and leukemia. Acta Med Scand 178:505, 1964
14. Sbarra AJ, Karnovsky M: The biochemical basis of phagocytosis. I. Metabolic changes during the ingestion of particles of PMN leukocytes. J Biol Chem 234:1355, 1959
15. Iyer GYN, Quastel JH: Biochemical aspects of phagocytosis. Nature 192:535, 1961
16. Strauss RR, Paul BB, Sbarra AJ: Effect of phenylbutazone on phagocytosis and intracellular killing by guinea pig PMN leukocytes. J Bacteriol 96:1982, 1968
17. Kvarstein B, Stormorken H: Influence of acetylsalicylic acid, butazolidine, colchicine, hydrocortisone, chlorpromazine, and imipramine on the phagocytosis of polystyrene latex particles by human leukocytes. Biochem Pharmacol 20:1, 1971
18. Mayer SE, Mayfield AC, Haas JA: Heart muscle hexokinase: subcellular distribution and inhibition by glucose-6-phosphate. Mol Pharmacol 2:393, 1966
19. Ward PA: Leukotactic factors in health and disease. Am J Patholol 64:521, 1971
20. Weissman G: Lysosomes and joint disease. Arthritis Rheum 9:834, 1966
21. Dimitrov NV, Stjernholm R, Weir DR: Metabolic deviations of polymorphonuclear leukocytes in rheumatoid arthritis. Blut 19:139, 1969
22. McCurrach PH, Park JK, Perry WLM: The effects of some drugs which induce agranulocytosis on the metabolism of separated human PMN leukocytes and lymphocytes. Br J Pharmacol 38:608, 1970
23. Dimitrov NV, Ellegaard J: Elevated lymphocyte adenosine triphosphatase activity in patients with gastrointestinal carcinoma. N Engl J Med 286:353, 1972
24. Scheurer-Karpin R: Phenylbutazone and leukemia. Z Ges Inn Med 13:416, 1958
25. Cast IP: Phenylbutazone and leukemia. Br Med J 2:1569, 1961
26. Garrett JV: Phenylbutazone and leukaemia. Br Med J 1:53, 1961
27. Cadman EFB, Limont W: Phenylbutazone and leukaemia. Br Med J 1:798, 1962
28. Thorpe GJ: Leukaemia and phenylbutazone. Br Med J 1:1707, 1964

29. Sen S, Hyder Siddique KK: Phenylbutazone and Leukemia. Bull Inst Post Grad Med Educ Res 6:23, 1964
30. Hart GD: Leukaemia and phenylbutazone. Br Med J 2:2569, 1964
31. Chalmers TM, McCarthy DD: Phenylbutazone therapy associated with leukemia. Br Med J 1:747, 1964
32. Woodliff HJ, Dougan L: Acute leukemia associated with phenylbutazone treatment. Br Med J 1:744, 1964
33. Chatterjea JB: Leukaemia and phenylbutazone. Br Med J 2:875, 1964
34. Golding JR, Hamilton MG, Moody HE: Monocytic leukaemia and phenylbutazone. Br Med J 5451:1673, 1965
35. Dougan L, Woodliff HJ: Acute leukaemia associated with phenylbutazone treatment: a review of the literature and report of a further case. Med J Aust 1:217, 1965
36. Perers D, Sjoberg SG: Akut leukemia leukemoid reaktion och leukocytes after behandling med oxifenylbutazon. Sv Lakartidn 63:53, 1966
37. Fraumeni JF: Bone marrow depression induced by chloramphenicol or phenylbutazone. Leukemia and other sequelae. JAMA 201:828, 1967
38. Dimitrov NV, Miller J, Ziegra SR: The effects of caffeine on glucose metabolism of polymorphonuclear leukocytes. J Pharmacol Exp Ther 168:240, 1969
39. Dimitrov NV, Douwes FR, Bartolotta B, et al: Studies of the metabolic activity of polymorphonuclear leukocytes in sickle cell anemia. Acta Hematol 47:283, 1972

Anthony V. Pisciotta

20 The Effect of Chlorpromazine on Peripheral Leukocytes

Agranulocytosis is a rare, though troublesome complication of treatment with phenothiazine derivatives.[1,2] In some forms of drug-induced granulocytopenia, an aberrant immunologic mechanism may play a role. In contrast, agranulocytosis attributed to phenothiazines appears to develop after decompensated cellular proliferation, when cells with limited proliferative potential come in contact with a toxic drug. Since phenothiazine-induced agranulocytosis is asymptomatic unless overwhelming infection gains a foothold, physicians who use these drugs in large quantities for prolonged time periods must be alert to its possible occurrence.

The incidence of phenothiazine-induced agranulocytosis was estimated at the Mental Health Center-North Division between 1960 and 1968 (Table 1). Six routine weekly leukocyte counts were made on all patients between the second and eighth week after treatment with phenothiazines was started. A total of 37,940 counts were made on about 6300 patients. Of this number, about 1851 episodes of leukopenia were recorded in 310 patients, or a ratio of 1 to 20 (Table 2). This was not agranulocytosis because granulocytes persisted in peripheral blood, and the patients recovered as treatment was continued. This experience is similar to that reported by Mandel and Gross[3] in which the degree of leukopenia was related to the dose of phenothiazine. In our own patients, 5 with agranulocytosis were identified while they were still asymptomatic. From 1960 to 1968, a ratio of 1 case of agranulocytosis per 1250 patients treated was estimated. Of these 5 patients, 4 recovered completely when the drug was discontinued, but 1 died from overwhelming infection. These results were compared to those obtained at the Mental Health Center-South Division, which is a nursing and custodial care facility for chronically ill mental patients. Phenothiazines are also used at this Hospital, but weekly leukocyte counts to monitor toxicity were not made. During this same time period, 10 patients with agranulocytosis were recognized after symptoms of sore throat, chills, and fever developed. Of these patients, 7 died of overwhelming infection, which gained a foothold during

Aided by Research Grant RO-1 Ca 05524 from the National Cancer Institute.

Table 1
Agranulocytosis Case Finding
Mental Health Center—North Division

Year	No. of WBC	No. with Leukopenia	No. with Agranulocytosis
1960	4702	275	0
1961	3905	214	0
1962	4734	243	2
1963	4228	213	0
1964	3707	182	2
1965	3594	192	0
1966	3477	211	1
1967	4872	162	0
1968	4721	159	0
Total	37,940	1851	5

White blood counts weekly from week 2 to 8 on all patients treated with phenothiozines.

the asymptomatic period of leukopenia. The importance of agranulocytosis is, therefore, related chiefly to the fact that if unrecognized in its early stages, it may terminate fatally (Table 3).

The clinical and hematologic changes characteristic of phenothiazine-induced granulocytopenia suggest a number of possibilities regarding the pathogenesis of this drug reaction. Agranulocytosis induced by phenothiazines involves a complete loss of all mature polymorphonuclear leukocytes from peripheral blood after a latent period of no less than 10 or 20 days, during which substantial amounts of the drug are given. In some cases, one may readminister phenothiazine in lower doses without an immediate recurrence of agranulocytosis, but this drug reaction would almost always recur provided enough drug is given for a sufficient period of time. In view of these relationships, one might surmise that the toxicity of phenothiazine is more closely related to a disturbance in the development of bone marrow precursors rather than to peripheral destruction of blood cells. To support this notion, the bone marrow in phenothiazine-induced agranulocytosis appears morphologically aplastic and consists only of fat spaces and a few scattered round cells, but neither granulocyte precursors nor normoblasts

Table 2
Incidence of Agranulocytosis: Mental Health Center-North Division

Approximate number of patients treated 1960–1968	6300
Estimated projected through 1972	9100
Number of leukopenic patients 1960–1968	310
Ratio of leukopenia to patients treated	1:20
Number of agranulocytosis	5
Ratio of agranulocytosis to patients treated 1960–1968	1:1260
Estimated ratio, projected through 1972	1:1820

Table 3
Results of Agranulocytosis Case Finding
1960–1968

	Number of Weekly WBC	
	North Division	South Division
No. with Agranulocytosis	5	10
No. of Deaths	1	7
Per cent Dead	20	70

(Figure 1). Infiltration with lymphocytes, occurring as it does 3 or 4 days after the drug is discontinued,[4] is interpreted as signifying an event in recovery hypothetically related to a stem cell function rather than as an expression of altered cellular immunity attributed to some lymphocytes. For these reasons, most of our studies were directed to the characteristics of bone marrow cell proliferation in phenothiazine-sensitive and normal patients.

THE EFFECTS OF CHLORPROMAZINE ON PERIPHERAL LEUKOCYTES

The effects of drugs on living cells in tissue culture must be interpreted with great caution. Many drugs are toxic and will damage or kill all living cells at a certain concentration. Furthermore, since mechanisms for detoxication or excretion to toxic products do not exist in tissue culture models, the cells are con-

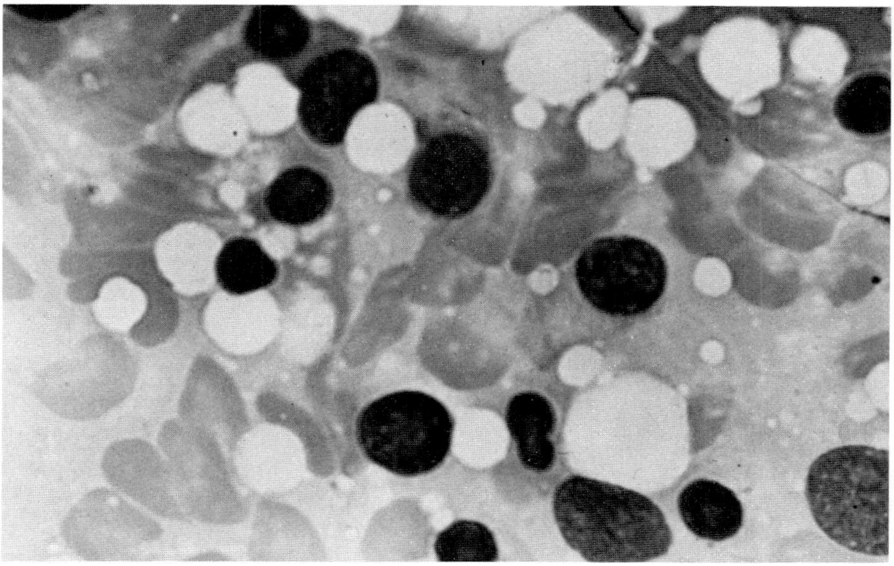

Fig. 1. Bone marrow during phenothiazine-induced agranulocytosis. Only cells present are lymphocytes and fat cells (× 1000).

Table 4
Effect of Chlorpromazine on Indices of Cell Viability

Function	Inhibitory Concentration	Noninhibitory Concentration
Motility	10^{-4}M	10^{-5}M
Incorporation of ^{35}S-L-cystine and L-methionine	10^{-3}M	2×10^{-4}M
Hemolysis	10^{-3}M	2×10^{-4}M
Redox	10^{-3}M	2×10^{-4}M
Trypan blue exclusion	10^{-3}M	10^{-4}M
WBC respiration	4×10^{-4}M	2×10^{-4}M
Phagocytosis-induced CO_2 release	10^{-4}M	10^{-5}M

tinually bathed in the drug. In addition, nonspecific changes, such as alterations in pH or binding of drug to cell or serum protein, might be manifested as drug toxicity. For these reasons, preliminary studies are necessary to define the limits of in vitro drug toxicity. Studies performed on the viability of living cells included observations on cell motility, phagocytosis, protein synthesis, redox potential, cellular respiration, and glycolytic metabolism (Table 4). Studies on cellular motility were performed, using phase contrast microscopy, by observing the number of motile cells which remained after 1 hour contact with varying molar concentrations of CPZ (Figure 2). At 10^{-5}M, cellular motility was the same as control values. At 10^{-4}M, 39% of the cells were motile. The toxic concentration for this white cell function is somewhere between these two points. The phagocytic index was estimated after heparinized whole blood was incubated with latex particles in the presence of various concentrations of CPZ (Table 5). No significant difference was observed in the number of cells containing particles in the controls and in preparations with CPZ, 10^{-3}M. Further preliminary studies disclosed that CPZ, 2×10^{-4}, did not affect the incorporation of ^{35}S-L-cystine or L-methionine into protein,[5] nor was there any change in the concentration of reduced glutathione at this dosage level.[6] A similar concentration of CPZ did not affect the rate of reduction of the redox dye, dichlorophenol-

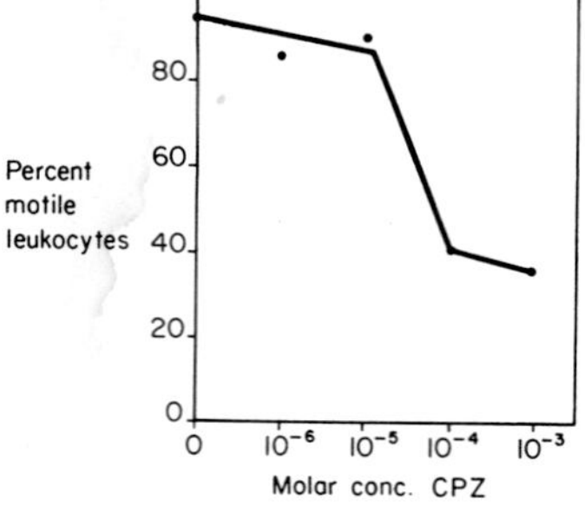

Fig. 2. Effect of various concentrations of CPZ on leukocyte motility. Observations made by phase contrast microscopy after 1-hour incubation at 37° with CPZ.

Table 5
Effect of CPZ on Phagocytic Index

Concentration of CPZ(M)	Leukocytes with Latex Particles (%)
No drug	68
10^{-6}	47
10^{-5}	57
10^{-4}	40
10^{-3}	60

indophenol, and the exclusion of trypan blue from viable leukocytes continued at control levels of 10^{-4}M.

Addition of chlorpromazine to a suspension of leukocytes had a slight effect on respiration at 2×10^{-4}M where about 15% of the O_2 consumption was suppressed. A concentration of 4×10^{-4}M had a more pronounced effect, since almost 30% of the O_2 consumption was inhibited (Figure 3). Related to this study is an experiment in which the effect of CPZ on the hexose monophosphate shunt (HMP) was evaluated. To accomplish this, human leukocytes were incubated with latex particles. As phagocytosis proceeds, the HMP shunt is activated with a burst of respiratory activity. If ^{14}C-1-glucose is added to the reaction mixture, $^{14}CO_2$ is released during phagocytosis, which can then be collected on filter paper strips impregnated with potassium hydroxide and counted in a liquid scintillation spectrometer. McIntyre[7] used this method to test serum for antileukocyte antibodies, since these substances may inhibit leukocyte function. In our study, a CPZ-sensitive patient's serum alone failed to inhibit the release of $^{14}CO_2$ under the conditions of this experiment. However, when CPZ 10^{-4}M was added in balanced salt solution or in combination with patient's or normal serum, a 38% inhibition of $^{14}CO_2$ release was observed (Table 6). Although these studies fail to demonstrate a humoral substance (antibody?) in

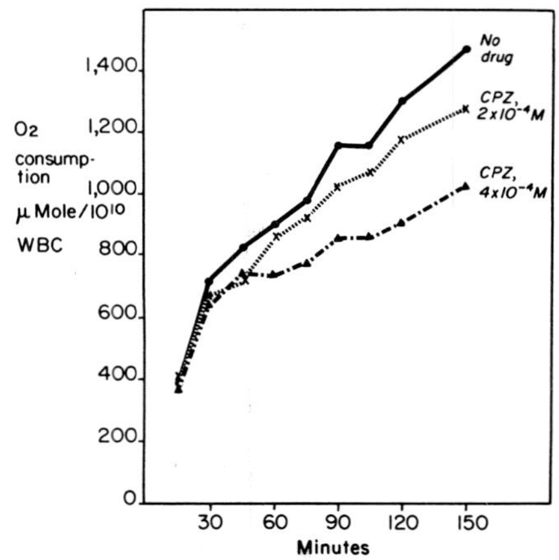

Fig. 3. Effect of CPZ on leukocyte respiration. Drug added at beginning of experiment.

Table 6
Effect of CPZ on $^{14}CO_2$ Release During Phagocytosis

CPZ Concentration (M)	CPM $^{14}CO_2$	Per cent Inhibition
0	845	0
1×10^{-5}	553	65
2.5×10^{-5}	458	54
5×10^{-5}	440	52
1×10^{-4}	498	59

Table 7
Effect of Serum-CPZ Combination on $^{14}CO_2$ Release During Phagocytosis

Combination	CPM	Per cent Inhibition
Patient Serum + No Drug	1491	
Patient Serum + CPZ (10^{-4}M)	566	38
Normal Serum + No Drug	1160	
Normal Serum + CPZ	136	12
Anti-WBC Serum + No Drug	309	27
Anti-WBC Serum + CPZ	25	8

serum from CPZ-sensitive patients, they confirm that at a concentration of 10^{-5}M, CPZ will significantly inhibit the release of $^{14}CO_2$ connected with activation of the HMP shunt during phagocytosis (Table 7). Increasing the concentration of CPZ to amounts greater than 10^{-3}M had a distinctive membrane effect, since erythrocytes were hemolyzed at this concentration. Accordingly, all subsequent studies were conducted at a concentration of 8×10^{-5}M or less, even though this exceeded therapeutic blood levels. Studies conducted on peripheral blood cells fail to disclose a specific effect of CPZ other than that explained by cellular toxicity. From an immunologic standpoint, serum from CPZ-sensitive patients, alone or in combination with the drug, failed to provide evidence of leukagglutination, leukolysis, or inhibition of phagocytosis-induced HMP activity.

EFFECT OF CPZ ON CELL DIVISION

The idea that CPZ retards cell division has found support in the delayed onset of agranulocytosis after treatment is started and the morphologically aplastic marrow characteristic of this disease, as well as of a number of experimental animal and tissue culture models. Again, the hazards of interpreting effects of CPZ in tissue culture models have been expressed in terms of its toxicity. Treatment of fertilized eggs with CPZ has slowed embryonic growth in chickens[8] and in axolotl embryos.[9] In intact animals, CPZ retards weight gain when given to newborn rats[10] and baby chicks; when given to pregnant mice, smaller litters with lower mean litter weights result.[11]

Our own experiments deal with the effects of CPZ on the proliferation of PHA-stimulated peripheral blood lymphocytes[12] and on human bone marrow cells in short-term[13] and 2-week culture systems. When phytohemagglutinin (PHA) is added to peripheral blood lymphocytes, they enlarge, undergo blast transformation, DNA synthesis, and mitosis. If CPZ is added, there is partial suppression of 'blast transformation and mitotic index,' which is restored to control values after dialysis of a CPZ–PHA mixture.[12] Sonicates prepared from PHA-stimulated lymphocytes show diminished DNA polymerase activity, which relates to drug concentration. Experiments with tritiated CPZ discloses adherence of CPZ to membranes of proliferating cells.[14]

In the presence of PHA, 8.7% of the added PHA was incorporated in a 72-hour culture and 6.2% after 1 hour. Where PHA was omitted, 5.5% was incorporated in a 72-hour culture and 4.6% in the 1-hour culture. Of this amount, half of the CPZ is recoverable in the acid soluble fraction. This is exclusively bound to protein with only a negligible amount bound to nucleic acids. Radioautographs of ^{3}H CPZ-treated white blood counts fail to disclose any accumulation of grains. These studies designate adherence of CPZ to proteins in proliferating cells.

SHORT-TERM MARROW CULTURE

When human bone marrow cells are first removed from the medullary cavity they continue to live for a short period of time. Cells engaged in DNA synthesis incorporate tritiated thymidine (^{3}H-TdR) into their DNA and become radioactive. This radioactivity can be measured by microradioautography, or by liquid scintillation spectrometry. Although the former technique is laborious, DNA synthesis in specific cell lines and even DNA synthesis in individual cells can be studied. Initial studies were reported on 35 randomly selected patients who were shown not to be sensitive to CPZ.[12,13] When marrow cells were incubated with CPZ (10^{-4}M), incorporation of ^{3}H-TdR was inhibited by 50% or more in half of these patients (Figure 4). The others were not so inhibited. All patients who had had agranulocytosis due to CPZ showed 50% or fewer labeled cells in CPZ-treated cultures. Since many normal people demonstrated fewer labeled

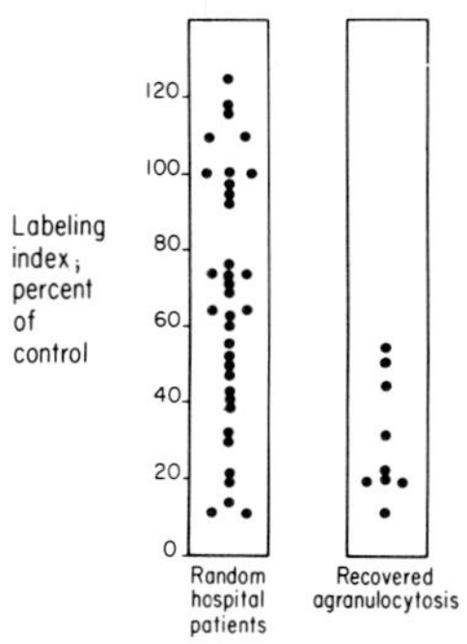

Fig. 4. Effect of CPZ on incorporation of ^{3}H-TdR into bone marrow of 35 random normal and 9 CPZ sensitive patients. Data expressed as per cent of no drug controls. Permission of JAMA.[2]

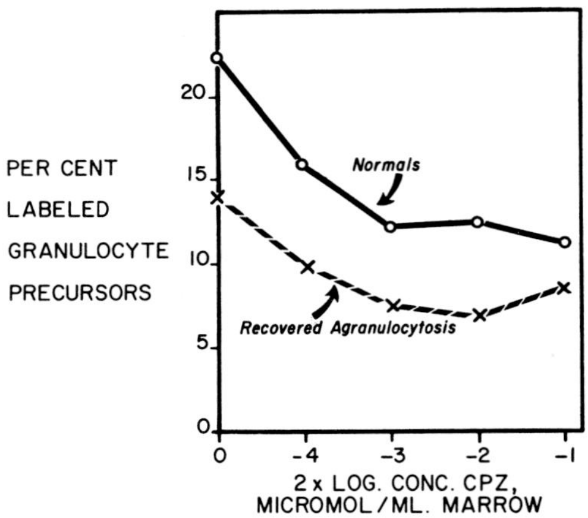

Fig. 5. Effect of four tenfold dilutions of CPZ on incorporation of ^{3}H-TdR into marrow cells. Mean values from 8 normals and 8 CPZ sensitive patients. Permission of JAMA.[2]

cells in the presence of CPZ, the question of a difference in reactivity between normal and drug-sensitive groups to various dilutions of CPZ was considered. When marrow cells from normal and from CPZ-sensitive patients were incubated with various concentrations of CPZ, all preparations were equally inhibited in various dilutions to produce an identical slope depicting inhibition (Figure 5). It appears that the toxicity of CPZ to many living cells suppresses DNA synthesis in culture, an effect that may be compensated for by nonsensitive patients. The unique characteristic that distinguishes CPZ-sensitive patients from normals may be identified in marrow culture even in the absence of CPZ, since this group shows significantly diminished incorporation of ^{3}H-TdR into marrow cells[15,16] (Figure 6). When marrow from normal patients are incubated with ^{3}H-TdR, about 20% of the granulocyte precursors become labeled in the first hour; this increases in linear fashion to about 40% labeling in 5 hours. Chlorpromazine-sensitive patients differ significantly from normal subjects in three respects. At the beginning of incubation, only 10% of the granulocyte precursors show a label.

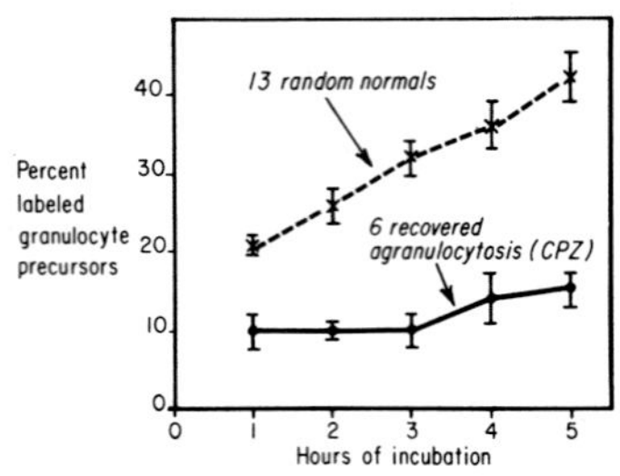

Fig. 6. Incorporation of ^{3}H-TdR into granulocyte precursors following incubation. No CPZ is included in incubation mixture. Data from 13 random normals and 6 CPZ-sensitive patients expressed as mean ± 1 SE. From J Lab Clin Med.[16]

At each time point, significantly fewer labels are observed than normals. At the end of 5 hours, only a negligible increase in labeling index has occurred. This is probably not the result of residual damage sustained from having had agranulocytosis, because patients who had agranulocytosis due to other drugs demonstrate a labeling index pattern similar to that of normal subjects.

Suppression of DNA synthesis involves a serious disturbance in one of the events that characterize the cell cycle. The cell cycle involves a short period of mitosis, followed by a rest period during which time apparently nothing demonstrable is going on in the cell (G_1). The cell may be totally dormant during this time (G_0) or it may be synthesizing enzymes required for DNA synthesis later on. The S phase of the cycle is characterized by DNA synthesis; at this period, cells acquire a ^3H label which represents the incorporation of ^3H-TdR into DNA. At the end of the S phase, the cell enters a second rest period, designated G_2, characterized by apparent quiescence but by doubled nuclear DNA content. This is soon followed by mitosis, with the distribution of equal amounts of DNA to each of the daughter cells. The diminished labeling index in CPZ sensitivity designates a disturbance in cell cycle kinetics interpreted in one of several ways. There may be fewer cells in cycle (G_0) or there may be a disturbance in DNA synthesis in individual cells because of enzymatic deficiency. An effect of cell cycle disturbance may be demonstrated by simply counting the number of mitotic figures per 1000 granulocyte precursors in direct marrow smears. In normal subjects, a mitotic index of 6–14 is obtained. In CPZ-sensitive patients, significantly fewer mitotic figures are noted; 2 to 6 per 1000 granulocyte precursors.[16] Additional studies were performed in cooperation with Dr. Ellen Raasch.[17] Microspectrophotometric observations were made on nonlabeled cells only (Table 8). In Feulgen-stained smears of marrow cells, after incubation with ^3H-TdR, preparations from normal individuals showed that 48% to 83% of the cells were in G_1 and 17% to 52% were in G_2 phase. In contrast, cells from CPZ-sensitive patients were 91% to 100% in G_1 and 0 to 9% in G_2 phase. The data, therefore, show that CPZ-sensitive patients have fewer S and M phase cells but more G_1 cells than normal. Further information depicting individual cellular synthesis of DNA was derived by making individual grain counts

Table 8
Microspectrophotometric Analysis of
Nonlabeled Granulocyte Precursors

Group	G_1(%)	G_2(%)
Normals	48	52
	62	38
	63	37
	83	17
	75	25
CPZ Sentitive	100	0
	91	9
	93	7
	92	8
	$p < .05$	

per cell after incubation with ^{3}H-TdR (0.3 μCi/per millimole) with film exposure time of only 3 days. The labeled cells were arbitrarily divided into lightly labeled (5–45 grains per cell), medium labeled (55–115 grains/cell), and heavily labeled (over 125 grains per cell, Table 9). The data indicate a predominance of medium-labeled cells in normals (59%) as compared with 37% in CPZ-sensitive patients. On the other hand, CPZ-sensitive patients demonstrate a predominance of lightly labeled cells, 41% compared with 20% in normal subjects. These data designate diminished DNA synthesis in individual CPZ-sensitive cells, which results in fewer cells in cycle.

It seems appropriate, at this point, to determine the stage at which the incorporation of TdR into DNA is retarded. Tritiated thymidine, as a starting point for TMP synthesis, is a minor salvage pathway. Under physiologic conditions, TMP is derived predominantly from dUMP, which is methylated in carbon 5 with tetrahydrofolic acid as methyl donor under the direction of thymidylate synthetase. From then on, both pathways for DNA synthesis are identical. With phosphate groups derived from ATP, TMP, TDP, and TTP are sequentially produced. TTP is then incorporated into DNA together with the other purine and pyrimidine triphosphates, with the release of pyrophosphate. To test which phase of DNA synthesis is compromised, bone marrow cells were incubated with ^{3}H-TdR for exactly 1 hour, then washed thoroughly, and sonicated into buffered sucrose. The sonicates were extracted three times with hot 5% perchloric acid. The acid-soluble supernate, consisting of unconverted TdR, its breakdown products, TMP, TDP, and TTP, were passed through a column, and separated from each other for counting in a liquid scintillation spectrometer. The total nucleotide counts were readjusted to relate to 10^{7} labeled cells and showed no difference between normal and CPZ-sensitive cells. Also, the yield of radioactive TMP, TDP, and TTP was similar in both groups. It may be concluded from these data that an adequate mechanism for nucleotide phosphorylation exists in CPZ-sensitive marrow cells (Figure 7a and b).

However, a striking difference was found when specific activity of radioactive DNA was extracted from acid insoluble residue. The preparation from CPZ-sensitive patients showed a mean incorporation of 19 $\mu\mu$ moles TdR into 100 μg DNA, as contrasted with 67 μg in normal subjects ($p<0.01$) (Figure 8a). Since cells that show a label are the only ones that synthesize DNA, a potential

Table 9
Classification of Labeled Cells According to Intensity of Labeling with ^{3}H-TdR

	Number of Cells That Show:			
	5–45 Grains (Lightly Labeled)	55–115 Grains (Medium Labeled)	Over 125 Grains (Heavy Labeled)	Totals
Normals	207	604	215	1,026
CPZ Sensitive	146	131	80	357

$X^2 = 69.32$; $DF = 2$; $p < 0.001$

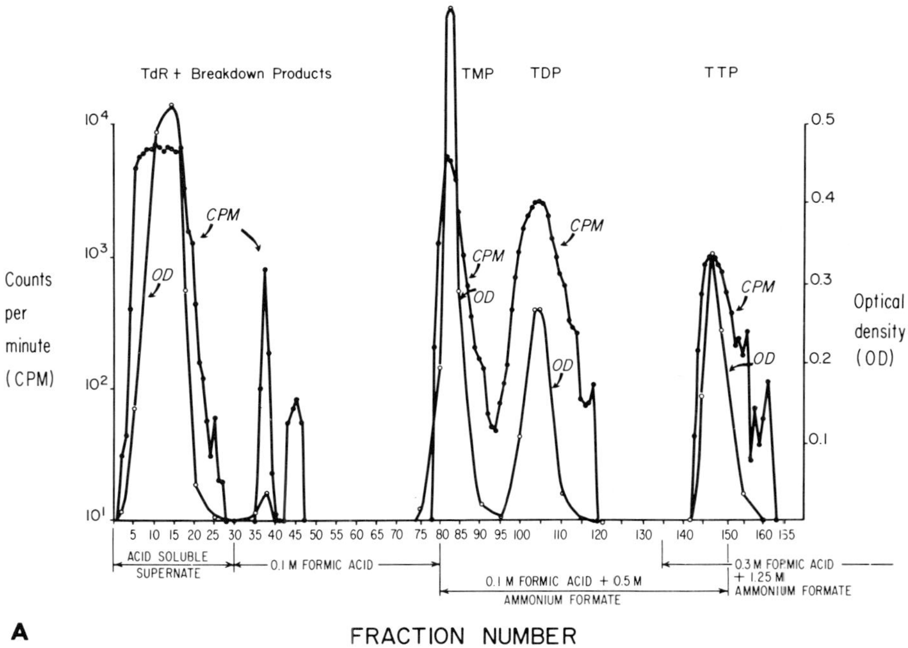

Fig. 7. Yield of intermediate substrates ^{3}H-TdR, TMP, TDP, and TTP after incubation of marrow cells with ^{3}H-TdR for 1 hour. **Fig. 7A.** Normal subject.

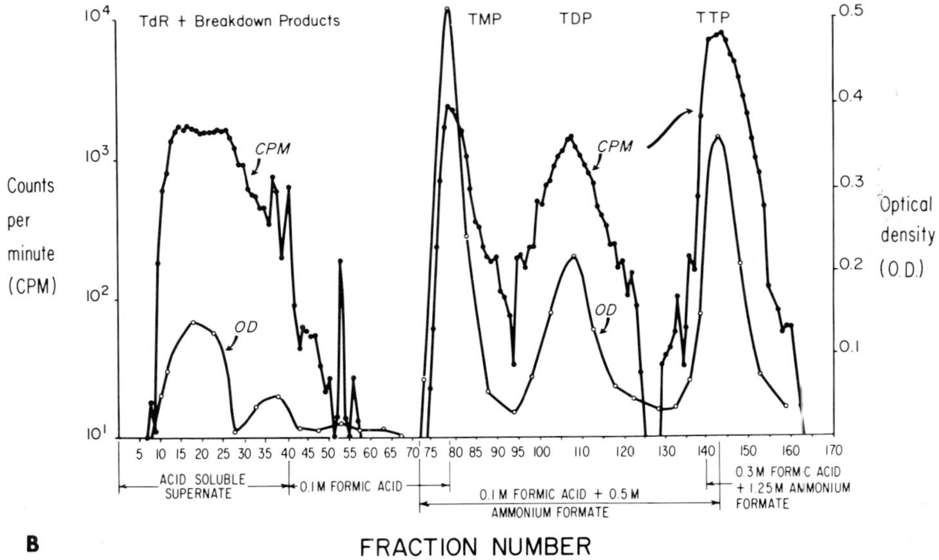

Fig. 7B. CPZ sensitive patient.

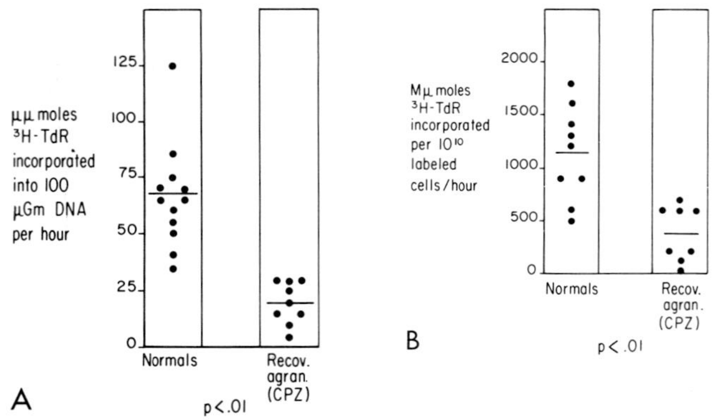

Fig. 8. Incorporation of ^{3}H-TdR into normals and CPZ-sensitive patients in 1 hour. **Fig. 8A.** Specific activity of DNA. **Fig. 8B.** Incorporation of ^{3}H-TdR per 10^{10} labeled marrow cells per hour. From J Lab Clin Med.[16]

source of error exists in the form of dilution with nonradioactive DNA from cells not in "S" phase. Even here, the data were recalculated in terms of TdR incorporated into 10^{10} labeled cells per hour (Figure 8b). There was a significant difference between both groups, depicting a disturbance in the final stages of DNA synthesis. Chlorpromazine-sensitive patients incorporated 382 mμ moles per 10^{10} labeled cells while normals yielded 1135 mμ moles per 10^{10} labeled cells ($p<0.01$). Since this stage is controlled by DNA polymerase, the data suggest that CPZ-sensitive patients are deficient in this enzyme.

LONG-TERM CULTURE OF MARROW CELLS ON AGAR GEL

A direct assay of DNA polymerase is not yet possible in marrow cell sonicates because contamination with nucleases preclude this procedure. For this reason, an indirect approach was taken to estimate repair function in marrow cells after ultraviolet irradiation and then cultured on agar gel over a feeder layer which consisted of normal human leukocytes. If DNA polymerase is deficient, then repair function after ultraviolet irradiation should be curtailed. Before incubation, some of the marrow cells were irradiated with ultraviolet, 88 ergs per square millimeter. Control preparations were subjected to room light for the same time period. The irradiated and nonmarrow cells were incubated with various dilutions of CPZ for 14 days. Granulocyte colonies were counted using the inverted phase microscope. The results are depicted in Figure 9. Normal individuals developed 35 colonies, which were not significantly diminished after ultraviolet irradiation but which were partially suppressed in CPZ, 5×10^{-5}M. A patient with agranulocytosis showed 12 colonies in the control preparation which was diminished further by ultraviolet irradiation to 3 and which were eliminated altogether by incubation in CPZ. These preliminary studies designate a limited

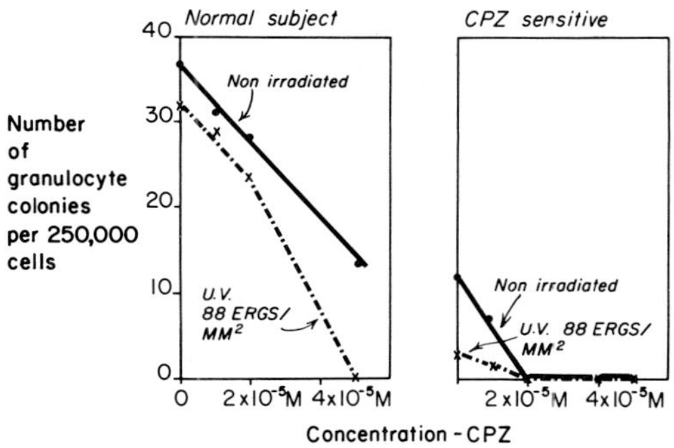

Fig. 9. Effect of CPZ and ultraviolet irradiation on development of granulocyte colonies on agar gel.

potential to form granulocyte colonies which is extremely sensitive to CPZ or ultraviolet irradiation, alone or in combinations. Since the CPZ-sensitive patient developed fewer colonies in the absence of drug, a smaller concentration of CPZ was adequate to eliminate colony formation altogether. This study also suggests that CPZ marrow cells have a limited ability to undergo repair from ultraviolet damage, especially in the presence of CPZ, suggesting a possible defect in repair enzyme activity.

DISCUSSION

Our studies confirm that a CPZ-sensitive population is incapable of regulated cell growth due to limited DNA synthesis. These patients apparently get along well apart from the infirmities of old age or of mental illness. They have a sufficient proliferative potential to resist infection and to develop leukocytosis on proper stimulation. Other sites, in which there is rapid turnover of cells, such as intestinal epithelium, apparently are normal in function. These patients get along well until they come in contact with a drug capable of tying up whatever little DNA synthesis they have. This would result in a proliferative standstill with loss of the most rapidly proliferative cells—the granulocytes. Chlorpromazine may affect many cellular functions, chiefly in a nonspecific manner. Any of these disturbances in cellular function may conceivably affect cell division. Chlorpromazine has a propensity to bind to soluble proteins derived from mammalian parenchyma to result in denaturation. If the protein happens to have enzymatic properties, that function may be lost. A large body of data has been published to show interference with enzyme function of various specificities in both in vitro and in vivo models. Chlorpromazine has a pronounced membrane effect which permits the enhanced passage of certain macromolecules through the membrane. Conceivably, certain substrates, vital to cell function, could be lost in this manner. At low pH, CPZ combines with polynucleotides to result in their precipitation and loss to participate in DNA synthesis. Finally, CPZ may uncouple oxidation phosphorylation and thereby inhibit functions dependent on this process.

SUMMARY

The clinical characteristics of a population sensitive to CPZ have been enumerated. Agranulocytosis is most apt to occur in sensitized women after treatment with large dosages of CPZ over a period of 20–40 days. Since the bone marrow in this reaction is characteristically aplastic, our attention was directed to a possible defect in cell division aggravated by CPZ. Indeed, this drug retarded or eliminated proliferation of normal as well as drug-sensitive bone marrow cells and PHA-stimulated lymphocytes from peripheral blood in culture. Toxic agranulocytosis is postulated to be the result of a proliferative defect inherent in a sensitive patient's marrow precursor cells, which leads to decompensated cell division when the patient is treated with a quantity of drug sufficient to retard what little DNA synthesis is present. The marrow cells of CPZ-sensitive patients have been uniquely characterized because they manifest a mitotic index lower than that of normal marrow cells. Furthermore, CPZ-sensitive myelocytes are predominantly in G_1 phase and incorporate less ^{3}H-TdR into DNA than do normal cells. Since the CPZ-sensitive marrow cells are capable of phosphorylating TdR through TTP, it is felt that kinase activity is not disturbed. However, the specific activity of DNA extracted after incubation with ^{3}H-TdR is lower than that of normals, indicating limited incorporation of TTP into DNA, a stage catalyzed by DNA polymerase. Preliminary studies, using the agar gel culture technique discloses the formation of fewer colonies using CPZ-sensitive cells than normals. These cells appear to be unusually sensitive to ultraviolet irradiation and to CPZ in the culture media.

REFERENCES

1. Pisciotta AV, Ebbe S, Lennon EG, et al: Agranulocytosis following administration of phenothiazine derivatives. Am J Med 25:210, 1958
2. Pisciotta AV: Agranulocytosis induced by certain phenothiazine derivatives. JAMA 208:1862, 1969
3. Mandel A, Gross M: Agranulocytosis and phenothiazines. Dis Nerv Syst 29:32, 1968
4. Pisciotta AV, Santos AS, Keller C: Studies on agranulocytosis. V. Patterns of recovery from drug-induced bone marrow damage. J Lab Clin Med 63:445, 1964
5. Pisciotta AV, Daly M: Studies on agranulocytosis. III. The reduced glutathione (GSH) content of leukocytes of normals and patients recovered from agranulocytosis. Blood 16:1572, 1960
6. Pisciotta AV, Ebbe SN, Ruwaldt M, et al: Studies on agranulocytosis. II. The effect of granulocytotoxic drugs upon the influx of S-35-L-cystine and L-methionine into human leukocytes. Blood 16:1456, 1960
7. McIntyre PA, Laleli Y, Wagner H Jr: Evidence for anti-leukocyte antibodies as a mechanism for drug induced agranulocytosis. Trans Assoc Am Physicians 84:217, 1971
8. Miller ZB, Pasciutto MC: Lethal effect of chlorpromazine on chick embryo. Proc Soc Exp Biol Med 114:398, 1963
9. Eyal-Giladi HJ, Eyal Z: The effect of chlorpromazine on the embryonic develop-

ment of the axolotl (Ambystroma mexicanum). J Embryol Exp Morphol 10:357, 1962
10. Burn JH: Pharmacology of chlorpromazine and promethazine. Proc R Soc Med 47:617, 1954
11. Ordy JM, Latanick A, Johnson R, et al: Chlorpromazine effects on pregnancy and offspring of mice. Proc Soc Exp Biol Med 113:833, 1963
12. Pisciotta AV, Westring DW, DePrey C: Studies on agranulocytosis. VIII. Inhibition of mitosis in phytohemagglutinin stimulated lymphocytes by chlorpromazine. J Lab Clin Med 70:229, 1967
13. Pisciotta AV, Kaldahl J: Studies on agranulocytosis. IV. Effects of chlorpromazine on nucleic acid synthesis of bone marrow cells in vitro. Blood 20:364, 1962
14. Cohen J, Pisciotta AV: Unpublished data
15. Pisciotta AV: Studies on agranulocytosis. VII. Limited proliferative potential of chlorpromazine sensitive patients. J Lab Clin Med 65:240, 1965
16. Pisciotta AV, Pawlowski N, Peterson L, et al: Studies on agranulocytosis. IX. A biochemical defect in chlorpromazine-sensitive marrow cells. J Lab Clin Med 78:435, 1971
17. Pisciotta AV, Walz K, Raasch E. Studies on agranulocytosis. X. The microspectrophotometric patterns of chlorpromazine sensitive granulocyte precursors. Unpublished data

Yeon S. Ahn
and Adel A. Yunis

21
Antithyroid Therapy and Leukocytes

The use of antithyroid drugs for the treatment of hyperthyroidism has been associated with a variety of untoward reactions. These included: fever, rash, urticaria, gastrointestinal disturbances, jaundice, arthralgia, lymphadenopathy, lupus-like syndrome, leukopenia, agranulocytosis, and bone marrow aplasia. Among these reactions, the most common is drug fever, and the most serious has been agranulocytosis.

Thiouracil, the first widely used antithyroid compound, was associated with a relatively high frequency of side reactions: 13% overall incidence and 1% agranulocytosis. Thus, thiouracil was discontinued in favor of the new agents, propylthiouracil (PTU) and methimazol (MTZ) (Figure 1), which have a lower incidence of toxicity. From among the various side effects of PTU and MTZ, leukopenia, agranulocytosis, and bone marrow aplasia will be reviewed in this report and the lupus-like syndrome considered briefly.

LEUKOPENIA AND AGRANULOCYTOSIS

Leukopenia in association with antithyroid therapy is well known and its incidence is variable. In their review of the literature in 1955, Vanderlaan and Storrie[1] reported an incidence of 1.1% leukopenia with PTU (27 of 2491 patients treated) and 0.84% with MTZ (8 of 831 patients). However, the incidence varied widely with the series: 0.1%–5.6% with PTU[2–5] and 0–1.5% with MTZ.[3,4,6] Much higher incidences have also been reported. In a study by Wing and Asper,[7] of 203 patients on PTU therapy (150–300 mg daily), leukopenia (WBC $<$ 4000/mm^3) was observed on one or more occasions in 12% of the cases. Most of the episodes were transient and did not require cessation of therapy. In a recently reported series of children receiving antithyroid medication,[8] leukopenia of less than 4000/mm^3 occurred in 26% and of less than 1500/mm^3 in 18%.

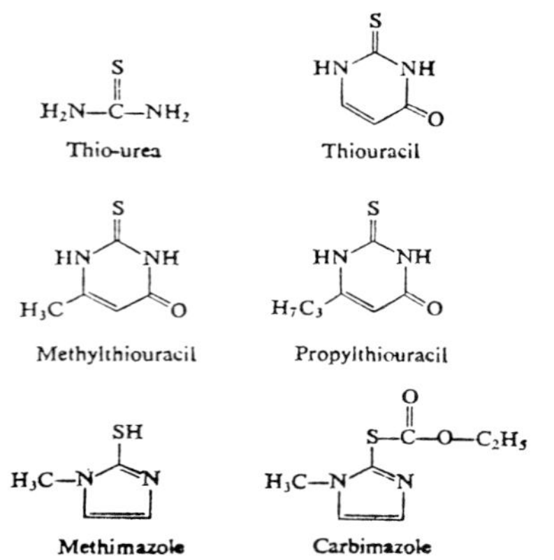

Fig. 1. Chemical structures of antithyroid drugs.

It is clear from all of these reports that mild leukopenia is quite a common occurrence with antithyroid drugs and is often transient. It is therefore expected that the incidence would vary, depending on how often a WBC count is performed during therapy. It should also be pointed out that in many studies, the terms leukopenia and agranulocytosis have been used interchangeably, an additional confusing factor.

Agranulocytosis is defined as a symptom-complex characterized by an acute onset of fever, agranulocytic angina, and profound granulocytopenia without changes in red cells or platelets. Not all reported cases of agranulocytosis from antithyroid drugs conform to this definition; most showed granulocytopenia of varying degree without sore throat or other signs of infection. As stated above, the term leukopenia is more applicable to such cases. The reported incidence of agranulocytosis has also varied: 0.44%—1.9% with PTU[1,4,5,7] and 0.12%—2% with MTZ.[1,4,6] Although there are many cases of agranulocytosis reported in the literature, relatively few have been described in detail. These are summarized in Table 1.

All patients were females, ranging in age from 25 to 85, with a mean age of 55 years. The clinical picture in most was typical and marked by sudden onset of sore throat, chills, and fever. In some subjects, the granulocytopenia was accompanied by nonspecific symptoms of lethargy, depression, and generalized aching. It is of interest that in 4 of 13 patients, the presenting symptom was jaundice. The peripheral blood picture was characteristic, with severe granulocytopenia, frequent monocytosis, and occasional eosinophilia. Mild anemia was present in one subject and one was thrombocytopenic. Bone marrow examination revealed the absence of mature granulocytes, decreased or absent myeloid precursors, or sometimes a decrease or absence of all myeloid elements.

Nine patients recovered completely in 5 days to weeks. In most cases, therapy consisted of penicillin alone or in combination with other antibiotics. Four patients died. The dosage of PTU and MTZ ranged between 100–300 and 10–30 mg per day, respectively. The duration from onset of therapy to the appearance of agranulocytosis ranged, in most cases, between 3 and 8 weeks; however, in some cases it appeared as early as 10 days or as late as 5 months after the initial dose.

Table 1
Cases of Agranulocytosis

Age Sex	Drug, Dosage, Duration	Presenting Symptoms	Hematologic Values	Bone Marrow	Therapy	Outcome Recovery	Other Complications (Reference)
55 ?F	PTU 75–150 mg/day × 60 days	Sore throat	WBC 1000	Not done	Penicillin	R 8 days	(2)
60 ?F	PTU 300 mg/day × 64 days	Sore throat	WBC 2400	Not done	Penicillin	R 2 wks	(2)
44 WF	PTU 300 mg/day × 5 mos	Fever, depression	WBC 1400 (15 seg, 78 lymph, 7mono)	Cellular Absence of poly	Penicillin	R 1 wk	(7)
68 WF	PTU 200 mg/day > 6 wks	Malaise, chills, fever, jaundice	WBC 1000 (0 poly)	Absence of granulocytic cells	Penicillin, Streptomycin	?recovered	Toxic hepatitis (13)
25 WF	PTU 200 mg/day > ?4 wks	Fever, sore throat	WBC 5700 (32 seg, 68 lymph)	Not done	Penicillin	Expired	(10)
60 WF	PTU 300 mg/day × 22 days	Chills, cough, jaundice, fever	Hb 11.5/WBC 2380 (7 seg, 47 lymph, 45 mono, 1 baso) platelets 64,000	Decreased granulocytic cells		Expired	Toxic hepatitis, acute appendicitis (11)
85 WF	PTU 200–250 mg × 3 wks	Cough, lethargy	Hb 8.5/WBC 3500 (26 seg, 73 lymph, 1 mono)	↓Cellularity ↓Granulocytic and red cell precursors	Penicillin	Expired	(14)
36 WF	MTZ 15–20 mg/day × 43 days	Sore throat, fever	WBC 2300 (2 seg, 95 lymph, 2 mono, 1 eos)	Not done	Penicillin Solu-B	R 3 days	(6)
62 WF	PTU 200 mg/day × 8 wks (D/C)	Jaundice	WBC 1150 (51 seg, 45 lymph)	Not done	Penicillin	R 5 days	(12)

Table 1 (continued)

Age Sex	Drug, Dosage, Duration	Presenting Symptoms	Hematologic Values	Bone Marrow	Therapy	Outcome Recovery	Other Complications (Reference)
65 WF	PTU 300 mg/day × 14 (D/C) MTZ 30 mg/day × 83 days	Chills, fever, diarrhea	WBC 1900 (70 lymph, 21 mono)	Not done	Penicillin, terramycin, cortisone, folic Acid	R 5 days	(9)
31 NF	Thiouracil ?mg/day × 5 (D/C) MTZ 60 mg/day × 9 days	Fever	WBC 2600 (23 poly) 1800 (48 poly)	Reactive	None	?	(15)
56 ?F	MTZ 15 mg/day (D/C) PTU 300 mg/day × 10 days	?	WBC 2000 (0 poly)	?	Penicillin, aureomycin	R 10–15	(16)
65 WF	MTZ 30 mg/day × 31 days	Weakness, aching, diarrhea, fever, jaundice	WBC 1300 (0 poly, 87 lymph, 13 mono)	Decreased cellularity, tumor cells	Penicillin, terramycin, whole blood, ACTH	Expired	Autopsy–broncho-pneumonia, metastatic adeno-carcinoma (17)

APLASTIC ANEMIA

Aplastic anemia in association with PTU and MTZ appears to be extremely rare. A total of 5 cases has been reported in the American literature.[18-22] These are summarized in Table 2. Although all patients had pancytopenia and bone marrow hypoplasia, in 3 the presenting symptom-complex, clinical course, and rapid recovery after the drug was discontinued are more in keeping with agranulocytosis. In one case,[21] explosive onset of aplastic anemia followed prolonged therapy with methylthiouracil. The presenting symptoms were fever and petechiae. Pancytopenia was severe, and bone marrow biopsy showed complete aplasia. The patient expired in 5 days despite supportive therapy. In another case,[22] the onset of weakness and epistaxis followed a 3-week course (total dose 4 g) of PTU. The patient had severe pancytopenia, bone marrow hypoplasia, and failed to respond to 2 months' therapy with transfusions, androgen, and corticosteroids. Thus, from among the 5 cases, 3 patients had reversible pancytopenia and bone marrow hypoplasia, presenting with symptoms of agranulocytosis, and 2 had a more classic clinical picture of aplastic anemia. Whether we are dealing with two types of aplasia—a mild reversible type and a severe fatal form—cannot be determined from the limited number of cases. It is also not clear what factors determine reversibility or irreversibility of bone marrow injury. Neither drug dosage nor duration of therapy appear to determine outcome. As can be noted in Tables 1 and 2, there was no difference in dosage or duration of therapy between the group with agranulocytosis and that with aplastic anemia. It is interesting to note that the mean age was 40 for the latter as compared to 55 years for the former.

MECHANISM OF BONE MARROW INJURY FROM ANTITHYROID DRUGS

Knowledge regarding the mechanism of hematologic toxicity from antithyroid drugs is meager. None of the hypotheses advanced in this regard has received conclusive experimental support. There is no substantial evidence to support an autoimmune process. Attempts to demonstrate drug-specific leukoagglutinin have given positive results in 2 reported cases[23,24] and negative results in others.[20,22] Waltzer, et al[23] described a 15-year-old girl who had been on propylthiouracil, 150 mg daily, for 3–5 years and developed fever, arthritis, purpuric lesions, leukopenia, leg ulcer, and splenomegaly. Her serum was positive for leukoagglutinins, and antigranulocyte antibody could be demonstrated by immunofluorescence techniques. In another study by Connell,[24] a 53-year-old woman, on methimazol, 60 mg daily for 26 days, developed rash, neutropenia, and eosinophilia. Her serum was positive for methimazol-specific leukoagglutinin. While these results are of interest, their general significance is difficult to assess. The presence of leukoagglutinins does not constitute conclusive evidence for an immune process, particularly when one considers the difficulties inherent in this problem—nonuniformity of the techniques used and leukoagglutinins in serum from patients without neutropenia. Neither does the absence of demonstrable antibodies rule out an immune mechanism.

Table 2
Summary of Reported Cases of Aplastic Anemia

Age Sex	Drugs, Dosage, Duration	Presenting Symptoms	Hematologic Values	Bone Marrow	Therapy	Outcome Recovery	Other Findings (Reference)
53 WF	PTU 400 mg/day × 40 digoxin, reserpine	Acute sore throat, chills, fever	Hb 9.7/Hct 31 WBC 950 (94 lymph, 6 eos), platelets 34,000	Hypoplastic (smear)	None	R 1 mo	(20)
37 WF	PTU D/C because of rash MTZ 20 mg/day × 43	Sore throat, fever	Hb 8.3/Hct 25 WBC 700 (90 lymph, 3 mono) platelets 131,000	Hypoplastic (smear) from 3 different sites	Cortisone 30 mg → 100 mg	R 13 days	(18)
21 ?F	MTZ 45 mg/day × 74	Fever, cough (pseudomonas, pneumonia, sepsis)	Hb 8.5/Hct 26, WBC 900 (100 lymph) platelets 18,000	Hypoplastic (aspiration and biopsy)	Tetracycline, penicillin, keflin, colomycin, gentomycin, cortisone, halotestin	R 20 days	(19)
51 WF	Methylthiouracil 100–200 mg/day > 82 days or year?	Fever, petechiae	Hb 4.4/Hct 11 WBC 1000 (100 lymph) platelets 0	No hematopoietic cells (biopsy)	Blood transfusions, penicillin, tetracycline	Expired	(21)
39 WM	PTU 50 mg tab × 80 in 3 wks	Weakness, epistaxis	Hb 3.5 WBC 2,600 (14 seg, 8 neutro, 10 mono, 68 lymph), platelets 10,000	Hypocellular (2 smears)	Transfusions, androgens, steroids, penicillin	No recovery 2 mos after D/C PTU	(22)

There are only few in vitro studies to test the metabolic effects of antithyroid drugs on bone marrow cells, and these have given variable results. Warren[25,26] reported inhibition of bone marrow respiration in vitro by thiouracil in a concentration of 1 mg/ml. He also noted that immature myeloid cells were more strikingly affected than erythroid cells. Paschkis[27] demonstrated inhibition of cytochrome oxidase activity of thyroid tissue by thiouracil but no inhibition of cytochrome oxidase of bone marrow or kidney tissue.

That bone marrow toxicity occurs only in some of the patients receiving antithyroid therapy suggests some form of individual predisposition. This possibility was recently examined[20] by studying bone marrow from a patient after full recovery from propylthiouracil-induced bone marrow aplasia. Attempts to demonstrate an immune mechanism or a metabolic effect of propylthiouracil on patient's bone marrow cells were unsuccessful.

It is clear, from what has been stated, that much more needs to be done to elucidate the pathogenesis of bone marrow toxicity from antithyroid drugs.

BRIEF COMMENTS ON PREVENTION AND MANAGEMENT

The treatment of antithyroid drug-induced agranulocytosis does not differ from that of agranulocytosis from other causes. Important considerations should be given to etiology, severity, and complications. The central problem is that of infection and its recognition. When suspected, infection should be treated promptly and vigorously, even when signs and symptoms are minimal. There is no specific therapy for neutropenia. Corticosteroids probably have no value and may increase susceptibility to infection. The value of androgen therapy is also uncertain.

Equally important as therapy is the prevention of agranulocytosis. Early recognition may be critical. Monitoring the leukocyte count is of definite value, but more so with some drugs than with others. For example: leukopenia in association with phenothiazine, when it occurs, does so in a relatively slow progressive fashion, and monitoring the leukocyte count is important in its early detection. While this may also be true for some patients on antithyroid drugs, in others the onset of agranulocytosis may be explosive. Not infrequently, a patient who on checkup has a normal leukocyte count may return a few days later with fully developed symptoms of agranulocytosis. It is therefore important to explain to patients the early signs and symptoms of this complication and to encourage them to report these promptly.

LUPUS-LIKE SYNDROME

Five cases of lupus-like syndrome have been reported in association with antithyroid therapy. These are summarized in Table 3. Common presenting signs and symptoms are fever, arthralgia or arthritis, leukopenia, and hypergammaglobulinemia. Other reported symptoms include pleuritis,[7,28] proteinuria,[8] leg ulcer, splenomegaly, and skin lesions.[23] In 4 patients, symptoms developed after

Table 3
Summary of Cases of Lupus-like Syndrome

Age Sex	Drug, Dosage, Duration	Presenting Symptoms	Laboratory Findings	Outcome after D/C PTU	Other Findings (References)
15 WF	PTU 150 mg/day × 3–5 yrs	Transient arthritis, fever, recurrent purpuric lesions on face, hands, ankles, feet; leg ulcers	Hb 12.4 WBC 3650 (50 lymph, 40 segs, 6 mono)	Symptoms disappeared	Splenomegaly (23)
14 NM	PTU 150–300 mg/day × 4 yrs	Afternoon fever, intermittent arthralgia without signs of arthritis	WBC 2800 (55 segs, 38 lymph, 5 mono, 2 baso) ⊕ ANA ⊕ LE prep proteinuria	Symptoms disappeared but maintained on prednisone 80 mg/day to suppress symptoms	⊖ Coombs, focal glomerular, mesangeal and membrane thickening, renal biopsy (8)
27 NF	PTU 100–300 mg/day × 27 mos	Migratory swelling and pain on joints, fever, pleuritic chest pain	Leukopenia, Hypergammaglobulinemia, ⊖ LE prep	Symptoms disappeared, placed on MTZ without recurrence	(7)
17 WF	PTU 300 mg/day × 6 wks	Fever, pleuritis, pericarditis, arthritis, edema	⊖ LE prep × 4	Disappeared but placed on prednisone, MTZ	(28)
14 ?F	PTU?	Arthralgia, recurrent febrile episodes, pleural and pericardial effusions, cutaneous eruption	WBC 3660, ANA ⊕, LE ⊖, Coombs ⊖, leukoagglutin ⊖	?	(30)

2–5 years of therapy with propylthiouracil; 1 developed symptoms after only 6 weeks of treatment.[28] All patients were in a young age group (mean: 17.6 years); females predominated. In only 1 of the 5 cases, was the LE test positive, as was the test for antinuclear antibody. In all cases, symptoms subsided after propylthiouracil was discontinued. However, 2 patients apparently required treatment with prednisone,[8,28] It is of interest that 2 of the subjects were subsequently given methimazol without relapse.[7,28] An unusual case report by McCormick[29] concerned a patient in whom therapy with propylthiouracil was discontinued after 15 days because of fever and atrial fibrillation. When, at a later date, propylthiouracil was resumed, the patient developed symptoms within 36 hours consisting of irritability, left facial paralysis, and a positive extensor reflex, all of which again subsided when the drug was discontinued. Fever, diarrhea, and confusion occurred 12 hours after a test dose of propylthiouracil and disappeared in 24 hours. Finally, when inadvertently the patient was placed on propylthiouracil, 200 mg daily for 6 days, he became unconscious and died of a cerebral hemorrhage. Autopsy revealed diffuse periarteritis. The course of this patient strongly suggests a hypersensitivity syndrome related to PTU therapy.

The lupus-like syndrome that occurred with propylthiouracil therapy appears to be extremely rare. A cause-effect relationship, although uncertain, is strongly suggested by the rapid improvement of symptoms after the drug was discontinued. In a recent review of drug-induced lupus syndrome, Alarcon-Segovia[31] classified drugs potentially capable of activating systemic lupus erythematosus into two groups: (a) those that do so through some postulated peculiar pharmacologic properties. (Lupus syndrome occurs with considerable frequency after prolonged therapy and large dosages.) Drugs in this group include: hydralazine, isoniazide, anticonvulsants, and procainamide. (b) The second group is said to induce allergic reactions, which, in turn, precipitate lupus. Sulfa drugs, various antibiotics, PTU, and other drugs fall into this category. This classification appears to be quite arbitrary, and some of the drugs may induce lupus by either of these mechanisms. For example: it would be hard to place PTU in either group because the incidence of lupus in association with its use is rare and seems to occur after prolonged therapy.

Cetina, et al[32] have recently reported serologic studies in 40 patients on long-term PTU therapy, using a microcomplement fixation method. They compared the results with those in patients on isoniazid, diphenylhydantoin, PTU, and controls. The incidence of antibodies to soluble nucleoproteins was higher in patients on INH and diphenylhydantoin than in controls; the incidence in patients on PTU was not. These authors concluded that SLE in association with PTU therapy is either incidental or is mediated by mechanisms other than those implicated for hydralazine, isoniazid, procainamid, or diphenylhydantoin.

SUMMARY

The use of antithyroid drugs for the treatment of hyperthyroidism has been associated with a variety of untoward reactions. These include fever, rash, urticaria, gastrointestinal disturbances, jaundice, arthralgia, lymphadenopathy, lupus-like syndrome, leukopenia, agranulocytosis, and bone marrow aplasia. The most common side reaction is drug fever and the most serious has been agranulocytosis.

Leukopenia of various degrees occurs rather frequently with antithyroid therapy, the incidence being as high as 25%. Leukopenia is more often transient and of no serious consequences. Agranulocytosis is uncommon, occurring in about 1% of the cases. Bone marrow aplasia in association with antithyroid therapy appears to be extremely rare, only 6 cases having been reported. Although in all 6 there was pancytopenia and bone marrow hypoplasia, in 4 the presenting symptom complex, clinical course, and rapid recovery after the drug was discontinued were more in keeping with agranulocytosis.

The mechanism of bone marrow injury from antithyroid drugs is unknown. None of the hypotheses advanced in this regard received conclusive experimental support. Evidence for an autoimmune process is fragmentary. An individual biochemical predisposition may be the underlying factor, but proof is lacking. In vitro studies testing the metabolic effects of antithyroid drugs on bone marrow cells have been noncontributory.

Lupus-like syndrome has been reported in 5 patients receiving propylthiouracil. In 4 of these the treatment was prolonged for 2–5 years. The LE test was positive in only 1 patient. In all, the syndrome was reversible when antithyroid treatment was discontinued. Prednisone was required in 2. The pathogenesis of this complication remains unknown.

REFERENCES

1. Vanderlaan WP, Storrie VM: A survey of the factors controlling thyroid function with special reference to newer views on antithyroid substances. Pharmacol Rev 7:301, 1955
2. Bartels EC: Agranulocytosis during propylthiouracil therapy. Am J Med 5:48, 1948
3. McGavack TH, Chevalley J: Untoward hematologic responses to the antithyroid compounds. Am J Med 17:36, 1954
4. Huguley CM Jr: Drug-induced blood dyscrasia. JAMA 188:817, 1964
5. Irwin GW, Van Vactor HD, Norris MS: Propylthiouracil and methimazole therapy. JAMA 149:1637, 1952
6. H'Doubler FT Jr, H'Doubler PB: Toxic reactions from methimazole. Missouri Med 51:888, 1954
7. Wing ES Jr, Asper SP Jr: Observations on the use of propylthiouracil in hyperthyroidism with special reference to long term treatment. Bull Hopkins Hosp 90:201, 1952
8. Amrhein JA, Kenny FM, Ross D: Granulocytopenia, lupus like syndrome and other complications of propylthiouracil therapy. J Pediatr 76:54, 1970
9. Croke AR, Berry JW: Agranulocytosis occurring during methimazole therapy. JAMA 148:45, 1952
10. Juliar B. Harris TL: Fatal agranulocytosis during propylthiouracil therapy. JAMA 139:646, 1949
11. Colwell AR Jr, Sando DE, Lang SJ: Propylthiouracil induced agranulocytosis, toxic hepatitis and death. Report of case. JAMA 148:639, 1952
12. Rosenbaum H, Reveno WS: Agranulocytosis and toxic hepatitis from methimazole. JAMA 152:27, 1953

13. Livingston HJ, Livingston SF: Agranulocytosis and hepatocellular jaundice, toxic reaction following propylthiouracil therapy. JAMA 135:422, 1947
14. Beebe RT, Propp S, McClintock JC et al: Fatal agranulocytosis during treatment of toxic goiter with propylthiouracil. Ann Intern Med 34:1035, 1951
15. Stone HH, Petit DW, Starr P: Therapeutic studies in hyperthyroidism: Methimazole. J Clin Endocrinol Metab 12:841, 1952
16. Bartels EC: Hyperthyroidism—An evaluation of treatment with antithyroid drugs followed by subtotal thyroidectomy. Ann Intern Med 37:1123, 1952
17. Specht NW, Boehme EJ: Death due to agranulocytosis induced by methimazole therapy. JAMA 149:1010, 1952
18. Levine B, Rosenberg DV: Aplastic anemia during the treatment of hyperthyroidism with tapazole. Ann Intern Med 41:844, 1954
19. Rosenberg AH: Methimazole induced aplastic anemia. Conn Med 34:32, 1970
20. Martelo OJ, Katims RB, Yunis AA: Bone Marrow Aplasia following propylthiouracil therapy. Arch Intern Med 120:587, 1967
21. Poate HRG: Death from aplastic anemia following methylthiouracil therapy. Med J Aust 2:208, 1957
22. Aksoy M, Erdem S: Aplastic anemia after propylthiouracil. Lancet 1:1379, 1968
23. Waltzer RA, Einbinder J: Immunoleukopenia as an aspect of hypersensitivity to propylthiouracil. JAMA 188:743, 1963
24. Connell JT: Abnormal eosinophils, eosinophilia and basophilia in methimazole neutropenia. Ann Allergy 27:595, 1969
25. Warren CO: The effect of thiouracil on the respiration of bone marrow and leukocytes in vitro. Am J Physiol 145:71, 1945
26. Warren CO: The effect of thiouracil on the respiration of bone marrow and leukocytes in vitro. Science 102:175, 1945
27. Paschkis KE, Cantarow A, Rakoff, AE, et al: The effect of thiouracil on tissue oxidase. Science 102:333, 1945
28. Best MM, Duncan CH: Lupus like syndrome following propylthiouracil administration. J Ky Med Assoc 62:47 62:47, 1964
29. McCormick RV: Periarteritis occurring during propylthiouracil therapy. JAMA 144:1453, 1950
30. Faber V, Preben E: Leukocyte-specific antinuclear factors in patient with Felty's syndrome, rheumatoid arthritis, systemic lupus erythematosus and other diseases. Acta Med Scand 179:267, 1966
31. Alarcon-Segovia D: Drug-induced lupus syndromes. Mayo Clinic Proc 44:664, 1969
32. Cetina JA, Fishbein E, Alarcon-Segovia D: Antinuclear antibodies and propylthiouracil therapy. JAMA 220:1012, 1972

PART IV

Drug Effects on Platelets and Coagulation

Jack Levin

22

Effects of Oral Antidiabetic and Diuretic Agents on Platelets

Oral antidiabetic and diuretic agents are well known to cause thrombocytopenia. These two broad groups of drugs are among those most frequently reported to the Registry on Blood Dyscrasias as being associated with thrombocytopenia.[1,2] Many are derivatives of the sulfonamides, compounds that can produce bone marrow depression.[3,4]

ORAL ANTIDIABETIC AGENTS

Figure 1 indicates the chemical structures of three drugs that produce hypoglycemia. All are sulfonylureas, and carbutamide is a sulfonamide with antibacterial activity. Carbutamide has been associated with a sufficient incidence of thrombocytopenia, along with other hematologic side effects, to preclude its current use.[5] Phemister[6] studied the hematologic effects of carbutamide in 40 patients. Seven developed a minimal decrease in platelet counts and 3 became definitely thrombocytopenic. One of the latter developed purpura, and rechallenge of this patient with carbutamide produced a gradual fall in her platelet count. Some of the patients, in whom only a mild reduction of platelets was observed, demonstrated rebound thrombocytosis after the drug was stopped. Bone marrow aspirations were performed on 5 patients with thrombocytopenia; in 4, megakaryocytes were reported as present and normal appearing, but questionably decreased. The drug was not shown to inhibit clot retraction, or to agglutinate or lyse platelets of affected individuals. Skin tests were negative. Nonthrombocytopenic purpura also was observed in this group of patients. Kirtley[7] reviewed the

Carried out under Contract COO-3014-7 between the United States Atomic Energy Commission and The Johns Hopkins University, and supported in part by Graduate Training Grant TI-AM-5260 from the National Institute of Arthritis and Metabolic Diseases, US Public Health Service.

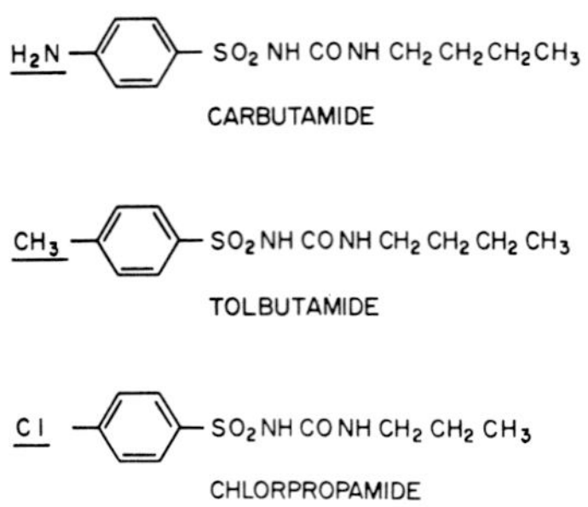

Fig. 1. Oral antidiabetic agents: the chemical structures of three sulfonylurea compounds.

case histories of 7000 patients who had received carbutamide; 2 developed thrombocytopenia and another 2 nonthrombocytopenic purpura.

Chlorpropamide has been reported to be associated with thrombocytopenia but the incidence is hard to ascertain. Although this drug is one of the more common of those reported to the Drug Registry as a cause of thrombocytopenia,[1] a compilation of papers that appeared in a symposium devoted to chlorpropamide failed to indicate significant hematologic abnormalities in any of 290 patients.[8–12] However, the tests used to detect platelet abnormalities were not always performed. Grace[13] reported the development of thrombocytopenic purpura in one patient after 7 days of therapy with chlorpropamide; he recovered rapidly after the drug was discontinued. The bone marrow aspirate was normal. Three other patients with thrombocytopenic purpura associated with the administration of chlorpropamide were reported by Meyler.[14]

Tolbutamide is reported to be less commonly associated with the development of thrombocytopenia than the two previously discussed drugs.[15] Dolger[16] and Fulmer, et al[17] did not observe thrombocytopenia or purpura in any of 167 patients who received tolbutamide. Balodimos, et al[18] observed 1 case of thrombocytopenic purpura and 1 of nonthrombocytopenic purpura in 3387 patients who received tolbutamide. O'Donovan[19] reviewed the toxicity of tolbutamide in over 9000 patients. Only 1 patient was reported to have developed thrombocytopenia; purpura did not occur. In neither of these reviews of experience with large groups of patients were specific data presented in regard to the rare patients with thrombocytopenia or purpura. Neonatal thrombocytopenia has been observed in the child of a mother who received tolbutamide during pregnancy.[20] The child gradually recovered. It is perhaps pertinent that congenital malformations also were present. The concentration of tolbutamide in the blood of this child was over twice that observed in his mother, and it was concluded that the thrombocytopenia was a direct toxic effect of elevated levels of tolbutamide. A bone marrow examination performed after recovery was within normal limits.

Consideration of the effects of drugs upon platelets should include potential metabolic and functional alterations, not necessarily reflected by changes in the platelet count. Tolbutamide has been shown to inhibit the aggregation of platelets by thrombin, decrease the release of calcium by thrombin, and inhibit phosphodiesterase activity in platelets.[21] The last effect is of potential physiologic significance because phosphodiesterase inactivates cyclic AMP, and cyclic AMP inhibits certain normal platelet functions, including aggregation. However, increased levels of cyclic AMP were not present in the platelets exposed to tolbutamide, and therefore the result of inhibition of phosphodiesterase activity is unclear. Nevertheless, these experiments indicate that tolbutamide and other drugs may produce functional damage to platelets, not associated with thrombocytopenia, and in such patients this mechanism might account for the development of nonthrombocytopenic purpura.

Another group of compounds that are administered orally to produce hypoglycemia are the biguanides. Phenformin (phenethyl biguanide) has not been reported to be associated with thrombocytopenia.[5,14,22]

ORAL DIURETIC AGENTS

The structural formulae of some of the thiazides used as oral diuretics are shown in Figure 2. They are benzothiadiazides. There are many reports that indicate that thiazides cause thrombocytopenia and purpura.[1,4,23,24] Böttiger and Westerholm[25] observed that 18% of 359 patients with thrombocytopenia had drug-induced thrombocytopenia and the largest single cause of drug-induced thrombocytopenia was the thiazides. In a more detailed study, they reported that 52 of 126 cases of drug-induced thrombocytopenia were attributable to oral diuretics.[26] Twenty-one of these 52 patients had been receiving thiazides. Björnberg and Gisslén[27] reported that 11 of 25 patients with purpura (primarily nonthrombocytopenic in type) were receiving thiazides at the time they developed purpura.

Antibodies against chlorothiazide or hydrochlorothiazide have been apparently detected in the blood of 7 patients who developed thrombocytopenia after receiving one of these drugs.[28–32] In vitro tests which indicated the presence of antibody that resulted in platelet damage included: platelet agglutination, platelet lysis, platelet factor 3 release, and inhibition of clot retraction. In one case,[29] reinstituting therapy with hydrochlorothiazide caused recurrent thrombocytopenic purpura. The patient reported by Eisner and Crowell[31] was shown to have an IgM antibody directed toward hydrochlorothiazide but not against chlorothiazide. Megakaryocytes have been present in bone marrow aspirates when they have been performed, and in almost all instances, recovery has been

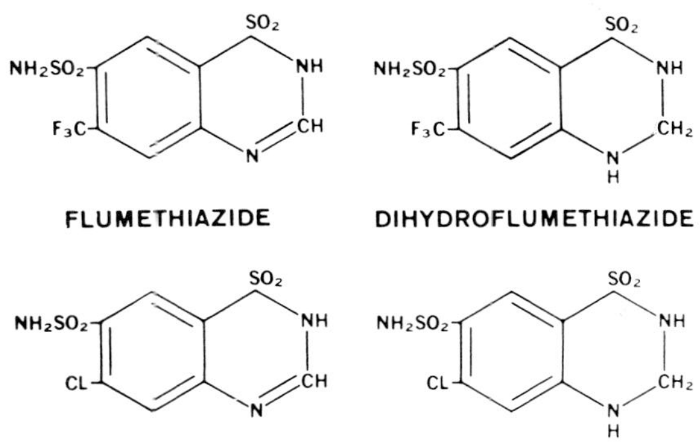

Fig. 2. Oral diuretic agents: the chemical structures of four benzothiadiazide compounds.

observed after the drug was discontinued. However, some of the patients in whom an immunologic mechanism was suggested by in vitro tests demonstrated a rate of recovery slightly slower than that usually seen in typical drug-induced thrombocytopenic purpura.[28] Nordqvist, et al[28] reported a patient rechallenged with chlorothiazide whose platelet count did not reach its nadir for 15 days. Perhaps a higher dose of the drug would have produced the more typical immediate development of thrombocytopenia.[33]

The thiazides also can cause nonthrombocytopenic purpura.[27,34–37] Björnberg and Gisslén[27] reported that almost all of their 11 patients who developed purpura while taking thiazides had normal platelet counts. Similar to patients who developed drug-induced thrombocytopenic purpura, patients with nonthrombocytopenic purpura also recovered when the drug was discontinued, and rechallenge with the offending drug caused recurrent nonthrombocytopenic purpura.[27,34–37] However, one patient became uremic and died, after the episode of nonthrombocytopenic purpura.[36]

Neonatal thrombocytopenia has been associated with the antepartum administration of thiazide drugs.[38] Seven newborn children, born to mothers who were taking thiazides, were observed to have thrombocytopenic purpura. All recovered but 1 who probably died of anoxia due to unrelated causes. The mothers were not thrombocytopenic and platelet isoantibodies and drug antibodies were not demonstrated in the mothers of the affected children. Bone marrow aspirations were performed in 5 children, and 4 demonstrated decreased or absent megakaryocytes. This finding, in association with thrombocytopenia, and the additional presence of pancytopenia in 1 child and leukopenia in another 2 children, suggested marrow depression secondary to the drug. The levels of drug in the children's blood perhaps were sufficiently elevated to cause this type of hematologic toxicity, in a manner similar to that observed in the child of a mother who was taking tolbutamide during pregnancy.[20]

Many other oral diuretic agents* also have been associated with the development of thrombocytopenia and purpura, including chlorthalidone,[25,27,39] furosemide,[26,40] acetazolamide,[41,42] and ethacrynic acid.[40]

The potential risk of purpura associated with oral diuretic agents is based, in part, on the true frequency of thrombocytopenia after the administration of these drugs. This is difficult to ascertain if one depends upon the development of clinical purpura to detect patients thus affected, since thrombocytopenia (or depression of red cell and white blood cell levels) may occur in the absence of pertinent signs or symptoms. Böttiger and Westerholm[26] reported that only 68% of 126 people with drug-induced thrombocytopenia had purpura, and therefore, in their population, many patients with thrombocytopenia due to oral diuretics would not have been detected without performing platelet counts. Their extensive study indicated that thrombocytopenia occurred in 1 of 15,000 patients who were using oral diuretics. Five per cent of their patients died with thrombocytopenia still present, but they concluded that only 2% of the patients had died as a direct cause of thrombocytopenic purpura. Furthermore, they estimated that only 33% of the patients with drug-induced thrombocytopenia

* The author does not intend to imply that the agents discussed in this paper are the only drugs in this therapeutic category that produce thrombocytopenia or purpura.

had been reported, which would indicate that the true incidence of thrombocytopenia is 3 cases per 15,000 users of oral diuretics. An even higher incidence of thrombocytopenia secondary to thiazides was reported by Kutti and Weinfeld[39] who reported that 26% of patients with heart disease who were receiving thiazides developed thrombocytopenia. Only 4% of the control group of patients in this series were thrombocytopenic; both groups apparently were taking equivalent amounts of other cardiac drugs. In some of their patients, rechallenge resulted in recurrent thrombocytopenia. It is noteworthy that none of their patients had purpura. The low incidence of purpura probably accounts for the failure of Dinon, et al[43] and Cohen[44] to observe isolated thrombocytopenic purpura in a total of 172 patients.

Although the mechanisms by which thiazides and other oral diuretic agents produce thrombocytopenia is not clear, in some instances it probably has been secondary to bone marrow depression and in others, it was apparently due to the formation of antibodies against the drug or one of its metabolic products. The specific mechanisms by which drug antibodies produce thrombocytopenic purpura have been described in detail,[45-47] and the general problem of drug-induced thrombocytopenia has been discussed (chap 7). Perhaps one of the mechanisms by which nonthrombocytopenic purpura is produced by oral diuretics is by qualitative effects upon platelet function, without a change in the circulating platelet count. Zieve and Solomon[48] have studied human platelets in vitro and demonstrated that ethacrynic acid causes the release of serotonin and potassium, inhibits amino acid uptake, increases platelet water, inhibits clot retraction, and also blocks platelet aggregation by thrombin. Acetazolamide caused the release of potassium from platelets, but interestingly, chlorothiazide had no demonstrable effects in the systems tested. While such studies indicate potential mechanisms by which nonthrombocytopenic purpura may occur in a person taking drugs, the authors pointed out that the concentrations of drugs used to produce these abnormalities in vitro, were much higher than those achieved after the administration of therapeutic doses to patients. However, they suggested that active uptake by platelets of a chronically administered drug might alter platelet structure and function.

DISCUSSION

Essentially all orally administered drugs used to lower blood sugar or produce diuresis have been associated with thrombocytopenia and/or purpura, but the mechanisms by which they produce these effects remain unclear. In some instances, there may be direct suppression of megakaryocytopoiesis or toxic effects directly upon platelets, and in others drug-induced antibodies apparently have been demonstrated. The true incidence of thrombocytopenia after the administration of certain drugs may not be recognized when dependence is placed on the development of overt purpura. The study of Kutti and Weinfeld,[39] in which 24% of the patients taking oral diuretics had thrombocytopenia, suggests that at least in their patient population an adequate dose of oral diuretics for a long enough period of time was capable of suppressing thrombopoiesis. However, the estimate by Böttiger and Westerholm[26] that thrombocytopenia occurs in 3 of 15,000 patients taking oral diuretics suggests that some patients may have an underlying genetic or metabolic abnormality that results in altered drug metabolism, making them susceptible to the development of thrombocytopenia. Perhaps some of the patients who developed thrombocytopenia secondary to these two categories of drugs have an as yet unrecognized enzymatic deficiency which makes their platelets susceptible to the actions of these drugs.[49] In this regard, they would be similar to patients with glucose-6-phosphate dehydrogenase deficiency who develop a hemolytic anemia when exposed to certain chemical substances or drugs. However, the evaluation of any drug-related alteration in hematopoiesis must take into account not only the possibility of occult enzymatic deficiencies but also the underlying disease state and the potential role of drug interactions.

AUTHOR'S NOTE

The reports cited have been limited to those in which isolated thrombocytopenia or nonthrombocytopenic purpura was present. Cases of aplastic anemia or thrombocytopenia in association with agranulocytosis have been excluded.

REFERENCES

1. Huguley CM Jr: Drug-induced blood dyscrasias. DM, October 1963.
2. Crosby WH, Kaufman RM: Drug-induced blood dyscrasias. IV. Thrombocytopenia. JAMA 189:417, 1964
3. Rinkoff SS, Spring M: Toxic depression of the myeloid elements following therapy with the sulfonamides; report of 8 cases. Ann Intern Med 15:89, 1941
4. Gynn TN, Messmore HL, Friedman IA: Drug-induced thrombocytopenia. Med Clin North Am 56:65, 1972
5. Duncan LJP, Baird JD: Compounds administered orally in the treatment of diabetes mellitus. Pharmacol Rev 12:91, 1960
6. Phemister JC: Thrombocytopenia and leukopenia following carbutamide. Br Med J 1:199, 1957
7. Kirtley WR: Occurrence of sensitivity and side reactions following carbutamide. Diabetes 6:72, 1957
8. Greenhouse B: Clinical experience with chlorpropamide. Ann NY Acad Sci 74:643, 1959
9. Hadley WB, Khachadurian A, Marble A: Studies with chlorpropamide in diabetic patients. Ann NY Acad Sci 74:721, 1959
10. Canessa I, Valiente S, Mella I: Clinical evaluation of chlorpropamide in diabetes mellitus. Ann NY Acad Sci 74:752, 1959
11. Hills AG, Abelove WB: Clinical experience with chlorpropamide in the management of diabetes mellitus. Ann NY Acad Sci 74:845, 1959
12. Serrano P, Chavez R: Clinicotherapeutic evaluation of chlorpropamide, a new sulfonylurea derivative for the treatment of diabetes mellitus. Ann NY Acad Sci 74:931, 1959
13. Grace WJ: Thrombocytopenia in a patient taking chlorpropamide. N Engl J Med 260:711, 1959

14. Side effects of drugs. Vcl 5. Edited by L Meyler. Amsterdam, Excerpta Medica, 1966, p 447
15. Side effects of drugs.[14] p 133
16. Dolger H: Clinical experience with orinase. Metabolism 5:947, 1956
17. Fulmer HS, Dube AH, Lloyd CW: Clinical experience with orinase. Metabolism 5:940, 1956
18. Balodimos MC, Camerini-Dávalos RA, Marble A: Nine years' experience with tolbutamide in the treatment of diabetes. Metabolism 15:957, 1966
19. O'Donovan CJ: Analysis of long-term experience with tolbutamide (Orinase) in the management of diabetes. Curr Ther Res 1:69, 1959
20. Schiff D, Aranda JV, Stern L: Neonatal thrombocytopenia and congenital malformations associated with administration of tolbutamide to the mother. J Pediatr 77:457, 1970
21. Roth J, Prout TE, Goldfine ID et al: Sulfonylureas: Effects in vivo and in vitro. Ann Intern Med 75:607, 1971
22. Travis RH, Sayers G: Insulin and oral hypoglycemic agents, The Pharmacological Basis of Therapeutics. Edited by LS Goodman, A Gilman. Fourth edition. New York, Macmillan, 1970, p 1581
23. Ball P: Thrombocytopenia and purpura in patients receiving chlorothiazide and hydrochlorothiazide. JAMA 173:663, 1960
24. Side Effects of Drugs.[14] p 224
25. Böttiger LE, Westerholm B: Thrombocytopenia I. Incidence and aetiology. Acta Med Scand 191:535, 1972
26. Böttiger LE, Westerholm B: Thrombocytopenia II. Drug-induced thrombocytopenia. Acta Med Scand 191:541, 1972
27. Björnberg A, Gisslén H: Thiazides: a cause of necrotising vasculitis? Lancet 2:982, 1965
28. Nordqvist P, Cramér G, Björntorp P: Thrombocytopenia during chlorothiazide treatment. Lancet 1:271, 1959
29. Gesink MH, Bradford HA: Thrombocytopenic purpura associated with hydrochlorothiazide therapy. JAMA 172:556, 1960
30. Bettman JW: Drug hypersensitivity purpuras. Arch Intern Med 112:840, 1963
31. Eisner EV, Crowell EB: Hydrochlorothiazide-dependent thrombocytopenia due to IgM antibody. JAMA 215:480, 1971
32. Karpatkin S, Strick N, Karpatkin MB, et al: Cumulative experience in the detection of antiplatelet antibody in 234 patients with idiopathic thrombocytopenic purpura, systemic lupus erythematosus and other clinical disorders. Am J Med 52:776, 1972
33. Shulman NR: Immunoreactions involving platelets. IV. Studies on the pathogenesis of thrombocytopenia in drug purpura using test doses of quinidine in sensitized individuals; their implications in idiopathic thrombocytopenic purpura. J Exp Med 107:711, 1958
34. Jaffe MO, Kierland RR: Purpura due to chlorothiazide (Diuril). JAMA 168: 2264, 1958
35. Horowitz HI, Shapiro B, Rubin IL: Athrombocytopenic purpura caused by chlorothiazide. NY State J Med 59:1117, 1959
36. Fitzgerald EW Jr: Fatal glomerulonephritis complicating allergic purpura due to chlorothiazide. Arch Intern Med 105:305, 1960
37. Reid JM, Stevenson JG, Orr M: Nonthrombocytopenic purpura due to chlorothiazide. Scot Med J 14:309, 1969
38. Rodriguez SU, Leikin SL, Hiller MC: Neonatal thrombocytopenia associated with ante-partum administration of thiazide drugs. N Engl J Med 270:881, 1964

39. Kutti J, Weinfeld A: The frequency of thrombocytopenia in patients with heart disease treated with oral diuretics. Acta Med Scand 183:245, 1968
40. Mudge GH: Diuretics and other agents employed in the mobilization of edema fluid, The Pharmacological Basis of Therapeutics. Fourth edition. Edited by LS Goodman, A Gilman. New York, Macmillan, 1970, p 839
41. Reisner EH, Morgan MC: Thrombocytopenia following acetazolamide (Diamox) therapy. JAMA 160:206, 1956
42. Bertino JR, Rodman T, Myerson RM: Thrombocytopenia and renal lesions associated with acetazolamide (Diamox) therapy. Arch Intern Med 99:1006, 1957
43. Dinon LR, Kim YS, Vander Veer JB: Clinical experience with chlorothiazide (Diuril), with particular emphasis on untoward responses. A report of 121 cases studied over a 15 month period. Am J Med Sci 236:533, 1958
44. Cohen BM: Clinical use of dihydroflumethizide in patients with high arterial pressure. Curr Ther Res 1:49, 1959
45. Shulman NR: Immunoreactions involving platelets. I. A steric and kinetic model for formation of a complex from a human antibody, quinidine as a haptene, and platelets; and for fixation of complement by the complex. J Exp Med 107:665, 1958
46. Shulman NR: Mechanism of blood cell destruction in individuals sensitized to foreign antigens. Trans Assoc Am Physicians 76:72, 1963
47. Shulman NR: Immunologic reaction to drugs. N Engl J Med 287:408, 1972
48. Zieve PD, Solomon HM: Effect of diuretics on the human platelet. Am J Physiol 215:650, 1968
49. LaDu BN: Pharmacogenetics: defective enzymes in relation to reactions to drugs. Annu Rev Med 23:453, 1972

Harvey J. Weiss

23
Aspirin and Platelets

EFFECTS OF ASPIRIN ON BLEEDING

The ingestion of aspirin in daily doses of 5–6 g for periods of about a week may prolong prothrombin time by 2–4 seconds.[1,2] It has been known for many years, however, that a mild bleeding tendency may occur after much smaller doses, which do not prolong the prothrombin time, have been ingested. For example: aspirin medication may be associated with excessive bleeding after tooth extraction,[3] biopsies,[4] and tonsillectomy.[5–7] It recently has been reported that hemorrhagic complications were more frequent in the newborn infants of women who had ingested aspirin during the last week of pregnancy.[8] Aspirin ingestion may also result in increased fecal blood loss in normal subjects,[9,10] but this may be due, at least in part, to a corrosive effect on the gut mucosa.[10]

French investigators were the first to demonstrate that aspirin does, in fact, interfere with the primary arrest of bleeding. They reported that ingestion of aspirin regularly prolonged skin bleeding time in normal subjects and, more dramatically, in patients with hematologic disorders, such as leukemia and hemophilia.[11,12] These observations were confirmed by Gast, in Holland, in 1964,[13] by Quick in the United States, in 1966,[14] and subsequently by many other investigators.[15,16] In general, bleeding time is prolonged by only a few minutes in normal subjects. It may, however, be markedly prolonged in an occasional normal subject[16] and in many patients with an underlying hemostatic defect, such as those with severe hemophilia or von Willebrand's disease.[17–20] In 1967, Weiss and Aledort reported that in man, aspirin ingestion impairs collagen-induced platelet aggregation[15] and, they suggested that these findings might explain the deleterious effect of aspirin on hemostasis. Before describing the effects of aspirin on platelets in more detail, the role of platelets in the primary arrest of bleeding and the mechanisms involved in platelet aggregation will be briefly reviewed.

Supported in part by Grant HE 14595 from The National Heart and Lung Institute, US Public Health Service.

PLATELET AGGREGATION AND THE ROLE OF PLATELETS IN HEMOSTASIS

Platelets ordinarily circulate in the bloodstream as disk-shaped cells, non-adherent to each other and to normal endothelium. Once the latter is broken, however, platelets adhere to collagen as well as to basement membranes and microfibrils present in the vessel wall (platelet adhesion).[21] Subsequently, platelets adhere to each other (platelet aggregation), and the formation of platelet aggregates constitutes the initial hemostatic plug which results in the primary arrest of bleeding. Adenosine diphosphate (ADP), in platelets in high concentration, has been shown to play a major role in platelet aggregation. Gaarder et al were the first to show that ADP can aggregate platelets.[22] Subsequent studies have shown that when platelets are exposed to collagen, some of the platelet ADP is released and results in platelet aggregation. The ADP released is derived from a special pool that does not participate actively in metabolism and which is stored along with ATP and serotonin in special electron-dense storage granules.[23] This "storage pool" of ADP plays an important role in the aggregation of platelets by a variety of other substances. For example: as seen in Figure 1A, when epinephrine is added to stirred, platelet-rich plasma, a small initial wave of aggregation, indicated by an increase in light transmittance, is caused by a direct effect of the drug. Subsequently, some or all of the ADP in the storage pool is released from the platelets, causing a second, larger wave of aggregation. A double-wave of aggregation may also be obtained with ADP.

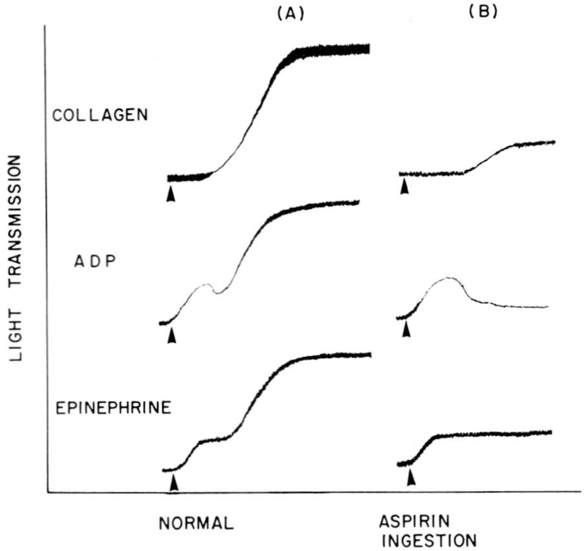

Fig. 1. Platelet aggregation in normal subjects before (**A**) and after (**B**) aspirin ingestion. The light transmittance through stirred platelet-rich plasma is recorded and platelet aggregation after addition (A) of collagen, ADP, or epinephrine is associated with an increase in transmittance. The abnormalities produced by aspirin are due to an impairment in the release of endogenous platelet ADP.

The first wave is due to a direct effect of ADP, while the second is the result of ADP released from platelets. The process by which the storage-pool of adenine nucleotides and other granule-bound substances, such as heparin-neutralizing factor (platelet factor 4, PF-4) are released from platelets by a variety of substances is known as the release reaction and has been compared with the secretory mechanism of endocrine cells. A more detailed discussion of mechanisms involved in both platelet aggregation and the release reaction may be found in several recent review articles.[23–25]

EFFECTS OF ASPIRIN ON PLATELETS

Platelet Aggregation

The amount of collagen-induced platelet aggregation in stirred platelet-rich plasma is diminished after aspirin ingestion in man[15,26,27] and other species.[28,29] Platelet aggregation may also be inhibited by the in vitro addition of aspirin to normal plasma.[26–28] The effects of aspirin on ADP-induced aggregation are more complex. It does not inhibit ADP-induced aggregation when this test is performed at room temperature[15] nor does it inhibit the first wave of ADP-induced aggregation, tested at 37°C.[26,27,30] However, aspirin completely blocks the second wave of aggregation, which may be obtained at 37°C[26,27,30] and which is due to the ADP released from platelets during the release reaction (see above). Aspirin, both in vitro and after ingestion, suppresses the second wave of epinephrine-induced platelet aggregation but has no effect on the first wave.[26,27] It also inhibits the aggregation of platelets by immune complexes and by low concentrations of thrombin.[28]

Release Reaction

The inhibitory effects of aspirin on platelet aggregation appear to be due entirely to its ability to prevent the release of ADP,[15,26,28] the agent ultimately responsible for platelet aggregation. As a consequence of this diminished release of storage pool ADP, collagen-induced aggregation and the second waves of epinephrine and ADP-induced aggregation are impaired (see above). In addition to inhibiting the release of ADP, however, aspirin, in vitro and in vivo, inhibits collagen-induced release of ATP,[26,31] serotonin,[32] and heparin neutralizing factor.[33] It also inhibits the release of these substances by epinephrine and ADP.[30,32,35,36] As these granule-bound substances are platelet constituents extruded during the release reaction, it seems highly likely that the most general effect of aspirin on platelets is to inhibit the release mechanism. Further evidence supporting this possibility are findings that aspirin prevents ultrastructural changes in platelets associated with early stages of the release reaction.[37]

Effects on Other Aspects of Platelet Function

The platelet coagulant activity (platelet factor 3, PF-3) cannot be demonstrated in intact platelet-rich plasma, but can be made available by incubating plasma with a variety of substances. Aspirin inhibits ADP[30] but not kaolin-induced[15] PF-3 availability. Breddin et al used a nonphotometric method to demonstrate that aspirin inhibits platelet aggregation.[38] Aspirin has been reported to decrease the adhesion of platelets to glass, as measured by the rotating bulb method,[13] but the retention of platelets in glass bead filters is not diminished.[39]

Dosage Requirements and Duration of Aspirin Effect

The concentration of aspirin which inhibits the platelet-release reaction in vitro appears to be of the same order of magnitude as that obtained in plasma in ordinary clinical usage. Weiss et al reported that the collagen-induced release of platelet ADP could be almost maximally suppressed by adding aspirin to platelet-rich plasma in a concentration of 50 μM. A tenfold increase in concentration resulted in only a modest increase in this inhibitory effect, and no further inhibition was obtained with concentrations of aspirin in excess of 500 μM.[26] Zucker and Peterson found that the collagen-induced release of platelet-bound ^{14}C-serotonin was maximally suppressed by aspirin in a concentration of 35 μM.[32] In man, oral doses of 600–2400 mg[40] and 300–3600 mg[41] of aspirin appeared to be equally effective in suppressing collagen-induced aggregation. The second wave of epinephrine-induced aggregation can be abolished by as small an oral dose as 150 mg.[27] There is no evidence that human platelets may become refractory to the inhibitory effects of aspirin after long-term administration of high doses.[42]

Comparison with Other Nonsteroidal Anti-inflammatory Agents

The effects of other nonsteroidal anti-inflammatory agents on platelets appear, in general, to be similar to those of aspirin.[32,43] Zucker and Peterson[32] and O'Brien[43] compared the relative potencies of these agents in inhibiting platelet aggregation. At equimolar concentrations, meclofenemic acid,[43] aspirin,[32,43] and indomethacin[32,43] were the most active. Phenylbutazone had only a weak inhibitory effect, while sulfinpyrazone, a pyrazole analog of this drug, had an activity similar to that of aspirin.[32] Among the anti-inflammatory agents, aspirin may be unique in that the inhibitory effects of a single oral dose may persist for a longer period of time. Thus, the effect of a single oral dose, in man, on both collagen-induced ADP release[26] (Figure 2) and epinephrine-induced platelet aggregation[27] may be detected for 4–7 days, when salicylate is no longer detectable in the blood.[26] These findings suggest that a single dose of aspirin may produce an irreversible injury which persists throughout the platelet's lifespan.[26] However, alternative explanations for the prolonged duration of aspirin-induced platelet defect have been suggested.[38,44]

Possible Mechanisms by which Aspirin Inhibits Platelet Function

Metabolic affects. Aspirin uncouples oxidative phosphorylation in many in vitro cell systems, but it has been difficult to demonstrate this in whole animal experiments.[46] Doery, et al have reported that aspirin, in a concentration of 55

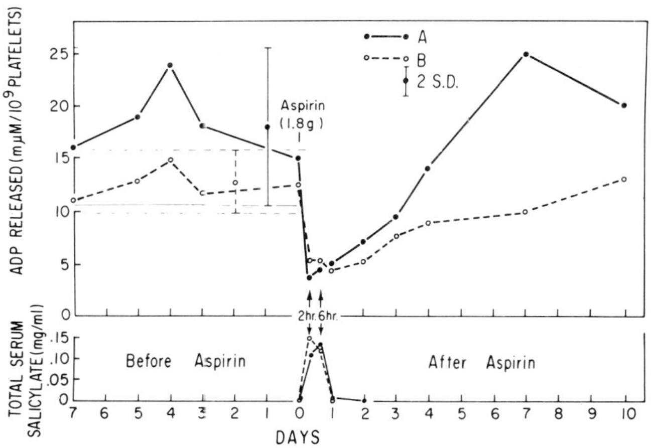

Fig. 2. Duration of aspirin-induced platelet defect. The amount of ADP released when 2.6 ml of citrated platelet-rich plasma was stirred with 0.1 ml of a connective tissue suspension (crude collagen) is shown for 2 normal subjects (**A** and **B**). The values for the mean ± 2 SD obtained 5 days before the ingestion of aspirin are indicated for each subject. The aspirin-induced defect is detectable for 4–7 days (Reprinted by permission from Weiss, et al.[26])

mM, inhibited glycolysis in washed platelets and produced a fall in platelet ATP.[47] More recently they have reported that a concentration of 0.05 mM resulted in a 17% fall in glucose uptake without, however, changing the rate of glycogen depletion.[48] This suggests that aspirin may have decreased glucose uptake in these experiments.[48] Ball et al reported that aspirin inhibits the conversion of ^{14}C-ATP in platelets to inosine monophosphate (IMP) and hypoxanthine, which normally occurs during collagen-induced aggregation.[31] Gaut and Solomon reported that aspirin inhibits the synthesis of nicotinamide adenine dinucleotide in washed platelets, but concluded that this effect was probably unrelated to its inhibitor effect on platelet aggregation.[49] The distribution of phospholipids and fatty acid in platelets remains unchanged in man after the ingestion of aspirin.[50]

Prostaglandins. Prostaglandin E_1 (PGE_1) has been shown to inhibit platelet aggregation and appears to be one of the most potent inhibitors of platelet aggregation studied. PGA_1 inhibits platelet aggregation to a much lesser degree than does PGE_1, whereas the B and F series of prostaglandins are inactive.[51,52] PGE_2, by contrast, stimulates platelet aggregation, and recent evidence suggests that this prostaglandin may play a role in platelet aggregation induced by a variety of stimuli. Thus, Smith and Willis[53] and more recently Smith, et al have shown that PGE_2 is synthesized and then released from platelets stimulated by thrombin, collagen, epinephrine, and ADP. Shio and Ramwell recently reported that PGE_2 potentiates both collagen-induced platelet aggregation and the second waves of epinephrine and ADP-induced aggregation.[55] These latter findings suggest that PGE_2, synthesized in the platelet, may play a role in the release reaction, and the findings of Smith and Willis that aspirin can inhibit PGE_2 synthesis in platelets[53] may, therefore, account for its inhibitory effect on the release mechanism. The production of PGE_2 in tissues is thought to be brought about by cyclization of arachidonic acid liberated by the action of phospholipase A. Findings that the production of PGE_2 in platelets was inhibited by aspirin, while the release of phospholipase A was unaffected, suggests that one action of aspirin on platelets may be to inhibit the conversion of arachidonic acid into prostaglandins.[53] The finding of Leonardi, et al that the inhibitory effect of aspirin on platelet aggregation can be prevented by prior preincubation of the platelet-rich plasma with arachidonic acid provides further support for this possibility.[56] However, Shio and Ramwell reported that the inhibitory effects of aspirin could not be prevented by the addition of PGE_2.[55] The entire relationship between prostaglandins and platelet abnormalities induced by aspirin requires further study.

Requirement of acetyl group. In contrast to the inhibitory effects of aspirin, sodium salicylate has little, if any, effect on either collagen-induced platelet aggregation,[26,27] the second waves of ADP and epinephrine-induced aggregation,[26,27] or the release of ADP[26] by platelet-bound ^{14}C-serotonin.[32] Neither does it prolong bleeding time.[14,16] It is not known why aspirin, but not sodium salicylate, is effective in inhibiting platelets, although the requirement of the acetyl group has been noted for some other biologic effects of salicylates.[26] The greater inhibitory effects of aspirin is probably not due to its more rapid diffusion into the cell or to a lesser degree of binding to albumin.[26] Hawkins, et al demonstrated that aspirin can acetylate albumin and other proteins.[58] Al-Mondhiry, et al incubated platelet-rich plasma with aspirin labeled with carbon-14 in either the carboxyl or acetyl group and found that only in the latter case did radioactivity become irreversibly bound to platelets.[59] However, they were unable to distinguish acetylation of platelets from incorporation of acetate into metabolically active pathways. Finally, it has been suggested that some of the long-lived effects of aspirin on platelets may be due to acetylation of a plasma protein which may be involved in platelet aggregation.[38,44]

Possible effects on platelet membrane. Holmsen, et al suggested that the induction phase of the release reaction may be directed at a receptor on the platelet membrane,[60] and it has been suggested that aspirin, as well as other anti-inflammatory agents, may "stabilize" the platelet membrane,[26] possibly by mechanisms involved in their stabilization of other membranes.[52,61] For example, many nonsteroidal anti-inflammatory agents protect red cells against both hypotonic and heat-induced lysis.[62–64] These agents also protect serum albumin and other proteins against heat denaturation,[65] and it has been suggested that the stabilization of erythrocyte membranes by anti-inflammatory drugs might be due to a stabilizing effect on certain proteins in the cell membrane.[64] A wide variety of other membrane-active drugs also affect platelets in a manner similar to that obtained with aspirin.[52] Mills and Roberts, for example, have shown that amitryptyline, a tricyclic antidepressant drug, blocks the release of adenine nucleotides and serotonin,[66] and Ball, et al showed that this drug, like aspirin, also blocks the conversion of ^{14}C-ATP in platelets to IMP and hypoxanthine, which normally occurs in association with the release reaction.[31] The phenothiazines and antihistamines, like the tricyclic antidepressants, also inhibit the second waves of epinephrine and ADP-induced aggregation.[66] All of these agents have been shown to stabilize biologic membranes. The phenothiazines, for example, stabilize red cells against hypotonic lysis[67] and may prevent mitochondrial swelling.[68] Antihistamines also appear to stabilize lysosomes,[69] while the tricyclic antidepressants inhibit the uptake of catecholamines by peripheral adrenergic neurons.[70] Thus, these drugs, as well as the nonsteroidal anti-inflammatory agents, appear to modify a wide variety of biologic membranes and their effects on platelets may be on a similar basis, the precise nature of which requires further clarification.

Jamieson, et al recently presented more direct evidence that aspirin may affect the platelet membrane.[71] They described the presence in the membrane of an enzyme, collagen glucosyltransferase, which can catalyze the transfer of glucose from uridine diphosphate glucose to incomplete heterosaccharide chains in collagen and suggested that the adhesion of platelets to collagen may be mediated by the formation of a complex between the enzyme and the incomplete carbohydrate chains. Aspirin inhibits glucosyltransferase,[71] and it was therefore suggested that the inhibitory effect of aspirin on platelet-to-collagen adhesion, reported in some[26,71] but not all[72] studies, was due to its inhibition of this membrane-bound enzyme. Finally, Barnhardt has reported that the surface configuration of platelets in circulating blood and after their exposure to formvar-coated surfaces is altered by aspirin.[73]

CLINICAL IMPLICATIONS

Hemostasis

Aspirin ingestion results in only a modest prolongation of the bleeding time in most normal subjects and, under most circumstances, the hemostatic defect is of no clinical significance. However, where maximum hemostasis is desirable, the deleterious effects of aspirin should be appreciated. For example: the effects of aspirin, either alone or in combination, on the amount of blood lost during surgical procedures requires further study. Its use should certainly be avoided in patients with bleeding disorders, such as hemophilia. Among analgesic agents with comparable potency, acetaminophen does not inhibit platelet aggregation or prolong bleeding time.[20,74] These effects also are not observed after the ingestion of codeine or propoxyphene.[20,43] The question has been raised as to whether aspirin should be proscribed in platelet donors, since platelets obtained from donors who have recently ingested aspirin are less effective in shortening bleeding time in thrombocytopenic patients.[75] It is possible, however, that platelet concentrates pooled from many donors may be hemostatically effective as long as some of these donors have not ingested aspirin. In vitro, it has been shown that the aspirin-induced defect in platelet aggregation in platelet-rich plasma (PRP) can be eliminated by adding as little as one-tenth volume of normal PRP.[27] Presumably, enough ADP can be released from normal platelets to cause the aggregation of aspirin-treated platelets. More clinical studies in this area are needed. Nevertheless, a history of recent drug ingestion should be obtained from prospective blood donors, and whenever a large yield of platelets is to be derived by plasmaphoresis of 1 or 2 donors, ingestion of aspirin within 5 days of blood collection should be avoided.

It has been suggested that an aspirin-tolerance test may be useful in detecting patients with mild bleeding disorders, particularly those with von Willebrand's disease.[14] While the bleeding time in such patients may be prolonged to a greater degree than in normal subjects, this effect is not specific for any one type of bleeding disorder.[19] The response of platelets to an in vitro challenge of aspirin has recently been shown to be different in patients whose defects in platelet aggregation are caused by a deficiency of the storage pool of adenine nucleotides (storage-pool disease) than in those with an "aspirin-like" defect.[76] This in vitro aspirin-tolerance test may be useful in studying patients with bleeding disorders due to defects in platelet aggregation.

Thrombosis

Since the formation of a platelet aggregate appears to be an early event in the formation of vascular thrombi, particularly those that occur in the arterial circulation, it has been suggested that drugs, such as aspirin, which inhibit platelet aggregation may be useful antithrombotic agents. When administered to dogs, aspirin significantly reduced the incidence of occlusive thrombi in peripheral arteries injured with a sclerosing agent or by endarterectomy.[29] Aspirin also reduced the size of electrically induced coronary thrombi[77] and modified both the lethal effects of endotoxin infusion[78,79] and the hyperacute rejection of renal allografts.[80] In rats, aspirin, as well as pyrazole compounds, conferred protection against hyperlipemia-induced thrombosis,[81,82] but not against thrombus formation in injured mesenteric arteries.[83] Aspirin also reduced both the amount of thrombotic deposit in extracorporeal shunts[28] and the incidence of morrhuate-induced thrombosis in the veins of rabbits.[84]

In clinical studies, aspirin has been reported to decrease the number of attacks of transient monocular blindness in 2 patients with amaurosis fugax[85] and produced dramatic improvement in 1 patient with microangiopathic hemolytic anemia.[86] It did not, however, appear to improve platelet survival in patients with cardiac prosthetic valves.[87] The results obtained with aspirin in venous thrombosis have been conflicting. In one study, aspirin significantly reduced the incidence of clinically detectable venous thrombosis after cup arthroplasty of the hip.[88] More recently, aspirin did not confer protection against the development of postoperative venous thrombosis, detected by the uptake of ^{125}I fibrinogen, in the calf.[89] The possibility that aspirin may confer protection against myocardial infarction and transient cerebral ischemic attacks associated with ulcerative lesion of the carotid artery is currently under investigation. When compared with defects in platelet aggregation in patients with idiopathic bleeding disorders, aspirin appears to be a rather weak platelet antiaggregant[89] and perhaps other, more potent, drugs may prove to be more useful antithrombotic agents.

REFERENCES

1. Quick AJ, Clesceri I: Influence of acetylsalicylic acid and salicylamide on the coagulation of the blood. J Pharmacol Exp Ther 128:95, 1960
2. Meyer OO, Howard B: Production of hypoprothrombinemia and hypocoagulability of the blood with salicylates. Proc Soc Exp Biol Med 53:234, 1943
3. Smith JM, MacKinnon J: Aetiology of aspirin bleeding. Lancet 2:569, 1951
4. Frick PG: Hemorrhagic diathesis with increased capillary fragility caused by salicylate therapy. Am J Med Sci 231:402, 1956
5. Neivert H: Late secondary tonsillar hemorrhage; studies of prothrombin and vitamin K. Arch Otolaryngol 42:14, 1945
6. Reuter SH, Montgomery WW: Aspirin vs acetaminophen after tonsillectomy: a comparative double-blind clinical study. Arch Otolaryngol 80:214, 1964
7. Singer R: Acetylsalicylic and a probable cause for secondary post-tonsillectomy hemorrhage. Arch Otolaryngol 42:19, 1945
8. Bleyer WA, Breckenridge RT: Studies on the detection of adverse drug reactions in the newborn. II. The effects of prenatal aspirin on newborn hemostasis. JAMA 213:2049, 1970
9. Stubbé L, ThFL: Occult blood in faeces after administration of aspirin. Br. Med J 2:1062, 1958
10. Smith MJH: Gastrointestinal bleeding, The Salicylates A Critical Bibliographic review. Edited by MJH Smith, PK Smith. New York, Interscience Publishers, 1966
11. Beaumont JL, Caen J, Bernard J: Influence de l'acide acetyl salicylique dans les maladies hemorragiques. Sangue 27:243, 1956
12. Blatrix C: Allongement du temps de saignement sous l'influence de certain medicaments. Nouv Rev Franc Hematol 3:346, 1963
13. Gast LF: Influence of aspirin on haemostatic parameters. Ann Rheum Dis 23: 500, 1964
14. Quick AJ: Salicylates and bleeding: the aspirin tolerance test. Am J Med Sci 252:265, 1967
15. Weiss HJ, Aledort LM: Impaired platelet/connective tissue reaction in man after aspirin ingestion. Lancet 2:495, 1967
16. Mielke CH Jr, Kaneshiro MM, Maker IA, et al: The standardized normal Ivy bleeding time and its prolongation by aspirin. Blood 34:204, 1969
17. Kaneshiro MM, Mielke CH, Kasper CK, et al: Bleeding time after aspirin in disorders of intrinsic clotting. N Engl J Med 281:1039, 1969
18. Quick AJ: Acetylsalicylic acid as a diagnostic aid in hemostasis. Am J Med Sci 254:585, 1967
19. Sahud MA, Cohen RJ: Aspirin-induced prolongation of the Ivy bleeding time. Calif Med 115:10, 1971
20. Kasper CK, Rapaport SI: Bleeding time and platelet aggregation after analgesics in hemophilia. Ann Intern Med 77:189, 1972
21. Baumgartner HR, Haudenschild C: Adhesion of platelets to subendothelium. Ann NY Acad Sci (In press)
22. Gaarder A, Laland S: Hypothesis for the aggregation of platelets by nucleotides. Nature 202:909, 1964
23. Holmsen H, Day HJ: Adenine nucleotides and platelet function. Ser Haematol 4:28, 1971
24. Mustard JF, Packham MA: Factors influencing platelet function: adhesion, release and aggregation. Pharmacol Rev 22:97, 1970

25. Michal F, Firkin BG. Physiological and pharmacological aspects of the platelet. Ann Rev Pharmacol 9:95, 1969
26. Weiss HJ, Aledort LM, Kochwa S: The effect of salicylates on the hemostatic properties of platelets in man. J Clin Invest 47:2169, 1968
27. O'Brien JR: Effects of salicylates on human platelets. Lancet 1:779, 1968
28. Evans G, Packham MA, Nishizawa EE, et al: The effect of acetylsalicylic acid on platelet function. J Exp Med 128:877, 1968
29. Danese CA, Voleti CD, Weiss HJ: Protection by aspirin against experimentally induced thrombosis in dogs. Thromb Diath Haemorrh 25:288, 1971
30. Zucker MB, Peterson J: Inhibition of adenosine diphosphate-induced secondary aggregation and other platelet functions by acetylsalicylic acid ingestion. Proc Soc Exp Biol Med 127:547, 1968
31. Ball G, Fulwood M, Ireland DM, et al: Effect of some inhibitors of platelet aggregation on platelet nucleotides. Biochem J 114:669, 1969
32. Zucker MB, Peterson J: Effect of acetylsalicylic acid, other nonsteroidal anti-inflammatory agents, and dipyridamole on human blood platelets. J Lab Clin Med 76:66, 1970
33. Youssef AH, Barkhan P: Inhibition by aspirin of release of antiheparin activity from human platelets. Br Med J 3:394, 1969
34. Weiss HJ, Rogers J: Platelet factor 4 in platelet disorders: storage location and the requirement of endogenous ADP for its release. Proc Soc Exp Biol Med 142:30, 1973
35. O'Brien JR, Finch W, Clark E: Platelet-bound and soluble platelet factor 4: effects of aggregating agents, of aggregation and of aspirin. Proc Soc Exp Biol Med 134:1128, 1970
36. Harada K, Zucker MB: Simultaneous development of platelet 4 activity and release of ^{14}C-serotonin. Thromb Diath Haemorrh 25:41, 1971
37. Weiss HJ, Ames RP: Ultrastructural findings in the platelets of patients with abnormalities of platelet function. Am J Path 71:397, 1973
38. Breddin K, Scharrer I, Schepping M: Acetylsalicylic acid and platelet function. Thromb Diath Haemorrh Suppl 42:241, 1970
39. Weiss HJ: Aspirin ingestion compared with bleeding disorders: search for a useful platelet antiaggregant. Blood 35:333, 1970
40. O'Brien JR, Tulevski V, Etherington M: Two in vivo studies comparing high and low aspirin dosage. Lancet 1:339, 1971
41. Stuart RK: Platelet function studies in human beings receiving 300 mg of aspirin per day. J Lab Clin Med 75:463, 1970
42. Atac A, Spagnuolo M, Zucker MB: Long-term inhibition of platelet functions by aspirin. Proc Soc Exp Biol Med 133:1331, 1970
43. O'Brien JR: Effect of anti-inflammatory agents on platelets. Lancet 1:894, 1968
44. Okonkwo P, Sise HS: Effect of aspirin in vivo and in vitro on plasma cofactors of platelet aggregation. Thromb Diath Haemorrh 25:279, 1971
45. O'Brien JR, Finch W, Clark E: A comparison of an effect of different anti-inflammatory drugs on human platelets. J Clin Pathol 23:522, 1970
46. Brody TM: Action of sodium salicylate and related compounds on tissue metabolism in vitro. J Pharmacol Exp Ther 117:39, 1956
47. Doery JCG, Hirsh J, de Gruchy GC: Aspirin: its effect on platelet glycolysis and release of adenosine diphosphate. Science 165:65, 1969
48. Doery JCG, Hirsh J: Divergent effects of aspirin and salicylate on glucose and glycogen metabolism in human platelets. Experientia 27:533, 1971
49. Gaut ZN, Solomon HM: Inhibition of 7-^{14}C-nicotinic acid metabolism in the

human blood platelet by anti-inflammatory drugs. Res Commun Chem Pathol Pharmacol 1:547, 1970
50. Safrit H, Weiss HJ, Phillips G: Platelet phospholipids and fatty acids in patients with primary defects of platelet function. Lipids 7:60, 1972
51. Kloeze J: Relationship between chemical structure and platelet aggregation activity of prostaglandins. Biochim Biophys Acta 187:285, 1969
52. Weiss HJ: The pharmacology of platelet inhibition, Progress in Hemostasis and Thrombosis. Edited by TH Spaet. New York, Grune and Stratton, 1972, p 199
53. Smith JB, Willis AL: Aspirin selectively inhibits prostaglandin production in human platelets. Nature (New Biol) 231:235, 1971
54. Smith JB, Silver MJ, Ingerman C, et al: Prostaglandin production during platelet aggregation. Third Congress of the International Society of Thrombosis and Haemostasis. Durham, Seeman Printery, 1972, p 246
55. Shio H, Ramwell P: Effect of prostaglandin E_2 and aspirin on the secondary aggregation of human platelets. Nature (New Biol) 236:45, 1972
56. Leonardi RG, Alexander B, White F: Prevention of the inhibitory effect of aspirin on platelets. Fed Proc 31:248, 1972
57. Hawkins DR, Pinckard RN, Farr RS: Acetylation of human serum albumin by acetylsalicylic acid. Science 160:780, 1968
58. Hawkins D, Pinckard RN, Crawford IP, et al: Structural changes in human serum albumin induced by ingestion of acetylsalicylic acid. J Clin Invest 48: 536, 1969
59. Al-Mondhiry H, Marcus AJ, Spaet TH: On the mechanism of platelet function inhibition by acetylsalicylic acid. Proc Soc Exp Biol Med 133:632, 1970
60. Holmsen H, Day HJ, Stormorken H: The blood platelet release reaction. Scand J Haematol Suppl: 8, 1969
61. Whitehouse MW: The molecular pharmacology of anti-inflammatory drugs: some possible mechanisms of action at the biochemical level. Biochem pharmacol Suppl p 293, 1968
62. Glenn EM, Bowman BJ: In vitro effects of nonsteroidal anti-inflammatory drugs (NAIFD). Proc Soc Exp Biol Med 130:1327, 1968
63. Kalbhen DA, Gelderblom P, Domenjoz R: Effects of antirheumatic drugs on human erythrocyte membranes. Pharmacology 3:353, 1970
64. Mizushima Y, Sakai, S, Yamaura M: Mode of stabilizing action of nonsteroid anti-inflammatory drugs on erythrocyte membrane. Biochem Pharmacol 19:227, 1970
65. Mizushima Y, Kobayashi M: Reaction of anti-inflammatory drugs with serum proteins, especially with some biologically active proteins. J Pharm Pharmacol 20:169, 1968
66. Mills DCB, Roberts GCK: Membrane active drugs and the aggregation of human blood platelets. Nature (Lond) 213:35, 1967
67. Seeman PM: Membrane stabilization by drugs: tranquilizers, steroids, and anesthetics. Int Rev Neurobiol 9:145, 1966
68. Judah JD, Ahmed K, McLean AEM: Possible role of ion shifts in liver injury, Ciba Foundation Symposium on Cellular Injury. Edited by AVS de Reuck, J Knight. Boston, Little, Brown, 1964
69. Judah JD: Protection against cellular injury by drugs, Drugs and Enzymes. Edited by JL Mongar, AVS de Reuck. Boston, Little, Brown, 1962, p 359
70. Malmfors T: Studies on adrenergic nerves. Acta Physiol Scand 64: Suppl, 248, 1965
71. Jamieson GA, Urban CL, Barber AJ: An enzymatic basis for platelet: collagen adhesion as the primary step in hemostasis. Nature (New Biol) 234:5, 1971

72. Spaet TH, Lejnieks I: A technique for estimation of platelet collagen adhesion. Proc Soc Exp Biol Med 132:1038, 1969
73. Barnhardt M, Walsh RT, Robinson JA: A 3-dimensional view of platelet responses to chemical stimuli. Ann NY Acad Sci 201:360, 1972
74. Mielke CH Jr, Britten AFH: Use of aspirin or acetaminophen in hemophilia. N Engl J Med 282:1270, 1970
75. Harker LA, Slichter SJ: The standardized bleeding time as a measure of platelet function in vivo. Abstracts of the Second Congress of the International Society on Thrombosis and Haemostasis, Oslo, 1971, p 78
76. Weiss HJ: Abnormalities in platelet function due to defects in the release reaction. Ann NY Acad Sci 201:161, 1972
77. Peter A, Regan TJ, Jesrani MU, et al: Effect of aspirin on experimentally induced coronary thrombosis. Clin Res 18:669, 1970
78. Hinshaw LB, Solomon LA, Erdos EG, et al: Effects of acetylsalicylic acid on the canine response to endotoxin. J Pharmacol Exp Ther 157:665, 1967
79. Erdos EG: Effect of nonsteroidal anti-inflammatory drugs in endotoxin shock. Biochem Pharmacol (Suppl), p 283, 1968
80. MacDonald A, Busch GJ, Alexander JL, et al.: Heparin and aspirin in the treatment of hyperacute rejection of renal allografts in presensitized dogs. Transplantation 9:1, 1969
81. Renaud S, Lecompte F: Thrombosis prevention by coagulation and platelet aggregation inhibitors in hyperlipemic rats. Thromb Diath Haemorrh 24:578, 1970
82. Renaud S, Godu J: Thrombosis prevention by acetylsalicylic acid in hyperlipemic rats. Can Med Assoc J 103:1037, 1970
83. Didisheim P: Inhibition by dipyridamole of arterial thrombosis in rats. Thromb Diath Haemorrh 20:257, 1968
84. Peterson J, Zucker MB: The effect of adenosine monophosphate, arcaine and anti-inflammatory agents on thrombosis and platelet function in rabbits. Thromb Diath Haemorrh 23:148, 1970
85. Harrison MJG, Marshall J, Meadows JC, et al: Effect of aspirin in amaurosis fugax. Lancet 2:743, 1971
86. Jobin F, Delage JM: Aspirin and prednisone in microangiopathic haemolytic anaemia. Lancet 2:208, 1970
87. Harker LA, Slichter SJ: Studies of platelet and fibrinogen kinetics in patients with prosthetic heart valves. N Engl J Med 283:1302, 1970
88. Salzman EW, Harris WH, DeSanctis RW: Reduction in venous thromboembolism by agents affecting platelet function. N Engl J Med 284:1287, 1971
89. Butterfield WJH, Br Med Res Council: Effect of aspirin on postoperative venous thrombosis. Lancet 2:441, 1972

Dale H. Cowan
and John D. Hines

24
Alcohol, Vitamins, and Platelets

An effect of ethyl alcohol on human blood platelets was first reported by Sullivan and Herbert[1] who documented thrombocytopenia in 3 subjects ingesting large quantities of whiskey and wine. Further evidence linking alcohol ingestion with thrombocytopenia was provided by Lindenbaum and Hargrove[2] who observed 10 episodes of thrombocytopenia in 5 patients admitted to hospital for acute alcoholism or alcohol withdrawal and by Post and Desforges[3] who documented thrombocytopenia on 20 occasions in 8 patients similarly hospitalized. This report will review clinical aspects of alcohol-related thrombocytopenia, the effect of ethanol and folic acid on thrombopoiesis and platelet survival, the effect of ethanol and folate deficiency on platelet function, and possible mechanisms by which ethanol affects platelets. The last portion of the article will review current knowledge of the relationship between ascorbic acid and platelets.

CLINICAL ASPECTS OF ALCOHOL-RELATED THROMBOCYTOPENIA

Thrombocytopenia, defined as platelet counts less than 100,000 per microliter, occurs in 20% to 35% of acutely ill alcoholic patients (patients admitted to hospital either because of acute intoxication, alcohol withdrawal, or complications of alcoholism)[4,5] and in 3% of nonacutely ill patients drawn from different socioeconomic classes in the community (Table 1).[6] Using this latter value and assuming an alcoholic population in the United States of 6,000,000,[7] alcohol-related thrombocytopenia is present in an estimated 180,000 individuals at any given time. This gives an overall incidence for the total population of 0.9 per 1000 and indicates that alcoholism is presently one of the most common single causes of thrombocytopenia in this country.

Supported by Grant 5 RO1 MH19558 from the National Institute of Alcohol Abuse and Alcoholism.

Table 1
Hematologic, Clinical, and Nutritional Abnormalities in Alcoholic Patients

			Incidence of*						
Authors	Status of Patients	No. of Patients	Anemia†	Leuko-penia†	Thrombo-cytopenia†	Folate Deficiency†	Megaloblastic Maturation	Hepto-megaly	Spleno-megaly
Cowan, Hines[4]	Acutely ill	43	51	5	35	67‡	60	63	9
Eichner, Hillman[5]	Acutely ill	65	62	8	20	40	50	55	—
Eichner, et al[6]	Chronic	112	9	4	3	20–25 50**	2	8–13	0

* Values listed are per cent (%) of total number of patients in study group.

† Definitions: Anemia–Hct < 38%; Leukopenia–WBC < 5000 per microliter; Thrombocytopenia–Platelets < 100,000 per microliter; Folate Deficiency–< 3.4 μg per milliliter.

‡Measurements done in 30 patients.

** 50% incidence seen in 1 of 4 groups studied; 20%–25% incidence present in the other 3 groups.

The incidence of thrombocytopenia in the different groups of alcoholic patients is one-third to one-half that of anemia (Table 1). No correlation exists between the presence of anemia and that of thrombocytopenia in acutely ill hospitalized patients (Figure 1).[4,5] Similarly, there is no correlation between the white blood cell and platelet counts in these patients.[4,5]

Alcohol-related thrombocytopenia may be quite severe; platelet counts as low as 10,000 per microliter have been reported in individual patients.[3–5] The clinical significance of the thrombocytopenia, however, is difficult to judge. No bleeding episodes were reported in the 108 acutely ill patients comprising the series reported by Cowan and Hines[4] and Eichner and Hillman.[5] By contrast, ecchymoses or other evidence of bleeding occurred with 7 of 10 episodes of thrombocytopenia reported by Lindenbaum and Hargrove.[2] Thrombocytopenia appears to be only one of several factors predisposing the alcoholic patient to bleeding, since the range of platelet counts in the groups of patients comprising these studies was similar.

Folic acid deficiency occurs in a large proportion of alcoholic patients (Table 1).[8] Although folate deficiency per se may cause thrombocytopenia, the

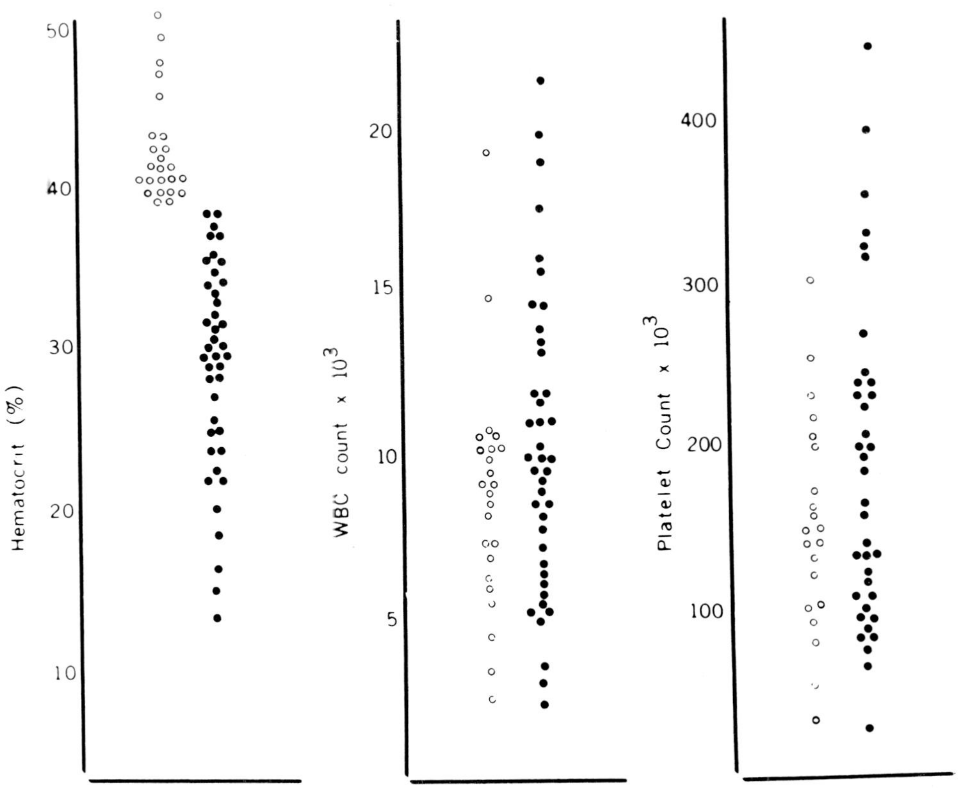

Fig. 1. Incidence of anemia, leukopenia, and thrombocytopenia in acutely ill hospitalized alcoholic patients. Open circles denote patients with Hct > 39% and closed circles denote patients with Hct < 39%. (Reproduced by permission from the publisher from Eichner, et al.[5])

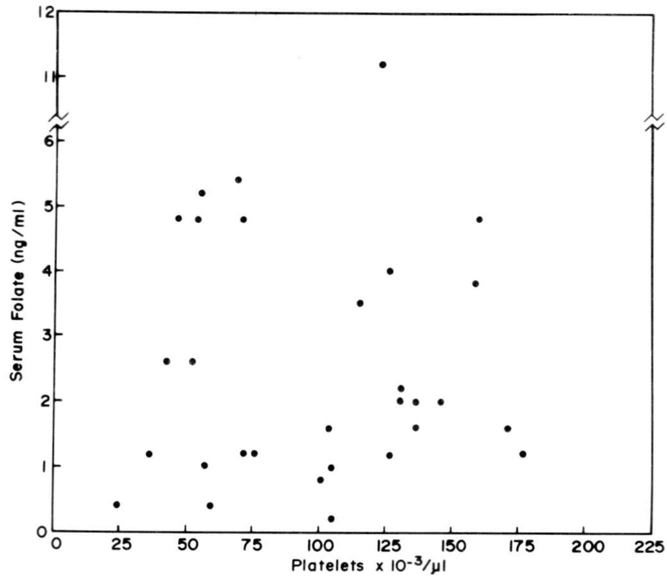

Fig. 2. Relationship between folate levels and platelet counts in patients admitted to hospital for acute alcoholism. (Reproduced by permission from the publisher from Cowan, et al.[4])

development of thrombocytopenia in the alcoholic patient may not be dependent upon the presence of a deficiency of this vitamin in the body (Figure 2). Indeed, there is evidence that thrombocytopenia can occur in alcoholic subjects who are not folate deficient and whose marrows show normoblastic cellular maturation. Lindenbaum and Hargrove[2] detected normal levels of serum folate with each of five episodes of thrombocytopenia in which folate was measured. Lindenbaum and Lieber[9] observed significant decreases in platelet counts in 4 of 9 patients given 1200 μg pteroylglutamic acid (PGA) orally every day and ethanol in doses equaling 46%–66% of their daily total caloric intake. Cowan[10] observed thrombocytopenia in 2 of 3 patients receiving 5 mg PGA orally every day and 30 ounces of 86 proof blended whiskey (constituting approximately 50%–60% of daily caloric intake). The bone marrows of these folate-supplemented patients did not show megaloblastic maturation.

Hepatomegaly and some degree of abnormality of liver function were present in the majority (55%–63%) of the acutely ill hospitalized alcoholic patients evaluated hematologically.[4,5] Since the degree of abnormality of liver function varies with the amount of ethanol ingested, the adequacy of the diet, and the degree of physical debility, it is understandable that a lesser incidence of hepatomegaly (8%–13%) and a lesser degree of liver dysfunction were observed in the nonacute patients seen by Eichner, et al[6] than in the acutely ill hospitalized patients (Table 1). There was no relation between the presence or severity of liver function abnormalities and the presence or severity of thrombocytopenia.

Splenomegaly was uncommon in each of the series of patients studied and appeared to be related to the severity of the derangement of liver function. Splenomegaly was not detected by physical examination in patients in whom thrombocytopenia occurred during the course of supervised alcohol ingestion.

Coagulation abnormalities have not been observed in association with alcohol-related thrombocytopenia.[3,4] Fibrinogen levels were normal, and fibrinogen-fibrin related antigens were not detected in the blood of volunteer subjects who developed thrombocytopenia while ingesting whiskey in the hospital.[11] Available data thus indicate that the thrombocytopenia associated with alcohol ingestion is not a manifestation of disseminated intravascular coagulation.

The platelet counts in patients with alcohol-related thrombocytopenia return towards normal spontaneously when ingestion of ethanol is discontinued.[2,4,5,9,12] Platelet counts in nonthrombocytopenic alcoholics also increase after alcohol ingestion ceases.[2,4] Although the concentration of circulating platelets may begin to increase before the ingestion of ethanol has been fully discontinued, often 2–3 days elapse after the last drink before the platelet counts start to rise. Thereafter, the counts increase rapidly, reaching a peak value that is often in the supernormal range ($>$ 450,000 per microliter) 5–18 days (mean 10.7 days) after ingestion has ceased. Subsequently, they decrease to a level within normal range for healthy individuals. The increase in platelet counts to supernormal values after ethanol ingestion has ceased, is analogous to that seen in other situations of recovery from thrombocytopenia (e.g., recovery from drug-induced thrombocytopenia) or from hematologic stress (e.g., after sickle cell crisis). The increase in platelets occurs whether or not vitamins are administered or adequate nutrition is resumed.[4] The onset and rate of recovery are unaffected by the administration of corticosteroids.[3]

EFFECT OF ETHANOL AND FOLIC ACID ON THROMBOPOIESIS AND PLATELET SURVIVAL

Megakaryocytes

Decreased numbers of adult megakaryocytes were observed in smears of marrow aspirates obtained from 4 folate-deficient alcoholic patients admitted to hospital with thrombocytopenia.[13] However, no decrease in the number of megakaryocytes in smears of marrow aspirates was detected in hospitalized patients whose platelet counts decreased during the course of supervised alcohol ingestion.[9] These patients were nutritionally replete and did not develop thrombocytopenia. In other studies, the total mass of megakaryocytes, measured in sections of bone marrow biopsies obtained from patients with dietary-induced folate deficiency associated with megaloblastic marrow maturation—increases in apparent size and relative numbers of basophilic and polychromatophilic erythroblasts, less compact chromatin network, presence of giant metamyelocytes and bands—was increased threefold over normal (Table 2).[14] The subjects were not thrombocytopenic. This increase was due largely to an increase in the number of megakaryocytes. A slight but not significant decrease in mean megakaryocyte volume was also observed. Similar alterations in megakaryocyte number, mean

Table 2
Thrombopoiesis and Platelet Survival in Alcoholism and in Folate Deficiency

	Platelet				Megakaryocyte		
Patients	Count (No./μliter)	Life-span (Days)	Recovery (%)	Turnover (No./μliter day)	Number ($\times 10^6$/Kg BW)	Volume (μ^3)	Total Mass ($\times 10^{10}$ μ^3/Kg BW)
Folate Deficient (7)*	282,000	8.6	52	62,300	40.6	3762	15.2
Folate Deficient Ingesting EtOH (3)	62,000	2.7	55	37,600	57.2	3347	18.6
Folate Supplemented Ingesting EtOH (2)	66,000	3.8	61	25,700	20.8	3627	7.7
Normal (9)	276,000±24,000†	8.5±0.2	62±3	49,200±3,600	13.0±4.3	3982±253	5.1±1.0

* Numbers in parentheses indicate numbers of patients or normals studied.
† Denotes 2 SE.
The numbers in this table are derived from data in references 10 and 14.

volume, and total mass were detected in 2 folate-replete subjects who developed thrombocytopenia with ingestion of alcohol.[10]* By comparison, the number and total mass of megakaryocytes in folate-deficient subjects in whom thrombocytopenia occurred with alcohol ingestion were greater and the mean megakaryocyte volume was less than in either of the other two groups of patients. The results are indicative of a synergistic effect between folate deficiency and ethanol on the megakaryocyte.

The mechanism by which ethanol affects the megakaryocyte is unknown. Since changes in megakaryocyte number, volume, and total mass occurred in patients with normal serum and erythrocyte folate levels whose marrows showed normoblastic maturation, the mechanism does not appear to relate to a tissue deficiency of folate per se. Conceivably, however, ethanol affects the utilization or intracellular metabolism of folate by megakaryocytes.

Platelet Survival

Unlike the effects of ethanol ingestion and folate deficiency on megakaryocytes, the effects of these situations on platelet survival are dissimilar (Table 2). The survival of ^{51}Cr-labeled autologous platelets in patients with folate deficiency is normal, whereas that in both folate-deficient and folate-supplemented subjects ingesting ethanol is 32%–45% of normal when thrombocytopenia supervenes and 68% of normal in the absence of thrombocytopenia.[10,14] Platelet turnover, i.e., the number of platelets entering and leaving the circulation per unit time, is normal or slightly elevated with ethanol ingestion and/or folate deficiency in the absence of thrombocytopenia and significantly decreased when thrombocytopenia supervenes. Although the total potential capacity of the marrow for platelet production is increased over normal in patients with alcohol-related thrombocytopenia, as determined from the total megakaryocyte mass, the actual delivery of platelets to the circulation is less than that seen in normal individuals. Thus, the effective production of platelets in these patients is impaired, indicating that ethanol ingestion can lead to relative bone marrow suppression even in the presence of adequate tissue levels of folate. A similar conclusion was also drawn by Sahud[15] from measurements of platelet size in patients admitted to hospital for acute alcoholism and thrombocytopenia.

The thrombocytopenia associated with ingestion of ethanol is related, therefore, to decreased platelet survival and impaired thrombopoiesis.

When ethanol ingestion ceases, a rapid increase in the effectiveness of thrombopoiesis in patients[44] with greater than normal platelet-producing capacity can lead to a rapid increase in the concentration of circulating platelets. Additionally, prompt recovery from thrombocytopenia is associated with a return to normal of the reduced platelet life-span.

* An apparent discrepancy exists between the finding of increased numbers of megakaryocytes in the bone marrow sections and decreased or unchanged numbers of megakaryocytes in smears of marrow aspirates from patients who are alcoholic and/or folate deficient. Since the numbers of erythroid precursors are usually increased several fold with megaloblastic maturation, a persistent net increase in megakaryocyte number may be present although inapparent when viewed on smears of marrow aspirates.

EFFECT OF ETHANOL INGESTION AND FOLATE DEFICIENCY ON PLATELET FUNCTION

Ethanol ingestion in amounts that produce high levels of blood ethanol (> 300 mg per 100 ml) can lead to impaired platelet function and produce a hemorrhagic diathesis in susceptible individuals. In studies done in folate-replete patients who ingested 30–34 ounces daily of 86 proof blended whiskey on a metabolic ward, the bleeding times were observed to increase four to fivefold over control values when thrombocytopenia (platelets 55,000–65,000 per microliter) supervened and to twice the control values when thrombocytopenia did not occur.[11]

The aggregation of platelets induced by adenosine diphosphate (ADP), epinephrine, thrombin, and collagen was also impaired during the period of ethanol ingestion (Figure 3).[11] Abnormalities of aggregation were greater in patients who became thrombocytopenic. In these patients, the rate of primary aggregation in response to ADP and epinephrine was decreased to one-half normal and secondary aggregation was absent. The interval between the addition of collagen to the platelets and the onset of aggregation was prolonged 1.5-fold, and the rate and maximal extent of collagen-induced aggregation were

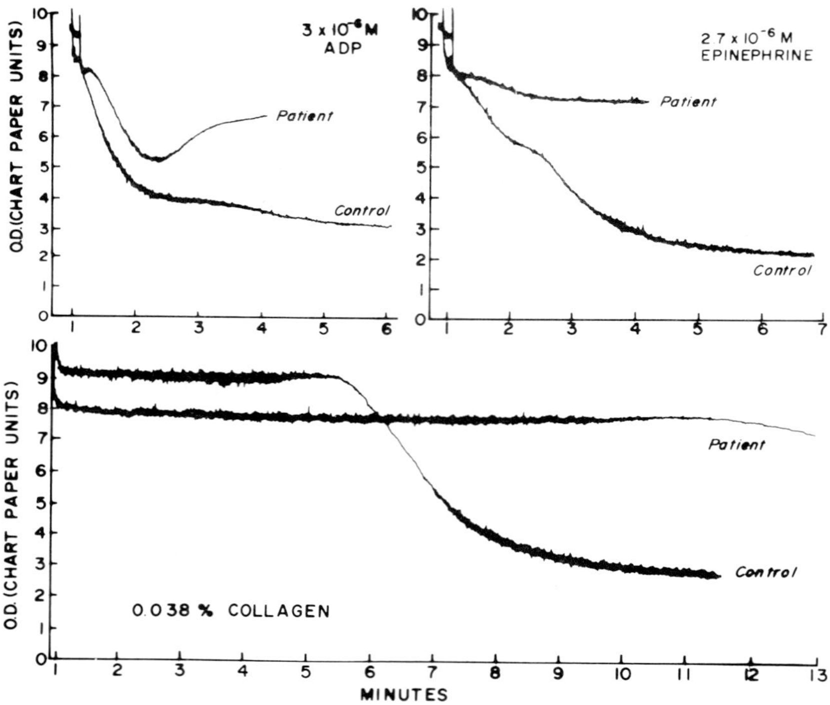

Fig. 3. Aggregation of platelets (citrated PRP) from a patient with alcohol-related thrombocytopenia (peripheral platelet count 60,000 per microliter) in response to ADP, epinephrine, and collagen. The concentrations of aggregating agents are shown. Measurements with normal and patient platelets were done the same day. The concentration of platelets in the normal PRP was made equivalent to that in patient PRP by dilution with autologous platelet-poor plasma.

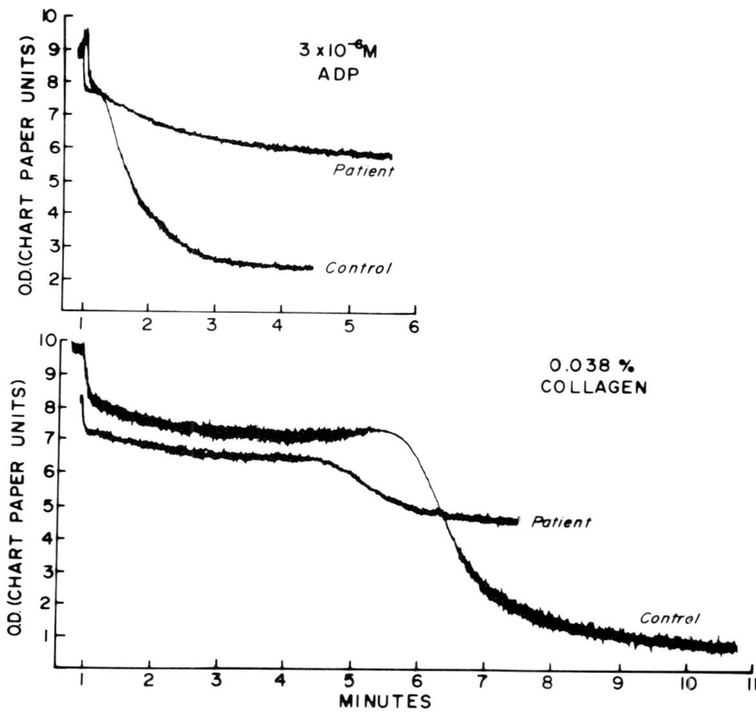

Fig. 4. Aggregation of platelets from a thrombocytopenic folate-deficient patient (peripheral blood platelet count 110,000 per microliter) in response to ADP and collagen at concentrations shown. All studies were done the same day. The platelet counts in the PRP from the patient and normal control were adjusted to 150,000 per microliter using autologous platelet-poor plasma.

decreased from normal by 20%–60% depending upon the concentration of collagen used. Additionally, platelets from the thrombocytopenic subjects showed a 50% decrease in platelet factor 3 (PF 3) availability and a 65% decrease in the release of endogenous adenine nucleotides after thrombin stimulation.[11] The latter appears related to a comparable decrease in the concentration of intracellular ADP.[16] The abnormalities in platelet function may be one factor causing the reduced platelet survival described earlier.

Alterations in platelet aggregation, similar to those mentioned above, may be seen in nonalcoholic patients with folate deficiency who are thrombocytopenic.[16] Representative results obtained in one patient are depicted in Figure 4. These observations are similar to those recently described in patients with pernicious anemia.[17] Normalization of platelet function occurs after appropriate replacement therapy is started.

MECHANISM OF THE EFFECT OF ETHANOL ON PLATELETS

The mechanism by which ethanol affects platelets is unknown. Results of several studies suggest that its affect may be a direct one. The intravenous administration of ethanol at rates leading to blood levels of 200 mg per 100 ml may induce a transient thrombocytopenia[18] and a reversible defect in platelet aggregation.[11] Addition of ethanol in vitro to normal citrated platelet-rich plasma in final concentrations of 240 mg per 100 ml or greater is associated with a 20%–25% decrease in collagen-induced aggregation and a reduction in secondary aggregation in response to ADP or epinephrine that varies with the relative concentrations of ethanol and the aggregating agent.[11,19] Significant reductions in PF 3 availability and in the rate of nucleotide release also occur with the addition of ethanol in vitro to normal platelets.[11]

It is possible that some of the effects of ethanol on platelets may result from increases in plasma osmolality, since appreciable increases in osmolality occur in plasmas containing ethanol in concentrations exceeding 300 mg per 100 ml.[20] Preliminary studies in our laboratory indicate that the addition to normal plasma of hypertonic sodium chloride in amounts which elevate plasma osmolality to levels associated with ethanol concentrations of 240 and 400 mg per 100 ml impairs platelet aggregation in a manner similar to that which occurs with in vitro addition of ethanol.

Another possibility is that ethanol may behave as a local anesthetic and alter the reactivity of platelet membranes.[21,22] Local anesthetic agents appear able to stabilize membranes,[23] and several drugs which are stabilizers of biologic membranes inhibit the secondary phase of ADP-induced platelet aggregation.[24] Additionally, local anesthetics, such as cocaine and tetracaine, inhibit ADP-induced aggregation.[25,26]

A third possibility is that ethanol increases the level of platelet adenylate cyclase (AC) activity. Recent studies have shown that ethanol can stimulate AC activity in both rat and human intestinal tissue.[27] There are considerable data which indicate that agents which produce increased levels of platelet AC activity resulting in increased levels of platelet 3′,5′-adenosine monophosphate inhibit platelet aggregation.[28] If ethanol has an effect on platelet AC activity, similar to that shown for jejunal AC activity, a decreased responsiveness to aggregating agents will result.

Conceivably, the effects of ethanol ingestion on platelets are due not to ethanol per se but to ethanol metabolites. For example, blood acetaldehyde concentrations of 0.11–0.15 mg per 100 ml (control 0.02 mg per 100 ml) occur after the ingestion of bourbon, when blood ethanol concentrations are 1–400 mg per 100 ml.[29] Concentrations of blood acetaldehyde do not correlate well with those of blood ethanol and remain relatively constant throughout intervals of long-term ingestion. Blood lactic acid levels increase two-to threefold with the ingestion of ethanol in amounts that produce blood ethanol levels of up to 75 mg per 100 ml.[30] The effects on platelet function of acetaldehyde, lactic acid, or other substances, which appear in the blood in increased concentrations as a result of ethanol ingestion, are as yet undetermined.

Finally, as mentioned earlier, it is probable that one mechanism by which ethanol affects platelets is by altering folate utilization. Presumably, some step in intracellular metabolism for which folic acid is required is deranged by the presence of ethanol (or a metabolite), since abnormalities in megakaryocytopoiesis occur in the presence of adequate tissue levels of this vitamin. It is possible that, as a result of a metabolic abnormality in the precursor cell, the adult cell has a biochemical and/or morphologic lesion which results in impaired functional activity and decreased survival. It is perhaps pertinent to recall that the abnormalities in platelet aggregation seen in patients with folic acid (or vitamin B_{12}) deficiency are very similar to those seen with ethanol ingestion. Conceivably, a common defect underlies the changes observed in each of these situations.

ASCORBIC ACID AND PLATELETS

Another nutritional disorder having an hemorrhagic diathesis is scurvy. The nature of the defect underlying the bleeding tendency in scorbutic individuals is not well understood. Platelet studies in scurvy have led to somewhat disparate results, but the evidence tends to indicate that some platelet defects are present in this situation. Although thrombocytopenia has been reported to occur in patients with scurvy,[31] normal platelet counts were detected in the patients comprising the few reports describing platelet abnormalities in human scurvy.[32–34] Slight thrombocytosis has been observed in scorbutic guinea pigs.[35,36] Hart, et al[33] reported that platelet morphology, bleeding time, and the tourniquet test were normal, and clot retraction was slightly prolonged in 3 patients with scurvy. Decreased or absent platelet agglutinability and adhesiveness were observed using phase-contrast microscopy by Cetingil et al in one patient.[32] Methods for assessing these events in the latter study were not, however, stated. Wilson, et al[34] observed reduced platelet adhesiveness to glass beads in two patients with scurvy and noted correction of the defect after administration of Vitamin C. Similar observations were made in experimental scurvy in guinea pigs by Born and Wright.[36] The latter authors also observed reduced platelet aggregation in response to ADP in scorbutic guinea pigs.[37]

The role of ascorbic acid in platelet physiology and the mechanism underlying platelet dysfunction in scurvy are not known. Platelets are known to contain a rather high concentration of ascorbic acid.[38,39] As expected, reduced platelet ascorbic acid levels are found in patients with scurvy.[34] Sahud and Aggeler[40] observed a direct correlation between the loss of ascorbic acid from platelets and platelet aggregation induced by ADP, epinephrine, thrombin, and collagen. No loss of ascorbic acid from platelets occurred when aggregation by collagen or epinephrine was impaired by prior ingestion of aspirin. Using analytic techniques, they did not detect the release of ascorbic acid from platelets into plasma during platelet aggregation. Based on these observations, they concluded that ascorbic acid has a definite physiologic role in platelet aggregation and is not merely being transported by the platelet to sites of tissue utilization.

Hornig, et al[41] reported that both (1-^{14}C) ascorbic acid and (1-^{14}C) dehydroascorbic acid were taken up by platelets from normal guinea pigs. Uptake of both of these substances was increased when platelets from scorbutic guinea pigs were used. After incubation with either of these substances, only (1-^{14}C) ascorbic acid was found within platelets. Release of (1-^{14}C) ascorbic acid from washed platelets occurred with incubation in the absence of aggregating agents. The significance of these observations with respect to the physiologic role of ascorbic acid in platelets remains to be determined.

It is pertinent that ascorbic acid deficiency is commonly associated with deficiencies of other vitamins and that, for example, when measured, serum folate levels in scorbutic patients have been subnormal and megaloblastic marrow maturation has been observed.[32,33] Although there is evidence that ascorbic acid participates in the reduction of folic acid to tetrahydrofolic acid,[42,43] the significance of the physiologic relationship between the metabolic functions of these two vitamins has not yet been established.[44] It is possible that some degree of platelet dysfuncton in the scorbutic patient, as in the alcoholic patient, may derive from a biochemical and/or morphologic defect caused by an abnormality in folate metabolism.

REFERENCES

1. Sullivan LW, Herbert V: Suppression of hematopoiesis by ethanol. J Clin Invest 43:2048, 1964
2. Lindenbaum J, Hargrove RL: Thrombocytopenia in alcoholics. Ann Intern Med 68:526, 1968
3. Post RM, Desforges JF: Thrombocytopenia and alcoholism. Ann Intern Med 68:1230, 1968
4. Cowan DH, Hines JD: Thrombocytopenia of severe alcoholism. Ann Intern Med 74:37, 1971
5. Eichner ER, Hillman RS: The evolution of anemia in alcoholic patients. Am J Med 50:218, 1971
6. Eichner ER, Buchanan B, Smith JW, et al: Variations in the hematologic and medical status of alcoholics. Am J Med Sci 263:35, 1972
7. Manual on Alcoholism. American Medical Association, 1968
8. Herbert V, Zalusky R, Davidson CS: Correlation of folate deficiency with alcoholism and associated macrocytosis, anemia, and liver disease. Ann Intern Med 58:977, 1963
9. Lindenbaum J, Lieber CS: Hematologic effects of alcohol in man in the absence of nutritional deficiency. N Engl J Med 281:33, 1969
10. Cowan DH: Thrombokinetic studies in alcohol-related thrombocytopenia. J Lab Clin Med 81:64, 1973
11. Haut MJ, Cowan DH: Effect of ethanol on hemostatic properties of human blood platelets. Unpublished data
12. Ryback R, Desforges JF: Alcoholic thrombocytopenia in three inpatient drinking alcoholics. Arch Intern Med 125:475, 1970
13. Sullivan LW, Lin YK, Talarico L, et al: Alcohol-induced thrombocytopenia in man. J Clin Invest 47: 95a, 1968 (abst)
14. Cowan DH, Hines JD: Thrombokinetics in dietary-induced folate deficiency in human subjects. J Lab Clin Med 81:577, 1973
15. Sahud MA: Platelet size and number in alcoholic thrombocytopenia. N Engl J Med 286:355, 1972
16. Cowan DH: Unpublished observations
17. Levine PH: A qualitative platelet defect in pernicious anemia. Observations on the development of thrombosis following vitamin B_{12} therapy, Third Congress of The International Society on Thrombosis and Haemostasis, Washington, DC, August 22–26, 1972, p 218 (abst)
18. Post RM, Desforges JF: Thrombocytopenic effect of ethanol infusion. Blood 31:344, 1968
19. Davis JW, Phillips PE: The effect of ethanol on human platelet aggregation in vitro. Atherosclerosis 11:473, 1970
20. Robinson AG, Loeb JN: Ethanol ingestion—commonest cause of elevated plasma osmolality? N Engl J Med 284:1253, 1971

21. Moore JW, Ulbricht W, Takata M: Effect of ethanol on the sodium and potassium conductances of the squid axon membrane. J Gen Physiol 48:279, 1964
22. Armstrong CM, Binstock L: The effects of several alcohols on the properties of the squid giant axon. J Gen Physiol 48:265, 1964
23. Seeman P, Kwant WO, Sanks T, et al: Membrane expansion of intact erythrocytes by anesthetics. Biochim Biophys Acta 183:490, 1969
24. Mills DCB, Roberts GCK: Membrane active drugs and the aggregation of human blood platelets. Nature (Lond) 213:35, 1967
25. O'Brien JR: A comparison of platelet aggregation produced by seven compounds and a comparison of their inhibitors. J Clin Pathol 17:275, 1964
26. Aledort LM, Niemetz J: Dissociation of platelet aggregation from clot retraction, potassium loss, and adenosine triphosphatase activity. Proc Soc Exp Biol Med 128:658, 1968
27. Greene HC, Herman RH, Kraemer S: Stimulation of jejunal adenyl cyclase by ethanol. J Lab Clin Med 78:336, 1971
28. Salzman EW: Cyclic AMP and platelet function. N Engl J Med 286:358, 1972
29. Majchrowicz E, Mendelson JH: Blood concentrations of acetaldehyde and ethanol in chronic alcoholics. Science 168:1100, 1970
30. Kreisberg RA, Owen WC, Siegal AM: Ethanol-induced hyperlacticacidemia: Inhibition of lactate utilization. J Clin Invest 50:166, 1971
31. Stefanini M, Dameshek W: The Hemorrhagic Disorders. Second edition. New York, Grune and Stratton, 1962
32. Cetingil AI, Ulutin ON, Karaca M: A platelet defect in a case of scurvy. Br J Haematol 4:350, 1958
33. Hart HC, Ploem JE, Panders JT, et al: Haemorrhagic diathesis and anemia in scurvy. Report on three cases. Acta Med Scand 176:497, 1964
34. Wilson PA, McNicol GP, Douglas AS: Platelet abnormality in human scurvy. Lancet 1:975, 1967
35. Barkham P, Howard AN: Some blood coagulation studies in normal and scorbutic guinea pigs. Br J Nutr 13:389, 1959
36. Born GVR, Wright HP: Platelet adhesiveness in experimental scurvy. Lancet 1:477, 1967
37. Born GVR, Wright HP: Diminished platelet aggregation in experimental scurvy. J Physiol 197:27P, 1968
38. Barkham P, Howard AN: Distribution of ascorbic acid in normal and leukaemic human blood. Biochem J 70:163, 1958
39. Denson KW, Richards JDM: Levels and uptake of ascorbic acid from plasma by white cells, platelets, and leukaemic cells. Nature 196:1218, 1962
40. Sahud MA, Aggeler PM: Utilization of ascorbic acid during platelet aggregation. Proc Soc Exp Biol Med 134:13, 1970
41. Hornig D, Weber F, Wiss O: Studies on the uptake of ($1\text{-}^{14}C$) ascorbic acid and ($1\text{-}^{14}C$) dehydroascorbic acid by platelets of guinea pigs. Clin Chim Acta 33: 187, 1971
42. Nichol CA, Welch AD: Synthesis of citrovorum factor from folic acid by liver slices. Augmentation by ascorbic acid. Proc Soc Exp Biol Med 74:52, 1950
43. Welch AD, Nichol CA, Anker RM, et al: The effect of ascorbic acid on the urinary excretion of citrovorum factor derived from folic acid. J Pharmacol Exp Ther 103:403, 1951
44. Stokstad ELR: Experimental anemias in animals resulting from folic acid and vitamin B_{12} deficiencies. Vitam Horm (NY) 26:443, 1968

Jan Koch-Weser

25
Drug Interactions During Oral Anticoagulant Therapy

Concomitant therapy with several drugs has become a common and necessary clinical practice.[1] The simultaneous use of multiple therapeutic agents frequently permits greater therapeutic effectiveness and fewer side effects than can be achieved with a single drug. Many diseases demand treatment with more than one drug, and many patients require treatment of more than one disease. During one hospitalization on acute medical services in the United States, the median number of drugs administered is 12, and some patients receive more than 30 drugs. At one time during their hospitalization, most patients take more than five drugs simultaneously. Ambulatory patients are also often treated with several therapeutic agents at the same time and, in addition, consume many drugs available without prescription.

Unfortunately, concurrent administration of two or more drugs may lead to unexpected interactions between them.[1–4] Such interactions are far more common than is generally appreciated and have been responsible for much serious morbidity and numerous deaths. Adverse drug interactions can impair the therapeutic action of drugs or can cause toxic drug effects.[1] One drug may change the activity of another either by altering its metabolic fate or by modifying its pharmacologic activity at the sites of action.[1]

The coumarin anticoagulants have been in therapeutic use for approximately 30 years. During the last 15 of these years their action has been shown subject to modification by certain other drugs.[5] Many therapeutic failures and hemorrhagic reactions during oral anticoagulant therapy have found their explanation in unexpected interactions of the coumarins with other drugs. Today it is clear that the coumarin anticoagulants are among the drugs most susceptible to therapeutically important drug interactions.[5] Their prominence in this regard results from three factors. First, many patients take oral anticoagulants over a long period of time and most of these patients receive one or more other drugs concurrently. Second, the pharmacokinetic fate and the pharmacologic action of the coumarins in the human body are complex and are altered by many drugs. Third, the exact intensity of the pharmacologic action of a coumarin anticoagulant is quite important during its therapeutic use. In other words, their therapeutic margin is narrow, and relatively small decreases or increases in the intensity of their action lead to therapeutic failures or to hemorrhagic reactions. For all these reasons drug interactions involving coumarins have become an important therapeutic problem with which all physicians should be familiar.

MECHANISMS OF DRUG INTERACTIONS WITH ORAL ANTICOAGULANTS

Drugs can modify the anticoagulant action of coumarins by a variety of mechanisms (Figure 1). They can change the concentration of the coumarin antagonist vitamin K at the hepatic site of synthesis of Factors II, VII, IX, and X. Other drugs can change the absorption of coumarins from the gastrointestinal tract, their binding to serum albumin, or their biotransformation in the liver to inactive compounds. Still other drugs interact with coumarin anticoagulants by exerting a direct effect on the synthesis or catabolism of the

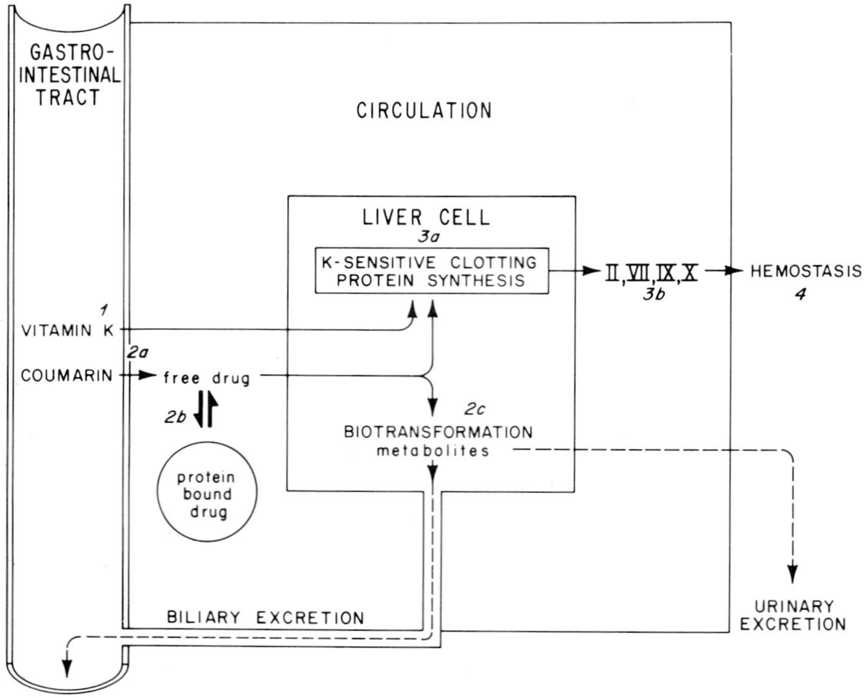

Fig. 1. Sites of drug interactions with the anticoagulant action of coumarins. **1-** Vitamin K bioavailability, **2a-** Coumarin absorption, **2b-** Coumarin binding to serum albumin, **2c-** Coumarin biotransformation, **3a-** Prothrombin-complex synthesis, **3b-** Prothrombin-complex catabolism, **4-** Hemostasis.

prothrombin complex. Finally, some drugs interact with the anticoagulant action of the coumarins by affecting non-prothrombin-complex-dependent hemostatic mechanisms, such as platelet function or vascular integrity. It should be emphasized that many drugs interact with coumarins by more than one mechanism.[5]

INTERACTIONS INVOLVING VITAMIN K

In normal persons, the rate of synthesis of vitamin K-dependent clotting factors is not limited by the availability of vitamin K in the liver. Drugs that decrease vitamin K bioavailability induce hypoprothrombinemia and prolong prothrombin time only if the effect is extreme. The situation is different in subjects who take coumarins. In such subjects, the prothrombin-complex content of plasma is determined by the opposing effects of the coumarin and of vitamin K on hepatic synthesis.[5] Thus, during coumarin therapy any change in the concentration of vitamin K in the liver will alter the plasma concentration of the vitamin K-dependent clotting proteins. Theoretically, the concentration of vitamin K at the site of prothrombin-complex synthesis could be changed by drugs that influence its intestinal synthesis or absorption, its distribution throughout the body, its transport in the blood, or its metabolism. Since the fate of vitamin K in man after absorption remains obscure, little is known about interactions after that stage.

Drug effects on intestinal synthesis of vitamin K are not important for its bioavailability. Antibiotic-induced reduction in synthesis of vitamin K by intestinal bacteria has little influence on prothrombin complex synthesis in anticoagulated patients, unless their dietary intake is grossly deficient.[5] Absorption of dietary vitamin K would theoretically be decreased by drugs that bind bile salts, increase intestinal motility, induce steatorrhea, or interfere with mucosal function. While many drugs have such actions, none has been convincingly shown to decrease vitamin K concentration in the body or to potentiate the hypoprothrombinemic action of coumarins. It seems possible that drug effects on vitamin K bioavailability are less important sources of fluctuation in the hypoprothrombinemia of coumarin-treated patients than the usual variations in the dietary intake of vitamin K.

INTERACTIONS INVOLVING COUMARIN METABOLISM

The ability of other drugs to alter the fate of coumarins in the human body is responsible for the most important drug interactions with coumarins. Any drug-induced change in the absorption, distribution, or disposition of a coumarin alters its hypoprothrombinemic effect. The clinical importance of such metabolic interactions of other drugs with coumarins has been amply confirmed. Although the pharmacokinetics of individual coumarins in man are similar, they are not identical (Table 1). Most importantly, bishydroxycoumarin is more slowly and incompletely absorbed from the gastrointestinal tract and ethylbiscoumacetate is less bound to serum albumin than other coumarins. For this

Table 1
Pharmacokinetics of Coumarins in Man

Coumarin	Gastrointestinal Absorption	Percentage Bound to Plasma Protein	Elimination	Plasma Half-life (Hrs)
Acenocoumarol	Rapid, complete	?	hepatic metabolism	20.0
Bishydroxycoumarin	Slow, incomplete variable	99	hepatic metabolism	24.0*
Ethylbiscoumacetate	Rapid, complete	90	hepatic metabolism	2.5*
Phenprocoumon	Complete	99	hepatic metabolism	160.0
Warfarin	Rapid, complete	97	hepatic metabolism	42.0

*Plasma half-life increases with plasma concentration.

reason, drug effects on absorption are most important with bishydroxycoumarin, and drug interactions related to serum albumin are least important with ethylbiscoumacetate.

Drugs that can decrease the rate and completeness of the gastrointestinal absorption of coumarins include compounds that increase gastric pH (e.g., antacids), alter gastrointestinal motility (e.g., laxatives, anticholinergics), interfere with normal mucosal function (e.g., neomycin, colchicine), form complexes with coumarins (e.g., cholestyramine), or are nonabsorbable materials that dissolve or adsorb coumarins (e.g., mineral oil, charcoal). However, these effects have rarely been shown to be of much therapeutic importance. Perhaps the same drugs interfere with the absorption of vitamin K and, therefore, cause little net change in prothrombin-complex synthesis. On the other hand, the effects of most other drugs on coumarin absorption have not been studied carefully and may be more important than they now seem.

Many drugs decrease the binding of coumarins to serum albumin. Drugs or drug metabolites that displace coumarins from serum albumin under clinical conditions are generally highly protein-bound, are administered in large doses, and accumulate to high levels in plasma.[6,7] Among the most important displacing drugs are acidic compounds.[8,9] Since all commonly used coumarins are highly bound to serum albumin, displacement of even a small amount of a coumarin from albumin causes a large increase in the concentration of free drug in serum. The resulting increase in the concentration of free, active drug at its hepatic receptor site enhances the depression of prothrombin-complex synthesis. In the case of warfarin, displacement of only 3% of the bound drug doubles the free warfarin concentration and greatly increases its hypoprothrombinemic effect.[9] Not surprisingly, administration of strongly displacing drugs to patients chronically treated with coumarins has commonly caused severe hypoprothrombinemia and bleeding.[5]

In contrast to other drug interactions with coumarin metabolism, those due to displacement of coumarins from serum albumin are transient.[5,10,11] The increase in the concentration of free coumarin in the serum not only potentiates the hypoprothrombinemic action of the drug but also makes more of it available for biotransformation. Thus, concentrations of total and free coumarin in serum fall progressively until a new equilibrium is reached. If coumarin dosage has not been changed, the new steady-state is characterized by a lower total coumarin concentration, the same free coumarin concentration, and the same degree of hypoprothrombinemia as before the addition of the displacing drug. The sequence proceeds in reverse when a drug that competes for binding sites on albumin is withdrawn.[5] Enhanced hypoprothrombinemia due to interference with albumin binding of coumarins during administration of other drugs always corrects itself spontaneously, but it may cause serious hemorrhage before it can do so. Clinical doses of important displacing drugs can potentiate the hypoprothrombinemic effect of warfarin within 24 hours and can cause maximum potentiation in 3 to 5 days. The stable lower plasma concentration of total warfarin and the original plasma concentration of free warfarin may be achieved in 7 to 10 days. The prothrombin time will not return to its predisplacement level in less than 2 weeks.

The coumarins are inactivated primarily through hydroxylation by hepatic microsomal mixed-function oxidase enzymes.[12,13] Any drug that increases or decreases the activity of the enzymes responsible for the biotransformation of coumarins can inhibit or enhance their hypoprothrombinemic action. Many drugs have been identified which increase the activity of hepatic enzymes that metabolize coumarins.[5,14,15] Such induction of enzymes increases the rate of metabolic inactivation of the coumarins, shortens their plasma half-life, decreases their total and free concentrations in plasma, and inhibits their hypoprothrombinemic effect.[5] In any given subject, the increase in the rate of coumarin metabolism when an inducing drug is administered is fairly reproducible.[16] However, the degree of inducibility varies considerably among individuals and may be in part genetically determined.[17] The extent to which coumarin metabolizing enzymes are induced in man also depends on the specific inducing drug, its dosage, and the duration of exposure. In some persons, a single therapeutic dose of a potent inducer can accelerate coumarin metabolism appreciably,[18] and 2 days of therapy have this effect on almost all subjects.[19] About 1 week of exposure to some inducing agents may be required for maximum enzyme induction. When the inducing drug is withdrawn, the rate of coumarin metabolism returns gradually to its original level, but this process may require several weeks.[20,21] Clinically, the most important consequence of the induction of coumarin metabolizing enzymes occurs in patients whose prothrombin time has been well controlled during the administration of an enzyme-inducing drug.[20] Such patients will gradually develop excessive hypoprothrombinemia and may bleed after the inducing drug is discontinued. Under these circumstances the coumarin maintenance dose must be reduced and its reduction should be guided by frequent determinations of prothrombin time.

In contrast to enzyme inducers are drugs which decrease the rate of biotransformation of coumarins, increase their plasma concentration, and potentiate their hypoprothrombinemic action. When such drugs are administered to patients on long-term anticoagulant therapy, the coumarin maintenance dose must be reduced to avoid excessive hypoprothrombinemia and bleeding. Drugs that inhibit the synthesis of coumarin metabolizing enzymes and drugs that interfere with the function of these enzymes have both been identified.[22,23] Interference with coumarin metabolism may be apparent within hours after the administration of the inhibiting drug.[23] Very possibly many drugs that inhibit protein synthesis or impair hepatic function nonspecifically also slow coumarin metabolism.

INTERACTIONS INVOLVING DIRECT EFFECTS OF OTHER DRUGS ON PROTHROMBIN-COMPLEX CONCENTRATION

Drugs that decrease or increase the plasma concentration of Factors II, VII, IX, and X directly will enhance or inhibit the hypoprothrombinemic action of coumarins. They may alter the concentration of vitamin K-dependent clotting factors in plasma by affecting their synthesis or their catabolism or both. Even drugs that change the one-stage prothrombin time of normal persons very little can have appreciable effects on the synthesis or catabolism of clotting factors.[5] The prothrombin time of persons not on anticoagulant therapy is an insensitive index of direct drug effects on these processes. In contrast, the rate of prothrombin complex of coumarin-treated patients is fixed at a greatly depressed level and cannot increase in response to further depression of plasma concentrations of clotting factors by other drugs that depress their synthesis or accelerate their catabolism. In anticoagulated patients, such drugs may cause major increases in the prolongation of prothrombin time.[5]

Drugs that potentiate hypoprothrombinemia in coumarin-treated subjects may depress clotting factor synthesis by specifically antagonizing the action of vitamin K in a coumarin-like fashion. Salicylates and cinchona alkaloids apparently act in this fashion, since their effects are overcome by the administration of high doses of vitamin K.[24–26] Less specifically, all drugs that are inhibitors of protein synthesis or impair hepatic function could decrease the rate of prothrombin complex synthesis in anticoagulated subjects. If the drug impairs liver function through a dose-related toxic effect, the potentiation of coumarin-induced hypoprothrombinemia is predictable and will occur in all persons sufficiently exposed. Doses of hepatic toxins that have no effect on the usual liver-function tests may markedly enhance the hypoprothrombinemia of coumarin-treated patients.[27] Drugs that cause liver damage by idiosyncratic or allergic mechanisms will potentiate hypoprothrombinemia only in occasional anticoagulated subjects. The only drugs thus far shown to increase the rate of catabolism of the vitamin K-dependent clotting factors are agents that produce hypermetabolic states, such as thyroid drugs.[28] Drug interactions with coumarins due to direct drug effects on prothrombin complex concentration are clearly of great clinical importance. Further investigations will likely identify additional drugs whose direct effects on prothrombin complex synthesis or catabolism become important in patients treated with coumarins.

INTERACTIONS INVOLVING EFFECTS OF OTHER DRUGS ON HEMOSTASIS

Normal hemostasis requires the unimpaired functioning of many intravascular, vascular, and extravascular mechanisms in addition to those dependent on the activity of Factors II, VII, IX, and X. These mechanisms are affected by many drugs.[29,30] Any drug that interferes with the normal function of parts of the hemostatic process unrelated to prothrombin-complex activity may interact with both the desired therapeutic effects and the hemorrhagic complications of coumarin therapy. Drug effects on platelet function and ulcerogenic action of drugs are the best studied examples. Many drugs that interact with coumarins in depressing prothrombin complex concentration also interfere with normal platelet function (e.g., aspirin, clofibrate, mefenamic acid, phenylbutazone).[30] Other drugs can induce low-grade bleeding or gastric ulceration (e.g., aspirin, phenylbutazone). All such drugs can cause serious bleeding in coumarin-treated patients, even when their prothrombin time remains in the desired therapeutic range.

INTERACTIONS OF INDIVIDUAL DRUGS WITH COUMARINS

During the past 15 years many drugs have been suspected of interacting with coumarin anticoagulants. Such suspicions have often been based on speculative interpretations of a single clinical event. Reports of such uncontrolled clinical impressions are useful leads but must be followed up by controlled investigations. It is unfortunate that some drugs have gained the false reputation of interacting with coumarins on the basis of a single anecdotal report. The clinical and experimental evidence relating to the interaction of individual drugs and drug groups with coumarins has recently been reviewed in detail.[5]

The number of drugs clearly shown to inhibit the hypoprothrombinemic action of coumarins in man in a therapeutically important fashion is relatively small (Table 2). All act either by inhibiting the gastrointestinal absorption of coumarins

Table 2
Inhibition of the Hypoprothrombinemic Action of Coumarins

Drug	Mechanism
Barbiturates	Acceleration of coumarin metabolism
Cholestyramine	Inhibition of coumarin absorption
Diphenylhydantoin	Acceleration of coumarin metabolism
Ethchlorvynol	Acceleration of coumarin metabolism?
Glutethimide	Acceleration of coumarin metabolism
Griseofulvin	Inhibition of coumarin absorption? Acceleration of coumarin metabolism?

or by accelerating their hepatic metabolism through enzyme induction. It is impossible to predict the amount of change in the relation of anticoagulant dosage to prothrombin time prolongation which will occur when intake of these drugs is started, changed, or stopped in a patient treated with coumarin anticoagulants. Chronic administration of inhibiting drugs may decrease plasma half-life and the average plasma concentration of coumarins by approximately 50% and may make it necessary to double the anticoagulant dosage to maintain the same hypoprothrombinemic effect. However, one cannot rely on this relation in any given patient. Frequent measurement of prothrombin time and appropriate adjustment of anticoagulant dose are essential when such drugs must be used in patients receiving a coumarin. Even with careful monitoring, optimal control of hypoprothrombinemia may be difficult in a patient receiving such drugs, and it is best to avoid them altogether.[31]

A large number of drugs have been found to cause clinically important potentiation of the hypoprothrombinemic action of coumarins (Table 3). This enhancement has a number of different mechanisms, the most important being displacement of warfarin from binding sites on serum albumin, inhibition of warfarin metabolism, and direct depression of clotting factor synthesis. Some drugs may potentiate coumarin action by several different mechanisms. For other drugs which clearly potentiate coumarin action, the mechanism of the

Table 3
Enhancement of the Hypoprothrombinemic Action of Coumarins

Drug	Mechanism
Allopurinol	Inhibition of coumarin metabolism
Anabolic steroids	Decrease in circulating vitamin K? Direct depression of clotting factor synthesis? Increase in clotting factor catabolism?
Chloral hydrate	Decrease in coumarin albumin binding
Chloramphenicol	Inhibition of coumarin metabolism
Clofibrate	Decrease in circulating vitamin K? Decrease in coumarin albumin binding? Inhibition of coumarin metabolism?
Dextrothyroxine	Decrease in circulating vitamin K? Increase in clotting factor catabolism?
Disulfiram	Inhibition of coumarin metabolism
Ethacrynic acid	Decrease in coumarin albumin binding
Glucagon	Decrease in clotting factor synthesis?
Neomycin	Decrease in vitamin K absorption?
Nortriptyline	Inhibition of coumarin metabolism
Phenylbutazone	Decrease in coumarin albumin binding
Quinidine	Direct depression of clotting factor synthesis?
Salicylate	Direct depression of clotting factor synthesis?
Sulfonamides, long-acting	Decrease in coumarin albumin binding
Thyroid drugs	Increase in clotting factor catabolism
Triclofos	Decrease in coumarin albumin binding

interaction has not yet been established. Both the time course of the interaction and the degree of enhancement of the hypoprothrombinemic actions of coumarins vary with the mechanism of the interaction, with the specific drug, and with its dose. Twofold or threefold enhancement of coumarin action within a few days occurs with usual doses of some potentiating drugs.[32] However, the time course and extent of interaction vary considerably among patients. Thus, in a given individual it is difficult to predict quantitatively the degree of enhancement of coumarin-induced hypoprothrombinemia when potentiating drugs are added to or withdrawn from therapy. The only safe course is to monitor prothrombin time closely and adjust coumarin dose according to the results obtained.

DETECTION AND INVESTIGATION OF DRUG INTERACTIONS WITH COUMARINS

Almost all drugs that interact with coumarin anticoagulants in man were dis covered to do so through fortuitous observations by astute clinicians.[5] Unfortunately, recognition of interactions has almost always been long-delayed, and this has resulted in many serious therapeutic accidents, including a number of deaths. In the case of barbiturates, detection of their interaction with coumarin anticoagulants came only after 15 years of their concomitant administration.[33] Another decade had to pass until the quantitative importance and mechanism of the interaction were understood.[18,34] Eight years were needed until a practicing clinician discovered the interaction of phenylbutazone with coumarins,[35] and it was not understood or quantitated until 11 years later.[32] These long delays occurred even though both barbiturates and phenylbutazone were very commonly administered together with coumarin anticoagulants and though their interaction is clinically important in every patient.[5] Morbidity and mortality due to such interactions, during the many years before their clinical recognition, must have been distressingly high.

The slow detection of drug interactions with coumarins through fortuitous observations by clinicians is not at all surprising. In the usual complex clinical situation, non-drug factors such as diet, activity, fever, circulatory state, hepatic function, transfusions, and many others continuously alter a patient's sensitivity to coumarins. Furthermore, frequent changes in coumarin dosage of hospitalized patients and the delay of several days until such changes are fully reflected in prothrombin time complicate the detection of changes in the relation of coumarin dose to hypoprothrombinemic response. It is fortunate, therefore, that chance clinical observations in this field are now being supplemented by faster and more predictably effective epidemiologic and experimental techniques.

These newer techniques have been employed only during the last several years, but their effectiveness is already clear.[36–38] Prospective epidemiologic studies of hospitalized or ambulatory patients can identify drug interactions with coumarin anticoagulants much more readily and reliably than random observations. Changes in a patient's sensitivity to coumarins can be detected by calculating the Coumarin Dose Index.[5,36,37] This index represents the ratio of prothrombin time prolongation to the cumulative coumarin dose. The number of days included in the calculation of the cumulative dosage depends on the duration of the action of the coumarin. In the case of warfarin, the cumulative dosage during the preceding 96 hours is used, and the daily doses are appropriately weighed. When the Coumarin Dose Index has been stable in coumarin-treated patients for a 3-day period and shows a statistically significant change when a potentially interacting drug is added, a drug interaction is likely.[5,37] Detection of such variations by appropriate computer programs is a relatively simple matter. Figure 2 shows a typical computer printout of the Warfarin Dose Index of a patient treated with warfarin. The hypoprothrombinemic response to warfarin is shown before, during, and after treatment with phenylbutazone, which the patient received from days 11 to 19. During the period of phenylbutazone administration, the Warfarin Dose Index increased from a mean of 0.2 to 0.6, indicating marked potentiation of the hypoprothrombinemic action of warfarin by phenylbutazone.

During the last 2 years, 500 patients hospitalized at the Massachusetts General Hospital have been prospectively monitored throughout the period during which they were treated with sodium warfarin.[36,37] Patients were seen daily by nurse surveillance officers who recorded detailed information concerning all patients' characteristics, underlying diseases, clinical course, diet, activity, prothrombin time, other laboratory data, warfarin dose, all other drug therapy, and adverse drug effects. The complete data on all patients were analyzed by appropriate computer programs and reviewed by clinical pharmacologists. This prospective epidemiologic study on a relatively small number of patients yielded quantitative data about the interaction or lack of interaction of 54 drugs with

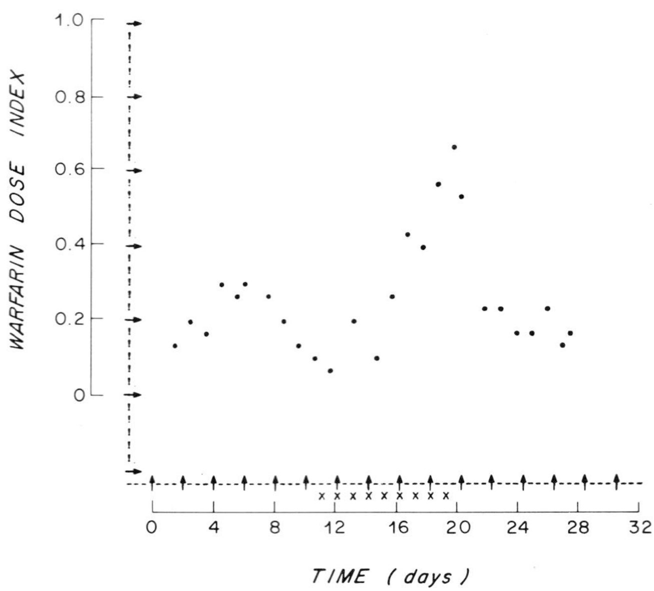

Fig. 2. Computer printout from prospective study of clinical drug interactions with warfarin. Potentiation of hypoprothrombinemic action of warfarin by concomitant administration of phenylbutazone.

warfarin. The most dramatic interactions, such as that between phenylbutazone and warfarin, were unequivocally detected even when only a few patients received the two drugs concomitantly. Several previously undescribed drug interactions with warfarin were uncovered.[37] Other interactions which had been suggested on the basis of animal experimentation or of uncontrolled clinical observations were shown to be clinically unimportant in all patients studied. Such epidemiologic techniques in the detection of drug interactions with coumarins are equally applicable to ambulatory patients. While these studies require considerable effort and are not inexpensive to perform, their effectiveness, and probably their information-cost ratio, is far higher than that of large-scale programs relying on spontaneous reporting of chance observations.

An alternative approach to the identification and understanding of drug interactions with coumarins in man is their prediction on the basis of pharmacologic action or metabolic fate of drugs involved.[6,11] Our understanding of the mechanism and quantitative aspects of absorption, distribution, binding at inactive sites, hepatic metabolism, and renal excretion of many drugs has advanced to such a point that their interactions with coumarins can be confidently predicted even before they have been observed in a single patient receiving the drugs for therapeutic purposes. Such predictions can be safely and conclusively verified and their quantitative characteristics established by controlled studies in a small number of normal volunteers or patients.[7,11,22,39–41] Alternatively, it can be established that in all usual patients clinically significant interactions between therapeutic doses of a coumarin and of another drug do not occur.[42–43] Screening in a few volunteers for drug interactions with coumarins is effective for most important drugs and should form part of the clinical evaluation of new drugs.

IMPLICATIONS OF DRUG INTERACTIONS FOR ANTICOAGULANT THERAPY

The number of drugs which modify the hypoprothrombinemic action of coumarins in a clinically important fashion is already large. As a result of ongoing studies, other drugs will surely be placed into this category. Such studies will also provide much needed information concerning the time course and intensity of the interaction of other drugs with coumarin anticoagulants. It seems doubtful that we shall ever be able to predict quantitatively the degree of interference with the hypoprothrombinemic action of coumarins which an interacting drug will exert in a given patient. The effects of individual differences, of multiple mechanisms of interaction for some drugs, of simultaneous administration of several interacting drugs, of drug dosage, and of sequence and duration of administration are likely to make this impossible. However, even with our present knowledge of drug interactions during oral anticoagulant therapy, therapeutic failures and adverse reactions due to these interactions are now largely preventable. As few simple precautions greatly increase the safety and effectiveness of coumarin therapy:

1. When first prescribing an oral anticoagulant, the physician should know all other drugs the patient is taking. He should then caution the patient

Table 4
Therapeutic Alternatives for Coumarin-Treated Patients

Interacting Drug	Substitute
Barbiturates	Flurazepam
Chloral hydrate	Flurazepam
Ethchlorvynol	Flurazepam
Glutethimide	Flurazepam
Triclofos	Flurazepam
Chloramphenicol	Appropriate antibiotic
Long-acting sulfonamides	Appropriate antibiotic
Allopurinol	Probenecid
Phenylbutazone	Indomethacin
Quinidine	Procainamide
Salicylate	Acetaminophen Indomethacin

not to take any drugs bought without prescription or prescribed by other physicians without first communicating with him.

2. Patients chronically treated with oral anticoagulants should avoid barbiturates and many other hypnotics, chloramphenicol, long-acting sulfonamides, allopurinol, phenylbutazone or its congeners, quinidine, and salicylates. Therapeutic alternatives that do not interact with the coumarins are available for all these drugs (Table 4).

3. Changes of drug therapy in patients taking a coumarin should be kept to the possible minimum. This precaution applies particularly to ambulatory patients whose prothrombin times are checked infrequently. When necessary changes involve known interacting drugs, some anticipatory alteration in coumarin dosage may be made. Most important is close monitoring of prothrombin time for some weeks after the change and appropriate adjustment of coumarin dosage on that basis. Drugs not yet shown to interact with coumarins are best regarded with suspicion, and when their administration is started or stopped, prothrombin time should be determined more often than usual.

SUMMARY

Therapeutic failures and adverse reactions due to interactions of other drugs with oral anticoagulants are common in clinical practice. The number of drugs known to diminish or enhance the hypoprothrombinemic action of coumarins in a clinically important fashion is large and constantly growing. At present, epidemiologic and experimental techniques are being applied successfully to the detection and investigation of such interactions. For many drugs, the varied and complex mechanisms underlying their interactions with coumarins have been established. Most adverse clinical events due to drug interactions with coumarins can be prevented by following simple precautions during oral anticoagulant therapy.

REFERENCES

1. Koch-Weser J: Drug interactions in clinical practice. The Science and Practice of Clinical Medicine. Edited by J Dietschy, L Early, H Fudenberg, A Renold, (Sanders and J Sandford). New York, Grune and Stratton (In Press)
2. Morrelli HF, Melmon KL: Drug interactions. Clinical Pharmacology. Edited by KL Melmon and HF Morrelli. New York, Macmillan, 1972
3. Hansten PD: Drug Interactions. Philadelphia, Lea and Febiger, 1971
4. Martin EW: Drug interactions, Hazards of Medication. Edited by EW Martin. Philadelphia, Lippincott 1971
5. Koch-Weser J, Sellers E: Drug interactions with coumarin anticoagulants. N Engl J Med 285:487, 547, 1971
6. Sellers EM, Koch-Weser J: Displacement of warfarin from human albumin by diazoxide and ethacrynic, mefenamic, and nalidixic acids. Clin Pharmacol Ther 11:524, 1970
7. Sellers EM, Koch-Weser J: Potentiation of warfarin-induced hypoprothrombinemia by chloral hydrate, N Engl J Med 283:827, 1970
8. Solomon HM, Schrogie JJ, Williams D: The displacement of phenylbutazone-^{14}C and warfarin-^{14}C from human albumin by various drugs and fatty acids. Biochem Pharmacol 17:143, 1968
9. Sellers EM, Koch-Weser J: Kinetics and clinical importance of displacement of warfarin from albumin by acidic drugs. Ann NY Acad Sci 179:213, 1971
10. Koch-Weser J, Sellers EM: Chloral hydrate and warfarin therapy. Ann Intern Med 75:141, 1971
11. Sellers EM, Lang M, Koch-Weser J, etal: Enhancement of warfarin-induced hypoprothrombinemia by triclofos. Clin Pharmacol Ther 13:911-915, 1972
12. Lewis RJ, Trager WF: Warfarin metabolism in man: identification of metabolites in urine. J Clin Invest 49:907, 1970
13. Lewis RJ, Trager WF: The metabolic fate of warfarin: studies on the metabolites in plasma. Ann NY Acad Sci 179:205, 1971
14. Conney AH: Pharmacological implications of microsomal enzyme induction. Pharmacol Rev 19:317, 1967
15. Kuntzman R: Drugs and enzyme induction. Ann Rev Pharmacol 9:21, 1969
16. Breckenridge A, Orme M: Clinical implications of enzyme induction Ann NY Acad Sci 179:421, 1971
17. Vesell ES, Page JG: Genetic control of the phenobarbital-induced shortening of plasma antipyrine half-lives in man. J Clin Invest 48:2202, 1969
18. Dayton PG, Tarcan Y, Chenkin T, et al: The influence of barbiturates on coumarin plasma levels and prothrombin response. J Clin Invest 40:1797, 1961
19. Corn M: Effect of phenobarbital and glutethimide on biological half-life of warfarin. Thromb Diath Haemorrh 16:606, 1966
20. MacDonald MG, Robinson DS: Clinical observations of possible barbiturate interference with anticoagulation. JAMA 204:97, 1968
21. Johansson SA: Apparent resistance to oral anticoagulant therapy and influence of hypnotics on some coagulation factors. Acta Med Scand 184:297, 1968
22. Vesell ES, Passananti T, Greene FE: Impairment of drug metabolism in man by allopurinol and nortriptyline. N Engl J Med 283:1484, 1970
23. Christensen LK, Skovsted L: Inhibition of drug metabolism by chloramphenicol. Lancet 2:1397, 1969
24. Shapiro S: Studies on prothrombin: VI. The effect of synthetic vitamin K on the prothrombinopenia induced by salicylate in man. JAMA 125:546, 1944

25. Pirk LA, Engelberg R: Hypoprothrombinemic action of quinine sulfate. JAMA 128:1093, 1945
26. Koch-Weser J: Quinidine-induced hypoprothrombinemic hemorrhage in patients on chronic warfarin therapy. Ann Intern Med 68:511, 1968
27. Luton EF: Carbon tetrachloride exposure during anticoagulant therapy. JAMA 194:1386, 1965
28. Loeliger EA, van der Esch B, Mattern MJ, et al: Biological disappearance rate of prothrombin, factors VII, IX and X from plasma in hypothyroidism, hyperthyroidism, and during fever. Throm Diath Haemorrh 10:267, 1964
29. Seegers WH: The influence of certain drugs on blood coagulation and related phenomena. Pharmacol Rev 3:278, 1951
30. Mustard JF, Packham MA: Factors influencing platelet function: adhesion, release, and aggregation. Pharmacol Rev 22:97, 1970
31. Robinson DS, MacDonald MG: The effect of phenobarbital administration on the control of coagulation achieved during warfarin therapy in man. J Pharmacol Exp Ther 153:250, 1966
32. Aggeler PM, O'Reilly RA, Leong L, et al: Potentiation of anticoagulant effect of warfarin by phenylbutazone. N Engl J Med 276:496, 1967
33. Avellaneda M: Interferencia de los barbituricos en la accion del tromexan. Medicina (Buenos Aires) 15:109, 1955
34. Cucinell SA, Conney AH, Sansur M, et al: Drug interactions in man. I. Lowering effect of phenobarbital on plasma levels of bishydroxycoumarin (Dicumarol) and diphenylhydantoin (Dilantin). Clin Pharmacol Ther 6:420, 1965
35. Sigg A, Pestalozzi H, Clauss A, et al: Verstärkung der Antikoagulantienwirkung durch Butazolidin. Schweiz Med Wochenschr 86:1194, 1956
36. Koch-Weser J: Potentiation by glucagon of the hypoprothrombinemic action of warfarin. Ann Intern Med 72:331, 1970
37. Koch-Weser J: Hemorrhagic reactions and drug interactions in 500 warfarin-treated patients. Clin Pharmacol Ther 14:139, 1973
38. Boston Collaborative Drug Surveillance Program: Interaction between chloral hydrate and warfarin. N Engl J Med 286:53, 1972
39. Robinson DS, Benjamin DM, McCormack JJ: Interaction of warfarin and non-systemic gastrointestinal drugs. Clin Pharmacol Ther 12:491, 1971
40. Hansen JM, Siersbaek-Nielsen K, Skoxsted L: Carbamazepine-induced acceleration of diphenylhydantoin and warfarin metabolism in man. Clin Pharmacol Ther 12:539, 1971
41. Hansen JM, Siersbaek-Nielsen K, Kristensen M, et al: Effect of diphenylhydantoin on the metabolism of dicoumarol in man. Acta Med Scand 189:15, 1971
42. Hague DE, Smith ME, Ryan JR, et al: The effect of methylphenidate and prolintane on the metabolism of ethyl biscoumacetate. Clin Pharmacol Ther 12:259, 1971
43. Bieger R, deJonge H, Loeliger EA: Influence of nitrazepam on oral anticoagulation with phenprocoumon. Clin Pharmacol Ther 13:361, 1972
44. Gould L, Michael A, Fisch S et al: Prothrombin levels maintained with meprobamate and warfarin. JAMA 220:1460, 1972

Sandor S. Shapiro

26
Drugs and Fibrinoysis

Pharmacologic modification of the activity of the fibrinolytic system is currently an area of great ferment. Thrombosis, in its various guises, is probably the major cause of death in much of the world today, and we have come to hope that a successful therapeutic attack might be mounted against this problem, either with the use of drugs capable of dissolving thrombi once formed or by some approach capable of achieving a sustained increase in "physiologic" fibrinolytic activity. Although neither of these aims has yet been achieved, much evidence has accrued suggesting that such goals eventually may be attainable. In addition, drugs have been introduced capable of inhibiting fibrinolytic activity and these have found limited but definite usefulness in those situations in which increased fibrinolytic activity has been found detrimental. This review will deal with some pertinent aspects of the physiology of the fibrinolytic system, points within the system that perhaps can be manipulated therapeutically, and some clinical and laboratory studies whose aims have been to alter the activity of this system.

THE PLASMINOGEN-PLASMA SYSTEM

Fibrinolytic activity in the bloodstream is the result of activation of the zymogen, plasminogen, to the proteolytic enzyme, plasmin. Human plasminogen, a single-chain polypeptide of molecular weight 75,000–80,000,[1] is present in plasma at a concentration of 15–20 mg per 100 ml.[2] It can be converted to plasmin by various activators (Figure 1), all of which apparently cleave a single arginine-valine bond, producing a two-chain enzyme.[3] Plasmin is a proteolytic enzyme resembling trypsin in substrate specificity,[4] and can hydrolyze proteins such as casein, in addition to fibrinogen and fibrin.[5] The light chain of plasmin,

Supported in part by grant HE-09163, from The National Heart and Lung Institute, National Institutes of Health.

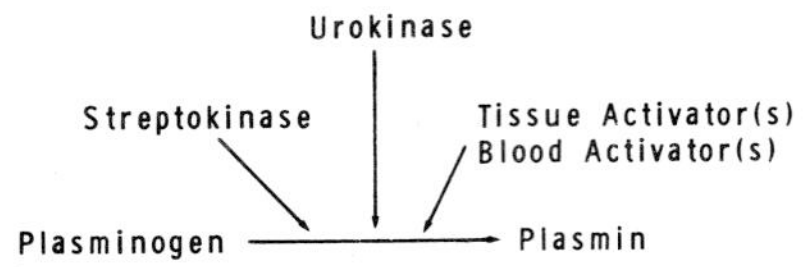

Fig. 1. Activation of plasminogen.

with a molecular weight 26,000, possesses the active enzymatic site,[6] and has many structural homologies to other DFP-sensitive "serine proteases," such as trypsin, chymotripsin A and B, thrombin, and elastase.[7,8]

Although the physiologic activation of the fibrinolytic system is poorly understood, currently available information suggests that one pathway is probably the release into the circulation of an activator from the endothelium of veins and, possibly, the pulmonary arteries.[9–12] Activator can be demonstrated in these locations by histochemical techniques,[11] and increased activator levels can be brought about by localized anoxia,[13] exercise,[14] and electroshock,[15] as well as by the administration of certain drugs, such as epinephrine,[14] nicotinic acid,[16] and bacterial pyrogens.[17] Such circulating activator activity is very transient, having a biologic half-life of less than 15 minutes.[18] Plasminogen activators are also present in lysosomal granules of many types of cells,[19] but this material is difficult to extract and may only reach the circulation as the result of tissue damage. Such release may be important clinically in the hyperfibrinolytic states seen after trauma and certain types of surgery.[20] Thus far, the mechanisms described are analogous to the so-called "extrinsic system" in blood coagulation. Whether an "intrinsic" fibrinolytic system actually exists, with a circulating "proactivator," is still problematic. Recently, Takada, et al have described the partial purification of a plasma protein, different from plasminogen, capable of being altered by streptokinase into a plasminogen activator.[21] Further work on this material will be awaited with great interest.

The two best-delineated activators of plasminogen, and those currently available for therapeutic trials, are streptokinase and urokinase (Table 1). Streptokinase, a product of the streptococcus,[22] is a protein of molecular weight 48,000,[23] capable of activating directly the plasminogen of man, monkey, and cat, but capable of activating plasminogen of all other species only in the presence of traces of human plasma.[24,25] Streptokinase itself appears to have no peptidase activity, but forms, under appropriate conditions, a 1:1 molar complex with human plasminogen, giving rise to an enzymatic activity capable of activating all plasminogens, regardless of source.[26–28] Urokinase is a product of the kidney, and can be purified from human urine.[29–31] This protein, of molecular weight approximately 55,000,[1,30] has proteolytic activity and, like

Table 1
Activators of Plasminogen

Streptokinase	Urokinase
Bacterial Product	Human Product
	Produced by kidney, excreted in urine
Molecular Weight 48,000	Molecular weight 55,000
Antigenic in man	Nonantigenic in man

Table 2
Large-molecule Fibrinolytic Inhibitors

	Molecular Weight
Inhibitors in Blood	
α_2-Macroglobulin	800,000
α_1-Antitrypsin	48,000
Inhibitors from Plants	
Soy bean	21,500
Kidney bean	10,000
Lima bean	9,000
Inhibitors from Tissue	
Pancreas (basic inhibitor)	6,500

trypsin and plasmin, can hydrolyze peptide bonds in which the carboxyl donor is arginine or lysine. Unlike trypsin or plasmin, however, urokinase has extremely restricted specificity and, although it can activate plasminogen, it has little or no proteolytic activity against, for example, casein or fibrin.[1]

Free plasmin has a very short life-span in the circulation, since its activity is quickly neutralized by several plasma proteins (Table 2), of which α_2-macroglobulin is probably the most important.[32,33] Plasma also contains inhibitors of activator activity,[34] accounting in large part for its very short life-span in blood. In addition, a large variety of plant and animal tissues contain plasmin inhibitors,[35,36] some of which have been purified, characterized, and used therapeutically in hyperfibrinolytic states.[37,38]

FIBRINOLYTIC DEGRADATION OF FIBRINOGEN AND FIBRIN

The clotting of fibrinogen (Figure 2) requires first the action of thrombin, cleaving two pairs of fibrinopeptides representing about 3% of the mass of the fibrinogen molecule, then the spontaneous polymerization of resultant fibrin monomers to the three-dimensional fibrin clot. Subsequently, the action of blood clotting Factor XIII converts this weak, hydrogen-bonded polymer into a strong, covalently bound structure. Plasmin is capable of hydrolyzing both fibrinogen and fibrin.

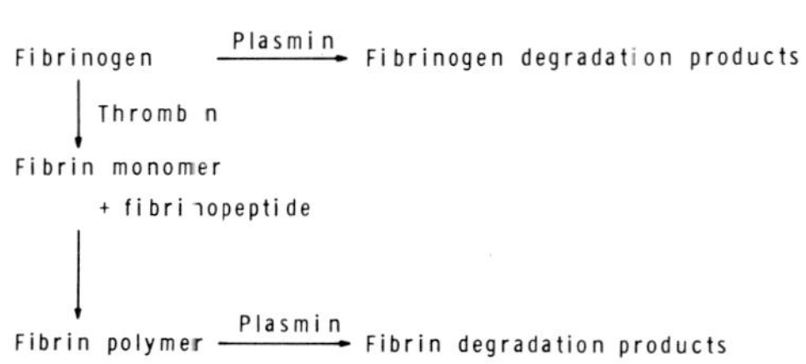

Fig. 2. Derivation of fibrinogen and fibrin degradation products.

Fibrinogen (M.W. 330,000)
↓
X (M.W. 250,000)
↓
Y (M.W. 155,000) + D (M.W. 85,000)
↓
D (M.W. 85,000) + E (M.W. 50,000)

Fig. 3. Plasmin degradation of fibrinogen.

The action of plasmin on purified fibrinogen and fibrin has been studied extensively,[39–41] and a general sequence of events has emerged (Figure 3). Although degradation is continuous, major stages are found, characterized by the formation of cleavage products identifiable by electrophoretic and immunologic techniques. The first major product, the so-called "X-fragment" has lost about one-fourth the mass of the parent molecule and, if derived from fibrinogen rather than fibrin, is still clottable, although slowly. With further degradation, the X-fragment is cleaved into two major parts, the Y and D fragments. Both of these fragments are anticoagulant, the former very strongly so, as evidenced by their ability to prolong the thrombin clotting time of normal plasma.[42–44] Each Y-fragment can be further degraded into an E-fragment and another D-fragment. The E-fragment is almost totally lacking in anticoagulant activity in thrombin time tests.[44] The D and E fragments represent the end-stages of plasmin action on fibrinogen or fibrin, being relatively resistant to further proteolysis by that enzyme. In addition to these large molecular products, a great number of smaller peptides, with molecular weights below 10,000, are released, some of which may inhibit other parts of the hemostatic mechanism, for example: ADP-induced platelet aggregation.[45]

Detection of the products of fibrinogen and fibrin degradation can be achieved by a variety of techniques (Table 3), although with differing degrees of sensitivity.[46] Thus the thrombin time is an easily performed clinical test, but is sensitive only to Y and D fragments. Probably the most sensitive technique available is the tanned red cell hemagglutination inhibition immunoassay (TRCHII) of Merskey,[47] which is sensitive to all fragments. Although the staphylococcal clumping reaction[48] is relatively insensitive to D and E fragments when purified materials are studied, it yields about the same number of positive results as the TRCHII when clinically suspect blood samples are examined.[46] Antibody-coated latex bead agglutination is a relatively insensitive test.[46] These tests, except for the thrombin time, must be done on clotted blood, since positive results due to the presence of fibrinogen must be avoided. As a result, fragment X, if derived from fibrinogen, will be incorporated into the clot, and hence not measured. In addition, some of the other fragments may complex

Table 3
Detection of Degradation Products of Fibrinogen and Fibrin

Thrombin time
Staphylococcal clumping
Tanned red cell hemagglutination inhibition (TRCHII)
Antibody-coated latex bead agglutination
Serial dilution protamine sulfate

with fibrin monomer and may also be incorporated into the clot. The serial dilution protamine sulfate (SDPS) test,[49,50] on the other hand, is performed on plasma. It is based on the observation that small amounts of protamine can enhance the spontaneous polymerization of fibrin monomer and fibrin degradation products. Fibrinogen and fibrinogen degradation products, on the other hand, do not give positive tests. The test is probably less sensitive than the TRCHII or staphylococcal clumping test, but since a positive test (in the absence of therapeutic thrombolysis) implies the proximate action of thrombin, it is a useful test for clinically significant intravascular coagulation.

FIBRINOLYTIC ACTIVITY AND THERAPEUTIC THROMBOLYSIS

In most situations in which increased fibrinolytic activity is observed, such as after electroshock or pneumoencephalography, with stress, or after the injection of epinephrine, proteolytic activity cannot be demonstrated in the circulation despite the fact that clots made from the subject's plasma may dissolve rapidly. Thus dilute whole blood and euglobulin clots lyse readily, although no activity is demonstrated against casein or plasminogen-free fibrin.[51] Further study has shown that such lytic activity is due to increased concentrations of blood activators of plasminogen, probably released from venous endothelium. By virtue of the fact that plasminogen tends to be found in close association with fibrin in thrombi in vivo and in blood clots in vitro, a mechanism operates which localizes proteolytic activity to the fibrin-containing thrombus itself.[52] Activators tend to diffuse relatively freely into the interstices of the thrombus, producing localized fibrinolysis, but the plasmin generated does not usually escape to any significant extent into the general circulation so that proteolysis of fibrinogen, coagulation Factor V, and other plasma proteins does not occur.

Therapeutic thrombolysis might be achieved, in theory, in several ways (Figure 1). Infusion of the active enzyme, plasmin, might be attempted. This approach is not practical, first because of the dangerous proteolytic state produced, and second because plasmin does not diffuse well into preformed fibrin clots.[52] A second approach would be to inject plasminogen activators, such as urokinase or streptokinase. Such an approach, of course, is currently undergoing worldwide trial. Another approach might involve increasing the level of "physiologic" blood activator(s). Although transient increases can be achieved with pyrogens,[17] nicotinic acid,[16] and other chemical compounds, sustained increases have been difficult to achieve. However, some promising results have been reported in recent years.[53] In any case, in vivo thrombolysis has not yet been demonstrated unequivocally by this approach. A fourth method of increasing fibrinolytic activity in vivo might involve interference with the action of natural fibrinolytic inhibitors. The value of this approach is presently unknown, although several in vitro fibrinolytic compounds, such as flufenamic acid and tretramethylbutylsalicylic acid, seem to operate by such a mechanism.[54]

Both streptokinase (SK) and urokinase (UK) are currently undergoing clinical trial as thrombolytic agents. Although older preparations of SK caused serious pyrogenic reactions in man, newer purification methods have eliminated this side-effect. A second problem associated with the administration of SK is its antigenicity. Since essentially the entire population has been exposed to streptococcal antigens to varying degrees, the range of concentrations of "naturally occurring" anti-SK antibodies is so wide, it was initially thought necessary to titrate each patient prior to therapy to determine an initial loading dose of SK that would neutralize natural antibodies. Further experience has made it possible to eliminate this practical problem by administering a fixed loading dose capable of neutralizing levels of anti-SK antibodies found in 80%–90% of the population.[55] An occasional patient, with very high anti-SK levels, may still need ttitration, however. Also associated with its antigenicity is the anamnestic rise in anti-SK antibodies seen in patients treated with SK. Thus it may be difficult or impossible to retreat a patient with SK within 6 months or a year after exposure to the drug.

Urokinase is not antigenic in man and is presently being produced from human urine—its only known source. Although the lack of antigenicity is a major advantage of this material, it is well to remember that the amount of UK needed to treat 1 patient arises from a volume of urine equivalent to the total yearly output of a single individual. Thus, unless other sources are found or purification yields are vastly improved, it seems likely that this drug would always be available in limited quantities.

At present, in the United States a large cooperative trial of the thrombolytic efficacy of urokinase and streptokinase is underway. The first part of this trial, comparing heparin alone with UK and heparin on the resolution of pulmonary emboli, has been completed.[56] Altogether, 160 patients were studied, approximately half in each group. Using rigid angiographic and hemodynamic criteria, it could be demonstrated that a 12-hour infusion of UK, followed by heparin, produced more rapid resolution of emboli than did heparin alone. However, when both groups were examined after 1–2 weeks, no differences were observed in therapeutic outcome. Furthermore, bleeding was a major complication in both groups, occurring in 45% of patients receiving urokinase and 27% of those receiving heparin, primarily at cutdown and arterial puncture sites necessitated by some of the study procedures. Since in vivo thrombolysis was clearly demonstrated in this study, the second phase is comparing 12-hour and 24-hour infusions of UK. A third group has been added as well, in which patients receive 24-hour infusions of SK. The amount of diagnostic work is being decreased, to avoid excessive bleeding. It is hoped that questions of therapeutic efficacy will be answered in this second phase.

The effectiveness of SK as an in vivo thrombolytic agent has been demonstrated in studies of acute, and even some cases of chronic, arterial occlusions.[57–59] A number of large studies of the effectiveness of SK in the treatment of myocardial infarction have produced conflicting results.[60–63] One study has shown that if treatment with SK is begun early, within 12 hours of the infarct, mortality with SK-heparin therapy is 15%, as compared with a mortality of 25% when heparin alone is used.[62] Bleeding occurred in 11% of patients receiving the drug combination and in 7% of those receiving only heparin. There is clearly a need for a cooperative study of thrombolytic therapy in myocardial infarction designed to exacting statistical standards.

In addition to acute therapy of thromboembolic episodes, the possibility is being pursued that sustained mild enhancement of blood fibrinolytic activity might prove efficacious in the long-term prevention of diseases, such as atherosclerosis, in which fibrin formation is thought to play a role. Thus it has been found that oral administration of the combination of the biguanide, phenformin, with the anabolic steroid, ethylestrenol, is capable of mildly enhancing fibrinolytic activity, which can be sustained for at least 2½ years, as evidenced by shortened euglobulin and dilute blood clot lysis times, as well as by other techniques.[53] Maximum effect is not seen until after 1–2 months of treatment,[53] and seems to be mediated by an increased turnover of the venous endothelial activator.[64] This drug combination is also reported to decrease platelet adhesiveness significantly,[64,65] although the mechanism of this effect is unknown. Perhaps because of the great variability in day-to-day results of such tests as the euglobulin lysis time, as well as the existence of a fibrinolytic circadian rhythm, these results have provoked some controversy. Nevertheless, Fearnley and others have reported beneficial results of long-term therapy with phenformin and ethylestrenol in rheumatoid arthritis and other conditions,[53] without significant side-effects due to treatment. Certainly, this novel approach merits careful and extensive study.

INHIBITION OF FIBRINOLYSIS

In situations in which plasmin activity cannot be contained by the biologic antiplasmin mechanisms, a dangerous generalized proteolytic state may develop. Such events have been seen after surgery,[20] particularly involving the lung and liver, with overdose of UK or SK, and, occasionally, spontaneously. In these situations, drugs that can inhibit the fibrinolytic system are useful. Other conditions exist in which inhibition of fibrinolytic activity may be advantageous even though the basic disease may have other causes. There is some evidence, for example, that inhibition of fibrinolytic activity may be beneficial to hemophilic patients undergoing tooth extraction[66,67] and to individuals with hereditary angioneurotic edema.[68–70]

In 1957, Okamoto and his colleagues, in a comprehensive study, found that basic amino acids, particularly lysine, inhibit clot lysis in vitro.[71] Investigating structural analogues of lysine, they found that removal of the α-NH_2 group from lysine, to produce epsilon aminocaproic acid (EACA, Figure 4), increased inhibitory potency tenfold.[71] Later, Okamoto and coworkers reported the synthesis of transaminomethylcyclohexanecarboxylic acid (trans-AMCHA),[72,73] with ten times the fibrinolytic potency of EACA. Both of these drugs inhibited the activation of plasminogen, several orders of magnitude better than they inhibited preformed plasmin activity,[74,75] and at the dose used in humans they no doubt operate by preventing further activation of the fibrinolytic system, allowing blood plasmin-inhibitors to neutralize any circulating plasmin. Both drugs have short half-lives in the circulation, in the order of 2–4 hours, and are excreted into the urine at least 50% unchanged.[72,76,77] Thus very high levels of drug build up in the urine, which may lead to unopposed clot formation in the urinary tract and serious renal dysfunction. Furthermore, use of these drugs in the presence of intravascular coagulation may result in serious throm-

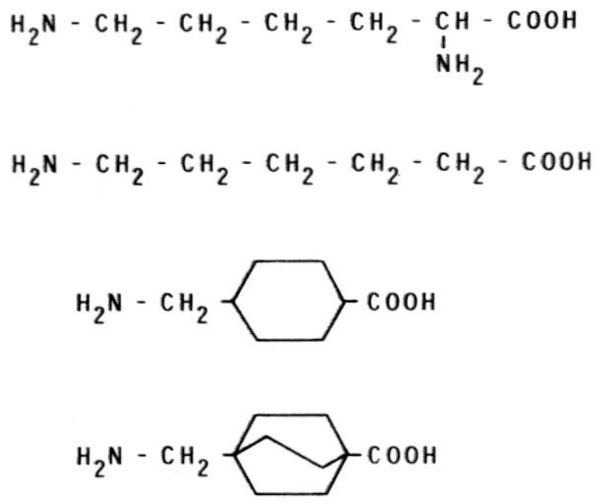

LYSINE

EACA

AMCHA

AMBCOCA

Fig. 4. Small-molecule fibrinolytic inhibitors.

botic episodes.[78–81] On the other hand, carefully used in appropriate situations, these drugs may be appropriate. For example: during prostatic surgery blood loss can routinely be decreased by as much as 75% by the administration of EACA[84,85] In the rare cases of generalized primary fibrinolysis, EACA and related drugs can be lifesaving.[86]

Recently, a still more potent analogue has been synthesized by Baumgarten and coworkers,[87] utilizing a chemical engineering approach. The need for a free amino group and free carboxyl group at opposite ends of the molecule had been established by Okamoto.[71–73] Furthermore, the optimal distance between the carbon atom of the carboxyl group and the carbon atom to which the free NH_2 group was attached appeared to be 5–7 Å. The EACA molecule, however, is not rigid, and the length of the molecule is not fixed. By introducing more rigid groups between the two ends of the molecule, the optimal distance for fibrinolytic inhibition could be better determined. Thus AMCHA has a distance of 5.82 Å between the relevant carbon atoms, while aminomethylbicyclooctane carboxylic acid (AMBCOCA) has a distance of 5.67 Å and is 10 times more potent than AMCHA and 100 times more potent than EACA. Studying a series of analogues, it could be shown that decreasing this distance to 4.8 Å abolished inhibitory activity, while increasing this distance to 6.4 Å, decreased inhibitory activity by a factor of 6.[86] Of course, in vitro potency alone does not promise greater therapeutic efficacy, and in vivo studies are necessary to determine whether significant therapeutic advantages will be found for such new compounds.

SUMMARY

Therapeutic manipulation of the fibrinolytic system is still in its infancy. Several approaches are theoretically possible to enhance fibrinolytic activity. Of these, only the administration of activators for acute thromboembolic episodes is currently under clinical trial. Although in vivo studies have established the thrombolytic potency of both SK and UK, definite evidence of therapeutic efficacy is still lacking. Other approaches, including preventive treatment by sustained, mild enhancement of fibrinolytic activity, are appealing, controversial, and unproven. Nevertheless such approaches will undoubtedly be pursued with vigor. The chemical engineering of small-molecular inhibitors of fibrinolysis is leading to more potent agents in vitro, but it is not clear whether they will be more useful clinically than agents already available. However, the ferment created by the enormous growth in our knowledge of the biochemistry of the plasminogen-plasmin system, its activators, and its inhibitors, gives promise for the discovery of better and more effective approaches to the treatment of thrombotic diseases.

REFERENCES

1. Robbins KC, Summaria L: Human plasminogen and plasmin, Methods in Enzymology. Proteolytic Enzymes. Edited by GE Perlman, L Lorand. New York, Academic, 1970
2. Schwick HG, Heimburger N: Biochemie der Fibrinolyse. Thromb Diath Haemorrh Suppl 32:9, 1969
3. Robbins KC, Summaria L, Hsieh B, et al: The peptide chains of human plasmin. Mechanism of activation of human plasminogen to plasmin. J Biol Chem 242:2333, 1967
4. Sherry S, Alkjaersig N, Fletcher AP: Activity of plasmin and streptokinase activator on substituted arginine and lysine esters. Thromb Diath Haemorrh 16:18, 1966
5. Johnson AJ, Kline, DL, Alkjaersig N: Assay methods and standard preparations for plasmin, plasminogen and urokinase in purified systems, 1967-1968. Thromb Diath Haemorrh 21:259, 1969
6. Summaria L, Hsieh B, Groskopf WR, et al: The isolation and characterization of the 5-carboxymethyl β (light) chain derivative of human plasmin. The localization of the active site of the β (light) chain. J Biol Chem 242:5046, 1967
7. Groskopf WR, Hsieh B, Summaria L, et al: Studies on the active center of human plasmin. The serine and histidine residues. J Biol Chem 244:359, 1969
8. Robbins KC, Summaria L.: Biochemistry of fibrinolysis. Thromb Diath Haemorrh Suppl 47:9, 1971
9. Kwaan HC, Lo R, McFadzean AJS: On the production of plasma fibrinolytic activity within veins. Clin Sci 16:241, 1957
10. Warren BA: Fibrinolytic activity of vascular endothelium. Br Med Bull 20:213, 1964
11. Todd AS: Localization of fibrinolytic activity in tissues. Br Med Bull 20:200, 1964
12. Kwaan HC, Astrup T: Fibrinolytic activity in thrombosed veins. Circ Res 17: 477, 1965
13. Kwaan HC, McFadzean AJS: Plasma fibrinolytic activity induced by ischaemia. Clin Sci 15:245, 1956
14. Biggs R, Macfarlane RG, Pilling J: Observations on fibrinolysis. Experimental activity produced by exercise or adrenaline. Lancet 1:402, 1947
15. Sherry S, Lindemeyer RI, Fletcher AP, et al: Studies on enhanced fibrinolytic activity in man. J Clin Invest 38:810, 1959
16. Weiner M, Redisch W, Steele JM: Occurrence of fibrinolytic activity following administration of nicotinic acid. Proc Soc Exp Biol 98:755, 1958
17. von Kaulla KN: Intravenous protein-free pyrogen. A most powerful fibrinolytic agent in man. Circulation 18:187, 1958
18. Fletcher AP, Biederman D, Moore D et al: Abnormal plasminogen-plasmin

system activity in patients with hepatic cirrhosis: its cause and consequences. J Clin Invest 43:681, 1964
19. Lack CH: Proteolytic activity and connective tissue. Br Med Bull 20:213, 1964
20. Ambrus JL, Ambrus CM, Stutzman L, et al: Therapeutic studies with fibrinolytic and antifibrinolytic agents, Chemical Control of Fibrinolysis-Thrombolysis. Edited by JM Schor. New York, Wiley, 1970
21. Takada A, Takada Y, Ambrus JL: Streptokinaseactivatable proactivator of human and bovine plasminogen. J Biol Chem 245:6389, 1970
22. Tillet WS, Garner RL: The fibrinolytic activity of hemolytic streptococci. J Exp Med 58:485, 1933
23. DeRenzo EC, Seiteri PK, Hutchings BL, et al: Preparation and certain properties of highly purified streptokinase. J Biol Chem 242:533, 1967
24. Niewiarowski S, Latallo Z: Comparative studies of the fibrinolytic system of sera of various vertebrates. Thromb Diath Haemorrh 3:404, 1959
25. Kline DL, Fishman JB: Improved procedure for the isolation of human plasminogen. J Biol Chem 236:3232, 1961
26. Ling CM, Summaria L, Robbins KC: Isolation and characterization of bovine plasminogen activator from a human plasminogen streptokinase mixture. J Biol Chem 242:1419, 1967
27. Summaria L, Hsieh B, Groskopf WR, et al: Direct activation of human plasminogen by streptokinase. Proc Soc Exp Biol 130:737, 1969
28. Kline DL, Ts'ao CH: Activation of human plasminogen by streptokinase in absence of plasmin-SK activator. Am J Physiol 220:440, 1971
29. von Kaulla KN: Urine adsorbate with fibrinolytic and thromboplastic properties. J Lab Clin Med 44:944, 1954
30. Lesuk A, Terminello L, Travez JH: Crystalline human urokinase. Some properties. Science 147:880, 1965
31. White WF, Barlow GH, Mozen MM: The isolation and characterization of plasminogen activators (urokinase) from human urine. Biochemistry 5:2160, 1966
32. Norman PS: Antiplasmins. Fed Proc 25:63, 1966
33. Ganrot PO: Inhibition of plasmin activity by α_2-macroglobulin. Clin Chim Acta 16:328, 1967
34. Aoki N, von Kaulla KN: Human serum plasminogen antiactivator: its distinction from antiplasmin. Am J Physiol 220:1137, 1971
35. Vogel R, Trautschold I, Werle E: Natural Proteinase Inhibitors. New York, Academic, 1968
36. Fritz H, Trautschold I, Haendle H, et al: Chemistry and biochemistry of proteinase inhibitors from mammalian tissues. Ann NY Acad Sci 146:400, 1968
37. Anderer FA, Hörnle S: Chemical studies on kallikrein inactivator from bovine lung and parotid gland. Ann NY Acad Sci 146:381, 1968
38. Ambrus JL, Ambrus CM, Stutzman L, et al: Treatment of fibrinolytic hemorrhage with proteinase inhibitors: a preliminary report. Ann NY Acad Sci 146: 625, 1968
39. Nussenzweig V, Seligmann M: Analyse, par des methodes immunochimiques de la degradation par la plasmine du fibrinogene humain et de la fibrine, a differents stades. Rev Hematol 15:451, 1960
40. Marder VJ, Shulman NR, Carroll WR: High molecular weight derivatives of human fibrinogen produced by plasmin. I. Physicochemical and immunological characterization. J Biol Chem 244:2111, 1969
41. Marder VJ: Identification and purification of fibrinogen degradation products produced by plasmin. Considerations on the structure of fibrinogen. Scand J Haematol Suppl 13:21, 1971

42. Niewiarowski S, Kowalski, E: Un nouvel anticoagulant derive du fibrinogene. Rev Hematol 13:320, 1958
43. Triantaphyllopoulos DC: Anticoagulant effect of incubated fibrinogen. Can J Biochem Physiol 36:249, 1958
44. Marder VJ: Physicochemical studies of intermediate and final products of plasmin digestion of human fibrinogen. Thromb Diath Haemorrh Suppl 39:187, 1970
45. Niewiarowski S, Gurewich V Senyi AF, et al: The effect of fibrinolysis on platelet function. Thromb Diath Haemorrh Suppl 47:99, 1971
46. Marder VJ, Matchett MO, Sherry S: Detection of serum fibrinogen and fibrin degradation products. Comparison of six techniques using purified products and application in clinical studies. Am J Med 51:71, 1971
47. Mersky C, Lalezari P, Johnson AJ: A rapid, simple, sensitive method for measuring fibrinolytic split products in human serum. Proc Soc Exp Biol 131: 871, 1969
48. Hawiger J, Niewiarowski S, Gurewich V, et al: Measurement of fibrinogen and fibrin degradation products in serum by staphylococcal clumping test. J Lab Clin Med 75:93, 1970
49. Niewiarowski S, Gurewich V: Laboratory identification of intravascular coagulation. The serial dilution protamine sulfate test for the detection of fibrin monomer and fibrin degradation products. J Lab Clin Med 77:665, 1971
50. Gurewich V, Hutchinson E: Detection of intravascular coagulation by a serial-dilution protamine sulfate test. Ann Intern Med 75:895, 1971
51. Fearnley GR: Fibrinolysis. London, Arnold, 1965
52. Sherry S, Fletcher AP, Alkjaersig N: Fibrinolysis and fibrinolytic activity in man. Physiol Rev 39:343, 1959
53. Fearnley GR: Pharmacologic enhancement of fibrinolysis. Chemical Control of Fibrinolysis-Thrombolysis. Edited by JM Schor. New York: Wiley, 1970
54. von Kaulla KN: On the in vitro mechanism of synthetic fibrinolytic agents.[53]
55. Hirsh J, O'Sullivan EF, Martin M: Evaluation of a standard dosage schedule with streptokinase. Blood 35:341, 1970
56. Urokinase pulmonary embolism trial. Phase 1 results. A cooperative study. JAMA 214:2163, 1970
57. Symposium on thrombolytic therapy with streptokinase. Aust Ann Med 19: Supp 1:1, 1970
58. Martin M, Schoop W, Zeitler E: Streptokinase in chronic arterial occlusive disease. JAMA 211:1169, 1970
59. Verstraete M, Mermylen J, Donati MB: The effect of streptokinase infusion on chronic arterial occlusions and stenoses. Ann Intern Med 74:377, 1971
60. Poliwoda H: Thrombolytic therapy in acute myocardial infarction. Aust Ann ed 19 Suppl 1:66, 1970
61. Amery A, Roeber G, Vermylen HJ: Single-blind randomized multicentre trial comparing heparin and streptokinase treatment in recent myocardial infarction. Acta Med Scand Suppl 505:5, 1969
62. Schmutzler R, Fritze E, Gebauer D, et al: Fibrinolytic therapy in acute myocardial infarction. Thromb Diath Haemorrh Suppl 47:211, 1971
63. Heikinheimo R, Ahrenberg P, Honkapohja H, et al: Fibrinolytic treatment in acute myocardial infarction. Acta Med Scand 189:7, 1971
64. Isacson S, Nilsson IM: Effect of treatment with combined phenformin and ethyloestrenol on the coagulation and fibrinolytic systems. Scand J Haematol 7:404, 1970
65. Chakrabarti R, Fearnley GR: Reduction of platelet stickiness by phenformin plus ethyloestrenol. Lancet 2:1012, 1967
66. Reid WO, Lucas ON, Francisco J, et al: The use of epsilon aminocaproic acid

in the management of dental extractions in the hemophiliac. Am J Med Sci 248:82, 1964
67. Walsh PN, Rizza CR, Matthews JM, et al: Epsilon-aminocaproic acid therapy for dental extractions in haemophilia and Christmas disease: a double-blind controlled trial. Br J Haematol 20:463, 1971
68. Lundh B, Laurell AB, Wetterquist H, et al: A case of hereditary angioneurotic edema successfully treated with EACA. Studies on C′1 esterase inhibitor, C′1 activation, plasminogen and histamine metabolism. Clin Exp Immunol 3:733, 1968
69. Donaldson VH: C′1 activation in hereditary angioneurotic edema plasma: role of urokinase and inhibitors. J Appl Physiol 25:416, 1968
70. Frank MM, Sergent JS, Kane MA, et al: Epsilon aminocaproic acid therapy in hereditary angioneurotic edema. N Engl J Med 286:808, 1972
71. Okamoto S: Plasmin and antiplasmin. Keio J Med 8:211, 1959
72. Okamoto S, Oshiba S, Mihara H, et al: Synthetic Inhibitors of fibrinolysis: in vitro and in vivo mode of action. Ann NY Acad Sci 146:414, 1968
73. Iwamoto M, Abiko Y, Shimizu M: Plasminogen plasmin activation and inhibition of plasminogen plasmin system by some synthetic inhibitors. J Biochem (Tokyo) 64:759, 1968
74. Ablondi FB, Hagen JJ, Philips M, et al: Inhibition of plasmin, trypsin, and the streptokinase activated fibrinolytic system by E-aminocaproic acid. Arch Biochem 82:153, 1959
75. Alkjaersig N, Fletcher AP, Sherry S: E-aminocaproic acid, an inhibitor of plasminogen activation. J Biol Chem 234:832, 1959
76. Thomas K, Stalder K, Stegemann H: Metabolic experiments with epsilon aminocaproic acid. Z Physiol Chem 317:276, 1959
77. Nilssen IM, Sjoerdsma A, Waldenstrom J: Antifibrinolytic activity and metabolism of epsilon amino caproic acid in man. Lancet 1:1322, 1960
78. Naeye RL: Thrombotic state after a hemorrhagic diathesis, a possible complication of therapy with epsilon aminocaproic acid. Blood 19:694, 1962
79. Gans H: Thrombogenic properties of epsilon aminocaproic acid. Ann Surg 163:175, 1966
80. Herschlein HJ, Steichele DF: Triggering of massive thrombus formation with epsilon-aminocaproic acid after previous activation of the coagulation system. Thromb Diath Haemorrh 17:568, 1967
81. Charytan C, Purtilo D: Glomerular capillary thrombosis and acute renal failure after epsilon aminocaproic acid therapy. N Engl J Med 280:1102, 1969
82. Gralnick HR, Greipp P: Thrombosis with epsilon aminocaproic acid therapy. Am J Clin Pathol 56:151, 1971
83. Bergin JJ: The complications of therapy with epsilonaminocaproic acid. Med Clin North Am 50:1669, 1966
84. Vinnicombe J, Shuttleworth KED: Aminocaproic acid in the control of haemorrhage after prostatectomy. Lancet 1:230, 1966, i:232, 1966
85. Schmutzler R, Fürstenberg H: The effect of epsilon-aminocaproic acid and trasylol on fibrinolysis and blood loss after operations on the prostate. Germ Med Mon 11:390, 1966
86. Sherry S, Aljaersig N, Fletcher AP: Fibrinolytic bleeding and its management. Ann NY Acad Sci 115:481, 1964
87. Baumgarten W: Synthetic antifibrinolytic agents, Hematologic Reviews. Edited by JL Ambrus. New York, Marcel Dekker, 1972

PART V

Therapy of Drug-induced Hematologic Disorder

Scott Murphy

27
Platelet Transfusion

Platelet transfusions are frequently used in the treatment of patients with drug-induced hypoplastic anemia and other disorders in which thrombocytopenia results from reduced platelet production. Research in this field, during the past five years, has lead to distinct improvements in our use of platelets but also it has raised new questions and problems. Three areas of interest will be discussed in this review: (a) the preparation and storage of platelet concentrates, (b) the selection of platelet donors, and (c) the indications for platelet transfusion.

PREPARATION AND STORAGE OF PLATELET CONCENTRATES

Preparation

In all but very rare circumstances, platelet concentrates (PC) will be used rather than platelet-rich plasma (PRP) or whole blood. The use of PC reduces the volume infused into the patient and allows recovery of other blood components for use in patients who specifically need them. In many centers, PC are prepared by plasmapheresis, returning red cells to the donor. In most instances, this should be unnecessary. In well-organized urban areas, the community's needs for platelets can be met by processing less than 20% of the routine blood donations. If this is done, plasmapheresis can be reserved for the preparation of PC from donors who are specifically matched for recipients refractory to platelets from random donors. Newer techniques of continuous-flow centrifugation[1] should allow the collection of 4–8 units of PC from these specially qualified donors.

In the routine preparation of PC, PRP is easily prepared from whole blood

Supported by grants from The John H. Hartford Foundation and the National Institutes of Health (HE 11047-06, NIH-70-2212, CA 12397-01A10).

by differential centrifugation. In past years, difficulties arose when PRP was centifuged and the platelet button was resuspended in small volumes of plasma; irreversible platelet clumping frequently occurred. A major advance was made by Mourad[2] who showed that clumping could be avoided if the entire procedure was carried out at room temperature (22°C) rather than at 4°C, and if the platelet button was allowed to rest undisturbed for 30 minutes after centrifugation. Subsequently, Kattlove and Alexander[3] reported that exposure of platelets to cold temperature followed by rewarming and agitation induced platelet aggregation; this helped to explain the superiority of working at 22°C. We also assume that some adenine nucleotides, capable of inducing platelet aggregation, are released during centrifugation to form a platelet button and that the 30-minute waiting period allows time for their degradation by plasma enzymes. Using the Mourad technique, PC can be prepared from blood anticoagulated with either acid-citrate-dextrose (ACD) or citrate-phosphate-dextrose (CPD). Our experience and that of others[4] has been that PC from ACD and CPD blood have equivalent in vivo viability.

Storage of PC

There is currently a lively controversy over the best temperature for PC storage. I would like to present data on which my current prejudices are based. The platelet circulates as a thin disc. This discoid shape is maintained by a continuous, circumferential bundle of rigid microtubles[5] which act as a cytoskeleton. The microtubules rapidly depolymerize at 4°C and the cell becomes spherical. After a few hours at 4°C, this change is irreversible. If such cells are labeled with radioactive chromium (^{51}Cr) and infused into their original donor, the half-life (T½) of their in vivo survival will be reduced to a degree proportional to the time of exposure to 4°C.[6] On the other hand, if platelets are maintained at 22°C, microtubules remain intact, the disc shape is well preserved, and no reduction in T½ occurs even after 48–72 hours of storage. Thus, exposure to 4°C appears to have a direct toxic effect on platelet viability. This concept was confirmed by Levin and Freireich in thrombocytopenic patients.[7] They found (Figure 1) that the rise in platelet count immediately after infusion of PRP was reduced by 37% and 62% after storage at 4°C for 24 and 48 hours, respectively. In addition, the platelet count always returned to baseline levels the day after transfusion. On the other hand, if platelets are stored at 22°C for 24–48 hours, it is common[6,8] for most platelets circulating immediately after infusion to still be present 24 hours later. An example of the normal survival of platelets stored at 22°C is presented in Figure 2.

One could envision that a storage procedure could preserve viability, i.e., ability to circulate, but not hemostatic efficacy. The only way to measure the in vivo hemostatic efficacy of a platelet transfusion is to demonstrate shortening of the prolonged bleeding time of thrombocytopenic patients. Figure 3 shows that fresh PC and PC stored for 24 hours at 22°C are equivalent in this regard.

Is storage at 22°C safe? Buchholz[9] reported two episodes of sepsis after infusion of platelets stored at 22°C. Other investigators [10,11] have reported on the absence of infection of PC, and I know of no other episode of clinical

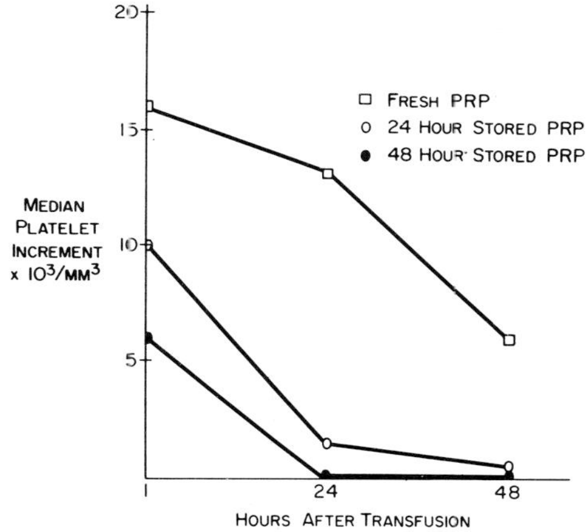

Fig. 1. Reduced platelet survival after refrigerated storage (4°C). Thrombocytopenic recipients received fresh PRP or PRP stored at 4°C. The response was measured as rise in platelet count (increment per 10^{11} platelets administered multiplied by the body surface area (M^2)). The initial rise in platelet count is reduced by storage and very few of the surviving platelets are still circulating 24 hours after infusion. (Redrawn from Levin, et al.[7])

sepsis related to the use of PC stored at 22°C. At the Children's Hospital of Philadelphia, during the past 2 years, 1500 units of PC stored at 22°C have been administered without septic sequelae.

Therefore, PC stored for 24 hours at 22°C appear to be safe and effective. Recently, Becker and Aster[12] reported that PC stored for 2–5 days at 4°C had acceptable viability and hemostatic efficacy, and that a large proportion of PC stored for more than 24 hours at 22°C had negligible viability. Their success with storage at 4°C is at variance with the experience of most investigators

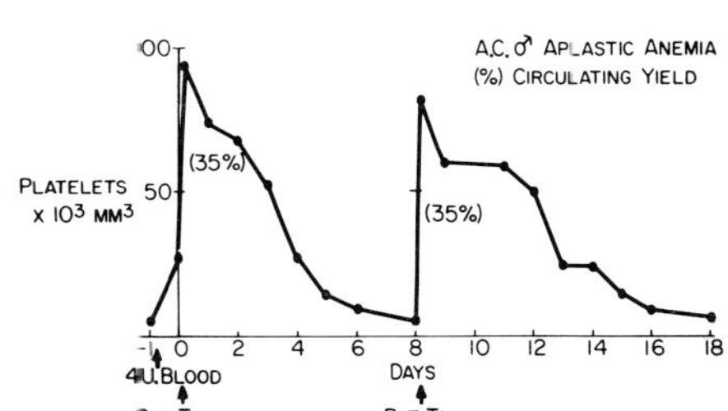

Fig. 2. Transfusion of platelet concentrates (PC) stored for 24 hours at room temperature (22°C). After both transfusions, 35% of the infused platelets were found in the circulation 1 hour after infusion. These platelets survived with a half-life (T½) of 3–4 days. The patient had an intact spleen. Normal or nearly normal survival of platelets stored at 22°C has been documented in several patients.[8] (I am grateful to Dr. James Bond who referred AC for study.)

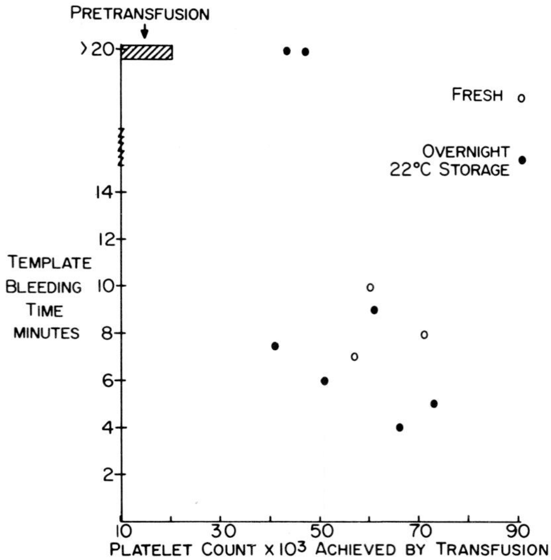

Fig. 3. Hemostatic efficacy of platelets stored at 22°C. Children with acute leukemia, platelet counts under 20,000 per mm^3, and bleeding times greater than 20 minutes, received fresh or stored PC. Repeat bleeding times were performed 1–3 hours after transfusion and related to the simultaneous platelet count. If the platelet count had been raised above 50,000 per mm^3, correction of the bleeding time was always observed. If the platelet count was elevated to less than 50,000 per mm^3, the bleeding time was not consistently corrected. We have observed the latter phenomenon even with fresh platelets. (These data were collected by Dr. Marie Stuart and Dr. Frank Oski.)

in the field and requires confirmation by other laboratories. Their poor results with storage at 22°C beyond 24 hours can probably be explained by the following considerations.

During PC storage at 22°C, platelet glycolysis produces lactate and pH falls. Figure 4 records simultaneous pH and lactate measurements in PC stored for 1–3 days. The nearly linear, inverse correlation between the two measurements indicates that at any given time, PC-pH is determined by the amount of glycolysis which has occurred since PC preparation. Since lactate production should be proportional to platelet count, one would expect that after a storage interval, PC-pH would be inversely correlated with the platelet count, and indeed this is the case (Figure 5). We have previously reported[8] that platelets undergo a dramatic morphologic change when pH falls to 6.0 or below; they become spherical, extend long, thin, rigid projections of cytoplasm, and frequently aggregate. This morphologic change is associated with an absolute loss of in vivo viability as judged by ^{51}Cr survival studies. Reference to Figure 5 will indicate to the reader the maximum platelet count for each storage interval which will allow PC storage without loss of viability due to pH fall. In practice, we have kept PC platelet counts relatively low by em-

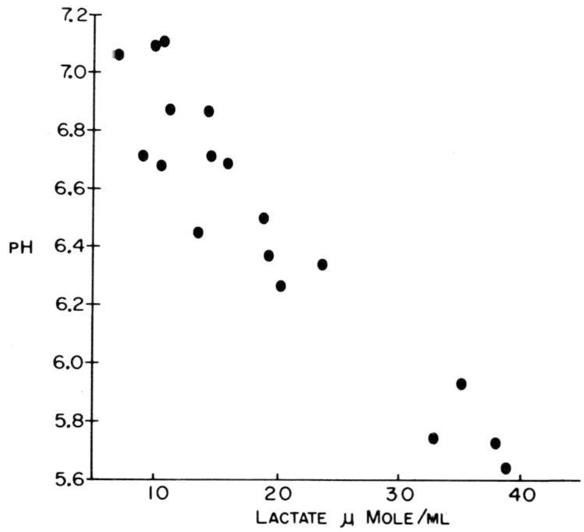

Fig. 4. Simultaneous pH and lactate measurements in platelet concentrates stored in polyvinylchloride bags for 1–3 days at 22°C. At any point in time during storage, PC-pH is determined by the amount of glycolysis which has occurred as reflected in the lactate concentration.

ploying a relatively large PC volume of 30 ml. If a blood bank wishes to store PC at 22°C for more than 24 hours, it should check the pH and platelet count of its product to be sure that units are not being lost due to pH fall. A major need in this field is to develop techniques by which this pH fall can be eliminated or minimized.

PC stored at 22°C should be agitated during storage to maintain a uni-

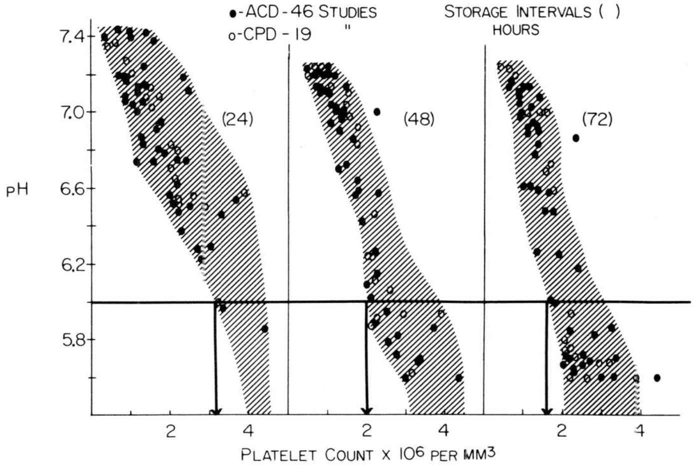

Fig. 5. Platelet concentrate (PC) stored in polyvinylchloride bags at 22°C. PC-pH was measured after storage for 24, 48, and 72 hours and related to the initial PC platelet count. The bags were agitated during storage. 46 PC were obtained from blood anticoagulated with ACD; 19 PC were from CPD blood. The pH after storage is inversely proportional to the platelet count. The arrows indicate that PC platelet count above which some PC will be nonviable due to fall of pH to below 6.0 during that storage interval.

form cell suspension. We have demonstrated[8] that this results in improved viability as measured in vivo. There have been no comparative studies to demonstrate the superiority of one method of agitation over another.

SELECTION OF PLATELET DONORS

ABO and Rh Compatibility

The ABO system significantly affects the results of platelet transfusion therapy. Aster reported[13] that the infusion of platelets from individuals whose red cells contained the A antigen into individuals whose plasma contained anti-A resulted in a poor in vivo recovery; an inverse correlation between recovery and titer of the isohemagglutinin was demonstrated. The same principle applied to the B antigen. Incompatibility in the Rh system did not adversely affect the results of transfusion. Furthermore, in clinical practice, the repeated infusion of platelets from Rh positive individuals into Rh negative patients results in a remarkably low incidence of isosentitization, i.e., the development of anti-Rh antibodies.[14] Therefore, the logical procedure for a well-organized urban area would be to harvest platelets from routine blood donations of A and O individuals in quantities sufficient to meet the area's needs.

The Refractory State

As patients are repeatedly transfused with blood products, their response to platelet transfusion is often compromised. During their first transfusion, they should have results similar to those seen in Figure 2. As the number of transfusions increases, the in vivo yield and life-span (T½) are reduced, and eventually the transfused platelets are removed from the circulation within minutes of infusion. Fresh or stored whole blood and PC transfusions are apparently equivalent in their ability to produce this refractory state. There is a surprisingly wide variability from patient to patient in the number of transfusions required. We have observed the refractory state in patients who have been transfused only once. On the other hand, patient AC continued to have results similar to those shown in Figure 2 after more than 200 units of blood products had been administered. We assume that antiplatelet isoantibodies with a broad range of specificities must be present in the plasma of these patients. Unfortunately, there is no in vitro test which is useful clinically in identifying these antibodies.

The recent work of Yankee and his colleagues[15,16] represents a significant advance in this field. They studied 5 patients with aplastic anemia[15] who had become totally refractory to platelet transfusions from random donors. The lymphocytes of the patients and their siblings were typed for histocompatibility antigens. As shown in Figure 6, transfusion of platelets from random donors or siblings who were not HLA-compatible resulted in no elevation of the platelet count of the patients. However, platelets from HLA-identical siblings produced in vivo yield and survival similar to what one sees with random platelets in patients who have never been transfused and are not refractory. Follow-up

Fig. 6. HLA-compatible donors in the refractory state. Five thrombocytopenic patients, refractory to platelets from unrelated donors, responded to platelets from HLA-compatible siblings. The platelet increments (rise in platelet count per unit infused multiplied by body surface area, M^2) 1 and 24 hours after transfusion were similar to results obtained with random platelets in recipients who are not refractory. (Graph drawn from data presented by Yankee, et al.[15])

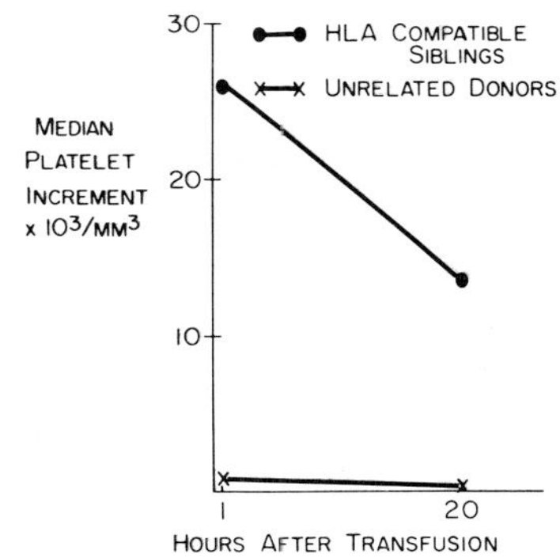

observations[16] of these patients has indicated that a good response to "matched" platelets persists indefinitely.

These results imply that all antigens responsible for inducing the refractory state are controlled by the same, single chromosomal pair which governs the synthesis of HLA antigens. We do know that most of the HLA antigens are represented on the platelet membrane, since HLA-typing by platelet complement-fixation yields results quite similar to those obtained by lymphocyte cytotoxicity. However, we do not know that the antibodies responsible for the refractory state are directed against the currently recognized HLA antigens. The success of HLA-typing in selecting compatible sibling donors may simply reflect the fact that HLA identity in siblings implies the inheritance of the same chromosomal pair. The HLA antigens as we now identify them may represent only a small fraction of the antigens coded by that chromosomal pair capable of inducing platelet isosensitization. The answer to this question will become available when refractory patients receive transfusions from *unrelated* donors who have the same four HLA antigens as the patient. Studies of this type are currently being carried out by several groups.

Our current practice is to begin the management of thrombocytopenic patients with platelets from random donors. If the patient becomes refractory, HLA-identical siblings are sought to support the patient. If none are available, a panel of normal donors whose HLA types are known is reviewed and platelets from the most compatible donors are obtained to determine if they will circulate in the patient. Most investigators[16] have found that immunosuppressive drug therapy and splenectomy have not improved the response of refractory patients to platelets from random donors. In one patient, we attempted to reduce the titer of the hypothesized antibodies by the infusion of 100 units of platelets over 5 days in preparation for a surgical procedure. On the day of surgery, the patient remained completely refractory to platelet transfusion. Improvements in techniques for plateletpheresis[1] and platelet storage by freezing[17] will have their most important applications in the management of refractory patients for whom one or more acceptable donors are found. Current plasmapheresis techniques yield a maximum of four units of platelets from a single donor; more may be required for an adult patient of large size. One can also envision freezing multiple units of platelets during periods when the patient is free from hemorrhage for use when the patient is symptomatic from thrombocytopenia.

THE EFFECT OF DRUG INGESTION BY DONORS ON THE HEMOSTATIC EFFICACY OF THEIR PLATELETS

A rapidly expanding literature has recently called attention to the inhibitory effect of many drugs on platelet function. In chapter 23, Dr. Harvey Weiss has reviewed the effects on platelets of aspirin, the most widely used and perhaps the best studied of these agents. In a recent survey,[18] 59% of routine blood donors had abnormal platelet aggregation studies, mostly related to the ingestion of aspirin or other medication. The figure was reduced to 2% when the donors specifically refrained from drug ingestion for 1 week prior to donation.

We recently carried out studies[19] designed to evaluate the importance of the widespread use of aspirin among blood donors. In our laboratory, 1 and 24 hours after the ingestion of 600 mg aspirin, the bleeding times of normal volunteers are significantly prolonged. The abnormal values return to normal 72 hours after ingestion. We questioned the value of platelets from donors during that 72-hour period. Donors were divided into three groups (Figure 7): Group I = no drug ingestion for 1 week prior to donation, Group II = aspirin ingestion 1 and 12 hours prior to donation, and Group III = aspirin ingestion

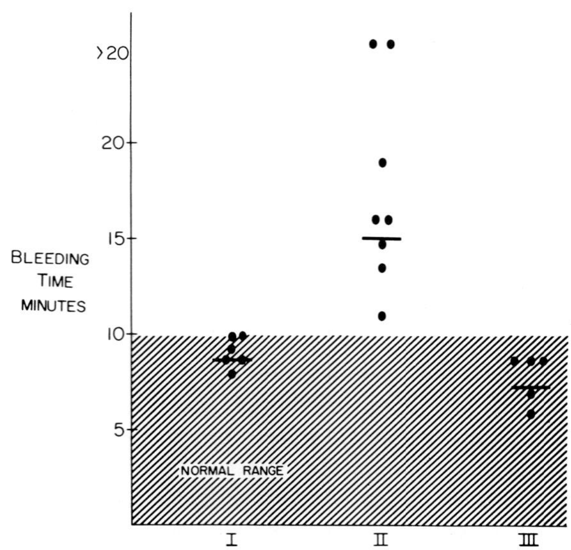

Fig. 7. Effect of aspirin ingestion by donors on the hemostatic efficacy of platelet transfusions. Children with acute leukemia, platelet counts less than 20,000 per mm^3, and bleeding times greater than 20 minutes, received platelets from three groups of donors: Group I= no drug ingestion for 1 week prior to donation, Group II= aspirin ingestion 1 and 12 hours prior to donation, Group III= aspirin ingestion 36 hours prior to donation. The recipient's bleeding time was measured again 1 hour after transfusion. Although the platelet counts achieved in the three groups were similar, platelets from Group II were hemostatically inferior. (Redrawn from Stuart, et al.[19])

36 hours prior to donation. Recipients were thrombocytopenic children with acute lymphatic leukemia and bleeding times greater than 20 minutes. Figure 7 indicates that platelet transfusions from Groups I and III returned bleeding times to the normal range, but transfusions from Group II did not. Presumably, in the Group III studies, the 36-hour interval was sufficient for the synthesis of enough new platelets free of the aspirin effect to allow normalization of the bleeding time. Analysis of the data in Group II indicated that some patients had a partial return of bleeding time toward the normal range while others had no shortening at all. Patients who had a partial response were those who contributed a significant number of their own platelets to the circulating platelet mass after transfusion, i.e., their platelet counts prior to transfusion were 10,000–20,000 per cubic millimeters. The patients who had no response had platelet counts near 0 per cubic millimeter.

We conclude from these data that aspirin-treated platelets can improve hemostasis if at least 20%–25% of the platelets circulating after transfusion are free of the aspirin effect. This is consistent with our current concepts that aspirin-treated platelets can respond to adenosine diphosphate (ADP) and contribute to the bulk of a platelet plug forming at the site of vessel injury, but sufficient numbers of unaffected platelets must be available at that site to release ADP. Aspirin interferes with the latter phenomenon only (Weiss H: chapter 23).

In practice, most patients receive pooled PC, and at least 20%–25% of each pool should be free of the aspirin effect. Nonetheless, we firmly discourage the ingestion of any medication by our donors within 36 hours of donation to reduce to a minimum the percentage of affected platelets in each pool. Furthermore, refractory, isosensitized patients and small children often receive platelets from a single donor. In these circumstances, particularly if the recipient's platelet count is very low, drug ingestion by the donor should be rigidly proscribed.

INDICATIONS FOR PLATELET TRANSFUSION

There are no data available to define indications for platelet transfusion. In past years, when platelets were in short supply, the decision to transfuse a patient was often made on the basis of availability in the Blood Bank rather than the needs of the patient. As urban areas are organized to utilize their blood donations properly and as techniques for short-term PC storage improve, it should be possible to make such decisions entirely on the basis of the patient's status. In patients with impaired platelet production, our policy is to give platelets only for specific clinical indications: central nervous system bleeding, gross hematuria, gross gastrointestinal bleeding, epistaxis requiring packing, oral mucous membrane bleeding. In addition, in some chemotherapeutic protocols, episodes of severe thrombocytopenia are so predictable that platelets are administered as the platelet count approaches its nadir. We find that we are often able to observe asymptomatic patients with platelet counts of 5000–20,000 per cubic millimeter for many months without the need for platelet transfusions. Other clinics prefer to transfuse such patients twice weekly to protect them against hemorrhagic complications. The major justification of our policy has been our desire to avoid sensitizing the patient so that he will not be refractory to platelets during future hemorrhagic episodes. A prospective protocol in which patients are randomized to one of these two therapeutic philosophies is currently in progress at the Children's Hospital of Philadelphia.

Platelet transfusions should rarely be given to patients whose thrombocytopenia results from accelerated platelet destruction. For example: in idiopathic thrombocytopenic purpura, patients with platelet counts greater than 15,000 per cubic millimeter are rarely symptomatic and have no need for transfusion. If the platelet count is lower than 15,000 per cubic millimeter, the survival time of both the patient's and the transfused platelets will be only a matter of minutes, and the therapeutic effect of the transfused platelets will be too short-lived to be worthwhile.

Since so many thrombocytopenic patients stop bleeding without platelet transfusions, it is really not possible to be certain that transfusions have been helpful by observing clinical events alone. One knows that hemostasis has been improved if the platelet count is elevated and the bleeding time shortened after transfusion. It has been our experience that the platelet count must be raised to 50,000 per cubic millimeter or higher to produce consistent shortening of the bleeding time to less than 20 minutes (Figure 3). If the patient has not been sensitized, this can be achieved by administering 0.1 unit per kilogram body weight. Larger doses will be required if the patient has fever or splenomegaly. Achieving less than this degree of platelet count elevation may help patients, but there is no way of demonstrating it objectively.

SUMMARY

Three areas of interest have received attention recently: (a) the preparation and storage of platelet concentrates (PC), (b) the selection of platelet donors, and (c) the indications for platelet transfusions.

Platelet concentrates from ACD and CPD blood can be prepared easily if processing is carried out at 22°C and suspension of the button is delayed for 30 minutes after centrifugation. Most data indicate that PC viability is best maintained at 22°C. The major problem with PC storage at 22°C is falling pH, which results in loss of viability when pH reaches 6.0. The rate of pH fall is directly related to the PC platelet count and rate of glycolysis.

The ABO system significantly affects the results of platelet transfusion. Platelets from A or B donors should not be given to recipients who lack these antigens. As patients are repeatedly transfused with blood products, they often develop isoantibodies which prevent transfused platelets from circulating. Such patients can be managed with platelets from HLA-identical siblings. It will be of great interest to determine if platelets from HLA-identical, unrelated individuals will be useful. Platelets from donors who have ingested aspirin immediately prior to donation do not have optimal hemostatic effect in thrombocytopenic recipients. Drug ingestion by donors should be discouraged.

There are no data available to delineate indications for platelet transfusion. As platelets become widely available for use, prospective studies should be done to answer this question.

REFERENCES

1. Tullis JL, Tinch RJ, Baudanza P, et al.: Plateletpheresis in a disposable system. Transfusion 11:368–377, 1971
2. Mourad N: A simple method for obtaining platelet concentrates free of aggregates. Transfusion 8:48, 1968
3. Kattlove HE, Alexander B: The effect of cold on platelets. I. Cold induced platelet aggregation. Blood 38:39–48, 1971
4. Tranum BL, Haut A: In vivo survival of platelets prepared in CPD anticoagulant. Transfusion 12: 168–174, 1972
5. White JG, Krivit W: An ultrastructural basis for the shape changes induced in platelets by chilling. Blood 30:625–635, 1967
6. Murphy S, Gardner FH: Platelet preservation: effect of storage temperature on maintenance of platelet viability—deleterious effect of refrigerated storage. N Engl J Med 280:1094–1098, 1969
7. Levin RH, Freireich EJ: Effect of storage up to 48 hours on response to transfusions of platelet rich plasma. Transfusion 4:251–256, 1964
8. Murphy S, Sayar SN, Gardner FH: Storage of platelet concentrates at 22°C. Blood 35:549–557, 1970
9. Buchholz DH, Young VM, Friedman NR, et al: Bacterial proliferation in platelet products stored at room temperature. N Engl J Med 285:429–433, 1971
10. Katz AJ, Tilton RC: Sterility of platelet concentrates stored at 25°C. Transfusion 10:329–330, 1970
11. Silver H, Sonnenwirth AC, Beisser LD: Bacteriologic study of platelet concentrates prepared and stored without refrigeration. Transfusion 10:315–316, 1970
12. Becker GA, Aster RH: Short-term platelet preservation. Clin Res 20:480, 1972
13. Aster RH: Effect of anticoagulant and ABO incompatibility on recovery of transfused human platelets. Blood 26:732–743, 1965
14. Goldfinger D, McGinniss MH: Rh-incompatible platelet transfusions—risks and consequences of sensitizing immunosuppressed patients. N Engl J Med 284: 942–944, 1971
15. Yankee RA, Grumet FC, Rogentine GN: Platelet transfusion therapy: the selection of compatible platelet donors for refractory patients by lymphocyte HL-A typing. N Engl J Med 281:1208–1212, 1969
16. Grumet FC, Yankee RA: Long-term platelet support of patients with aplastic anemia: effect of splenectomy and steroid therapy. Ann Intern Med 73:1–7, 1970
17. Handin RI, Valeri CR: Improved viability of previously frozen platelets. Blood 40:509–513, 1972
18. Schwartz AD: Platelet aggregation in blood donors. Transfusion 12:344–347, 1972
19. Stuart MJ, Murphy S, Oski FA et al: Observations on platelet function in the recipients of platelets from donors ingesting aspirin. N Engl J Med 287:1105–1109, 1972

Harold A. Wurzel

28
Red Cell and Plasma Transfusions in Drug-induced Disorders

In general, most patients who require blood transfusions do not need whole blood.[1] Except for acute blood loss, patients usually do better with red cells. The plasma thus salvaged can be used for preparing other components patients may need; for example: platelets, cryoprecipitate for Factor VIII deficiency, serum albumin, and others. Likewise, the patient who has drug-induced anemia rarely requires whole blood.

The decision to transfuse or not should be based on the patient's symptoms and not on laboratory values. Most patients can tolerate a moderate degree of anemia and may even, if inactive, tolerate a marked degree of anemia.

PLASMA TRANSFUSIONS

The requirements for plasma transfusions are usually minimal in patients who have drug-induced hematologic disorders. Drugs that cause severe liver damage prevent the production of many clotting factors. Patients with liver disease secondary to these drugs may require replacement of these clotting factors. Usually fresh plasma or fresh frozen plasma will supply the missing clotting factors.

AVAILABLE COMPONENTS AND USES FOR TREATMENT OF ANEMIA

Whole Blood

Its use should be restricted to those patients who are also volume depleted (e.g., after acute blood loss).

Red Cells

Red cells are administered to replenish the oxygen carrying capacity of the blood. Either "banked" red cells or leukocyte-free red cells obtained by: (a) nylon filtration, (b) differential centrifugation, (c) "washed" red cells, or (d) "frozen" red cells, may be used.

"Banked" Red Cells

For patients who require blood to correct symptomatic anemia, especially that secondary to aplasia of the bone marrow, red cells are available. Any blood bank that has a refrigerated centrifuge can separate the red cells from whole blood without difficulty. In fact, the red cells can be separated by simple sedimentation in the blood bank refrigerator.

One of the major problems after repeated transfusions is the febrile transfusion reaction. This type of reaction is usually due to the formation of leukoagglutinins in recipients, which agglutinate leucocytes of transfused blood. The reaction may occur shortly after the beginning of the transfusion to several hours post-transfusion. Because of the symptoms (chills and fever), the transfusion must be stopped and studies undertaken to rule out a hemolytic transfusion reaction. Although the incidence of this type of reaction is less with red cells than with whole blood, it still occurs. In some patients, pretreating with aspirin, antihistamines, or corticosteroids may prevent or alleviate the symptoms.

A better way of preventing febrile reactions is to remove the white blood cells from the blood. This can be accomplished in several ways.

Leukocyte-Free Red Cells

FILTRATION OF BLOOD[2]

Filtration through a nylon filter will remove most of the granulocytes but allows the lymphocytes to remain. Fresh blood collected in heparin must be used. The blood is then filtered through the nylon into ACD solution. By this method, almost all granulocytes will be removed.

DIFFERENTIAL CENTRIFUGATION

A less effective method is to invert the blood and allow it to sedimentate by gravity or centrifugation. The red cells are then expressed into another bag, leaving the plasma, platelets, and white cells in the original container.

WASHED RED CELLS

"Washed" red cells can be prepared by adding saline to the red cells, centrifugating, removing the saline, and repeating the process two more times. Washing can also be done with a continuous flow system.[3]

The former method is much less expensive but, because the blood bag must be entered often, the chance of contamination with bacteria is a danger. We have found that to remove most of the white blood cells, five washings are actually required.

Table 1
Primary Uses of Frozen Blood

Routine source of red blood cells
To prevent sensitization of the recipient by leukocytes
Autotransfusions
Rare donors

The latter method, because it is a "closed system," reduces the chance of bacterial contamination. The original equipment and bowls used are expensive. At present, this method has not been used widely and more general experience is needed to evaluate it.

"FROZEN" RED CELLS

There are at present two different systems in general use. In both, glycerol is used as a cryoprotective agent. One method is rapidly freezing with liquid nitrogen and a low concentration of glycerol.[4] The other is mechanical slow freezing at $-85°$ using a high concentration of glycerol, as described by Huggins.[5] The glycerol is removed after thawing and prior to transfusion. In the process of freezing and then thawing the red cells, the white cells are destroyed.

In our experience, the high glycerol-slow freezing method of preparing leukocyte-poor blood has been very successful in preventing febrile transfusion reactions.

The Huggins method of freezing and thawing red cells has also been used in our laboratory for many other reasons than just preparing leukocyte-free red cells (Table 1).

RBC COMPATABILITY—ANTIHUMAN GLOBULIN (AAG) REACTIONS

The biggest problem of hemotherapy related to drug-induced anemia is caused by those drugs that produce a positive direct antihuman globulin test [(Coombs test) AHG]. Among these drugs are such commonly used ones as penicillin,[6] cephalothin,[7] and α-methyldopa.[8,9] The last drug causes the greatest difficulty. About 20% of the people taking this drug develop a positive direct AHG test, but only a small number actually develop a hemolytic anemia.

The positive direct AHG test is frequently accompanied by a positive indirect AHG and gives serologic reactions similar to those found in many autoimmune hemolytic anemias.

The problem arises when the laboratory tries to find compatible blood for the patient. Even the results obtained from such routine testing as ABO grouping and Rh typing may be difficult to interpret. If the indirect AHG is positive, it may be impossible to find compatible blood for transfusion; if only the direct AHG test is positive, it is usually not difficult to find compatible blood.

A positive indirect AHG usually signifies the formation of an isoantibody after exposure to a foreign antigen due to previous transfusions or pregnancies. Usually it is easy to delineate the specificity of the antibody in these cases.

In autoimmune hemolytic anemia and/or drug-induced hemolytic anemia a positive indirect AHG test may not be due to previous exposure to a foreign antigen. The positive indirect AHG test in these circumstances probably represents excess antibody formation, with saturation of the antigenic sites on the erythrocytes. The excess antibody therefore "spills over" into the plasma. In some patients with autoimmune hemolytic anemia or drug-induced hemolytic anemia the antibody is found to be a panagglutinin with no blood group specificity. In other patients, the antibody may seem to react specifically with one of the blood group systems. These specific antibodies seem to be directed against antigens in the Rh system, usually hr′(c̄) and hr″(ē).

Recently, von dem Borne, et al[10] reported that in patients with autoimmune hemolytic anemia with anti-hr″(ē) specificity, cell survival with transfused hr″(ē) negative cells is slightly longer than the patient's own cells, but hr″(ē) positive cells have a much shorter cell survival.

The decision then, whether or not to transfuse, requires consultation between the clinician and director of the blood bank. The blood bank director can suggest methods to determine if blood transfusion will be helpful or harmful to the patient.

One method is the "biologic test." A small amount (25–50 ml) of the least incompatible blood can be given and bilirubin, haptoglobin, and hemoglobin in urine measured pre- and post-transfusion. As the patients already have laboratory evidence of hemolytic anemia, it may be difficult to ascertain the significance of change in these parameters.

Recently, in our hospital we have been using a modification of Mollison's method[11] to study the survival of transfused cells. Usually 1.0 ml of the most incompatible cells is labeled with ^{51}Cr. The survival of these cells in the recipient is followed for at least the next 24 hours. This method has helped us to decide which patients can be safely transfused.

Not all patients who have a positive direct AHG due to drugs, will have hemolytic anemia. Recently, with the advent of surgical procedures, such as those to correct stenosis of the coronary artery, we have had patients taking α-methyldopa for hypertension who require corrective operations. Some of these patients also have had positive AHG tests without hemolytic anemia. Because compatible blood could not be found, we used the ^{51}Cr survival test to decide whether or not to proceed with the operation.

Another complication of repeated transfusions is the formation of isoantibodies due to red cell antigens lacking in the recipient. Many patients develop several isoantibodies after multiple transfusions. It probably is a good idea to type the red cells of the patient for as many antigens as possible prior to the first transfusion. It is almost impossible to find enough donors who will be compatible with all antigens of the recipients. However, if multiple antibodies are found, personnel in the blood bank will have some idea as to which antibodies could be present. Blood lacking the corresponding antigen should be transfused. As noted in Table 1, frozen blood can be stockpiled for these patients as it has a shelf life of at least 2 years instead of the usual 21 days for regular blood.

Modern blood-banking techniques have now reached the stage of development in which patients with drug-induced anemia can be treated for long periods of time with the hope that bone marrow function can be restored. Red cells usually should be used, and special procedures are now available to overcome many of the complications of repeated transfusions.

HEMOSIDEROSIS

The main complication still not resolved, however, is hemosiderosis. Perhaps in the near future a good, easy-to-use drug will be found to chelate the iron given with each transfusion so that transfusion hemosiderosis will not occur in patients who require multiple transfusions over long periods of time.

SUMMARY

Indications for blood transfusions for drug-induced anemia are similar to those of other patients. Whole blood is only indicated when active bleeding is being treated. The need for transfusion should be based on medical evaluation of the signs and symptoms of the patient and not on the results of laboratory tests.

Many complications that follow the transfusion of multiple units of red cells, e.g., febrile reactions, isoimmunization, can now be handled by most banks.

Finding compatible blood for patients with drug-induced autoimmunization is still a difficult problem.

REFERENCES

1. Westphal RG: Rational alternatives to the use of whole blood. Ann Intern Med 76:987, 1972
2. Greenwalt TJ, Gajewski M, McKenna JL: A new method for preparing buffy coat-poor blood. Transfusion 2:221, 1962
3. Meryman HT: Washing erythrocytes in a centrifugal system with particular reference to glycerolized cells. Transfusion 8:348, 1968
4. Rowe AW, Eyster E, Kellner A: Liquid nitrogen preservation of red blood cells for transfusion: a low-glycerol rapid freeze procedure. Cryobiology 5:119, 1968
5. Huggins CE: Frozen Blood: Principles of practical preservation. Monogr Surgical Sci 3:133, 1966
6. Petz LD, Fudenberg HH: Coombs positive hemolytic anemia caused by penicillin administration. N Engl J Med 274:171, 1966
7. Gralnick HR, Wright LD, McGinniss MH: Coombs positive reactions associated with sodium cephalothin therapy. JAMA 199:135, 1967
8. Worlledge S: Autoantibody formation associated with Methyldopa (Aldomet) therapy. Br J Haematol 16:5, 1969
9. Wurzel HA, Silverman JL: The effects of alpha-methyl-3,4-dihydroxyl-1-phenylalanine (Methyldopa, Aldomet) on erythrocytes. Transfusion 8:84, 1968

10. von dem Borne AEG Kr, Engelfriet CP, Beckers Do, et al: Autoimmune haemolytic anaemias. IV. Biochemical studies of red cells from patients with autoimmune haemolytic anaemia with incomplete warm autoantibodies. Clin Exp Immunol 8:377, 1971
11. Mollison PL: Blood Transfusion in Clinical Medicine. Philadelphia, Davis, 1967, pp 721–722

Robert G. Graw, Jr.

29
Bone Marrow Transplantation for the Therapy of Aplastic Anemia

Aplastic anemia is a hematologic disorder characterized by an impairment of effective hematopoiesis. A precise diagnosis of this disease depends on the confirmation of bone marrow hypoplasia as demonstrated with bone marrow aspiration and bone marrow biopsy (Figure 1). Many etiologies have been postulated for aplastic anemia, including congenital and inherited forms of hematopoietic dysfunction, toxic or infectious injury to bone marrow stem cells and supporting stroma (i.e., infectious hepatitis), and manifestations of systemic diseases, such as leukemia, and paroxysmal nocturnal hemoglobinuria (PNH). Since the etiology of pancytopenia cannot be discriminated simply on the basis of bone marrow morphology, it does not seem surprising that many different therapies have been practiced for patients with this disorder. Although many unique therapies have been proposed, such as treatment with phytohaemagglutinin, immunosuppressive drugs, bone marrow curettage, androgens, and corticosteroids, no particular modality has demonstrated reproducible benefit. Most certainly, the variable severity of each patient's disease course and complications have confused the interpretation of the results of any new regimen. This paper will attempt to place in perspective the role for bone marrow transplantation in the treatment of patients with aplastic anemia.

EVALUATION AND CLASSIFICATION OF PATIENTS

To appropriately treat patients with profound pancytopenia, it is most important that the disease be confirmed by bone marrow aspirations and biopsy. Every attempt must be made to distinguish patients with mild bone marrow hypoplasia from those with complete aplasia, a disease with a uniformly poor survival. Some authors believe that the differential leukocyte count on a bone marrow aspirate is very helpful in prognosticating the course of any individual patient. Li, et al have proposed that bone marrow lymphocytosis in excess of 85%, together with a relative absence of hematopoietic elements, identifies patients with a poor prognosis.[1] The variable nature of this disease

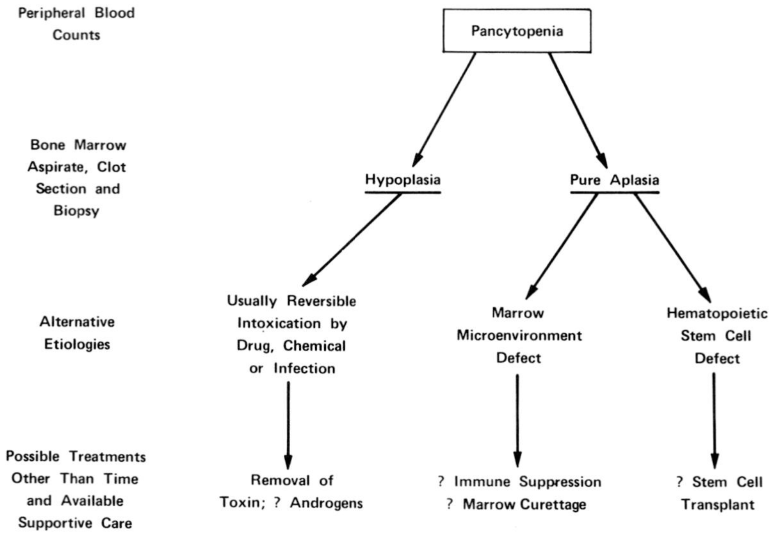

Figure 1

necessitates that bone marrow aspirations be performed on several occasions and that the natural history of bone marrow activity be correlated with the patient's clinical course. If at all possible, an attempt should be made to distinguish a defect in hematopoietic stem cells from that of a microenvironment malfunction. Assays which examine the proliferative capacity of bone marrow cells in vitro, such as bone marrow agar colony culture, may be useful in distinguishing a selective hematopoietic cell defect from that of microenvironment.[2,3] The ability to culture normal numbers of agar colonies from peripheral blood leukocytes of patients with aplastic anemia may serve to distinguish a defect in bone marrow microenvironment from that of hematopoietic precursor cells.[4] Histopathologic examinations of large bone marrow biopsies may offer an opportunity to visualize the vasculature and other essential structures of bone marrow stroma. Clearly, a patient who is shown to have a deficiency in a single cellular element or a mildly impaired functional capacity of bone marrow will respond better to management with drugs and supportive care than will patients with no bone marrow function. The history of all patients must be examined thoroughly for common etiologies of aplastic anemia in order that the most appropriate therapy can be instituted, as judged from similar patients treated within any etiologic classification. In the case of patients with marrow hypoplasia resulting from chemical toxins, it is interesting and perhaps helpful to attempt analysis of body tissues and bone marrow fat for any residual chemical agent.

MEDICAL MANAGEMENT WITH DRUGS AND SUPPORTIVE CARE

Since most patients, even after a comprehensive medical evaluation, are relegated to an idiopathic etiologic classification, interpretation of the results of therapeutic maneuvers has been most difficult. In general, most confusion has resulted from the failure to classify patients in categories as to the extent of marrow dysfunction. Table 1 summarizes the most recent attempts at treatment of aplastic anemia using various methods of supportive care, often in combination with androgens and/or corticosteroids. In the review of treatment of 780 patients with aplastic anemia, 302 (39%) recovered. Notable among those studies is that reported by Heyn, et al who documentated a 51% survival without androgen therapy.[14] Most recently two studies from the United States have shown a uniformly poor survival rate (26% and 25% survival, respectively) for patients treated with oxymetholone and combinations of androgen and corticosteroids.[1,17]

Other adjuncts in the supportive care of patients, such as patient protective isolation,[21,22] frozen red blood cell transfusions,[23] and splenectomy performed in an effort to alter the course of alloimmunization to random donor blood products,[24] and a generally improved blood component transfusion support capability have had a variable influence on patient survival.[25] Laminar airflow rooms, developed to purify the hospital environment, can be used in conjunction with oral nonabsorbable antibiotics to reduce the incidence of hospital-acquired infections of enteric origin. As yet, there is no evidence that there is a reduced incidence of fungal or viral infections.[22] Splenectomy after partial alloimmunization to blood products can temporarily improve the circulation of transfused platelets, but, in general, will not prevent or delay sensitization to platelet and leukocyte antigens. The small potential benefits observed in patient management after splenectomy should be carefully weighed against risks of surgical complications for individual patients. Splenectomy should not become a routine procedure to be performed thoughtlessly on all patients with aplastic anemia. The use of HL-A matched sibling platelets for the long-term transfusion requirements of patients with severe thrombocytopenia refractory to random donor platelet transfusions can significantly alter their survival.[26] Frozen red blood cells to replenish hemoglobin can further delay the time to complete alloimmunization to leukocytes contained in random donor blood components. Recent technologic developments in the collection of leukocytes from single normal donors can be used to provide these patients with granulocyte transfusions during episodes of overwhelming bacterial infection.[27]

EARLY MARROW TRANSPLANTATION STUDIES

Bortin, in his review of human bone marrow transplants in 1970, reported 73 attempted marrow transplants for aplastic anemia.[28] Sixty-six of these failed to engraft and 5 patients developed graft-versus-host disease (GVH). These early studies serve to emphasize major obstacles in early marrow transplantation studies—failure of marrow engraftment or subsequent development of fatal graft-versus-host disease in those patients successfully engrafted.

To avoid problems associated with histoincompatibility, a number of bone marrow transplants were performed from identical twin siblings to patients with aplastic anemia. Table 2 summarizes the 12 isogeneic bone marrow transplants reported. It is interesting that in 4 patients (33%) engraftment failed, as documented by a lack of hematopoietic cell function. In 2 of these patients, the authors speculated that a defect in marrow microenvironment may have been

Table 1
Results of Recent Attempts at the Medical Management of Aplastic Anemia

Year	No. of Patients	Drug Therapy	Surviving No.	Surviving %	Comment	Author	Reference
1961	17	Testosterone	9	51	—	Shahidi, Diamond	5
1965	60	Various drugs	9	15	No benefit from testosterone–50% dead by 6 mo	Lewis	6
1967	43	Androgens, corticosteroids	16	37	Sustained benefit from drugs evident in one-third	Vincent, DeGruchy	7
1968	5	Oxymetholone	5	100	2 children refractory to testosterone prior to oxymetholone	Allen, et al	8
1969	117	ACTH/corticosteroids	59	50	1953–1969	Hiraki, Arimori	9
1969	37	Various drugs	9	19	No apparent influence of androgen	Nora, Fernbach	10
1969	19	Androgens/corticosteroids	9	47	Improvement best correlated with marrow hypocellularity	Killander, et al	11
1969	3	Oxymetholone	3	100	Oxymetholone effective in diseases with high level of erythropoietin	McCredie	12
1969	69	Oxymetholone	33	48	Patients with varying severity of disease	Sanchez-Medal, et al	13

1969	33	No androgen therapy	17	51	Only supportive care (1951–1968)	Heyn, et al	14
1970	172	Various drugs	65	38	—	Keiser	15
1971	18	Androgens/ corticosteroids	9	50	"Androgens appeared beneficial; cortico-steroids were ? dangerous"	Corneo, et al	16
1972	58	All but 1 given androgens and and corticosteroids	15	26	11 of 11 admitted since 1965 died within 6 mo	Li, et al	1
1972	24	Oxymetholone/ corticosteroids	6	25	5 of 6 survivors received 6 mos of drug therapy	Davis, Rubin	17
1972	32	Various drugs	24	75	Varying severity of disease	Aksoy, et al	18
1972	20	Androgens	9	45	Idiopathic aplasia	Giralt, et al	19
	20	No androgen therapy	2	10	Idiopathic aplasia	Giralt, et al	19
1972	33	Oxymetholone/ corticosteroids	3	9	—	Speck	20
Totals	780	—	302	39	—		

Table 2
Isogeneic Bone Marrow Transplants for Refractory Aplastic Anemia

Year	No. of Patients	No. of Takes	No. of Failures	Postulated Reason for Failures	Reference
1961	1	1	0	—	29
1962	2	1	1	? Microenvironment	30,31
1964	4	3	1	? Microenvironment	32–35
1966	4	2	2	Not stated in reference	36–40
1968	1	1	0	Transplanted on 3 occasions	41
Totals	12	8(66%)	4(33%)		

responsible.[30,34] In this regard, Knospe and Crosby[42,43] have recently discussed the sinusoidal microcirculation as a possible etiologic factor in aplastic anemia, as had Trentin.[30,44] The experience of Knospe, et al with damaged marrow microcirculation secondary to radiation, which was responsive to curettage of the bone marrow space is most fascinating. The definition of hemopoietic inductive microenvironment (HIM), by Trentin and associates, and the elucidation of the deficiency present in the Sl/Sl^d mouse anemia, which is corrected by infusion of spleen cell stroma but not by the infusion of spleen cells, may have a bearing on failures to engraft histocompatible bone marrow in patients with idiopathic aplastic anemia.

RECENT BONE MARROW TRANSPLANT STUDIES USING HL-A MATCHED DONORS

Recognition of the importance of the HL-A lymphocyte antigen system for determining success in organ transplantation prompted many attempts to improve the success rate for human bone marrow transplant studies.[45] The combination of mixed leukocyte culture analysis to confirm HL-A identity within families further convinced hematologists that bone marrow transplantation could be attempted from siblings matched for histocompatibility antigens.[46] Initial studies using HL-A and mixed leukocyte culture (MLC) identical siblings involved transplantation of bone marrow to patients with lymphopenic forms of immunologic deficiencies. This group of patients required no form of immunosuppression in preparation for marrow transfer because of deficiencies in cellular immunity.

The next category of patients in whom marrow transplantation was attempted were those with acute leukemia refractory to conventional chemotherapy. These patients were transplanted after total body x-ray[47,48] or after cyclophosphamide.[49–51] In general, experience with HL-A and MLC identical bone marrow transplantation for the treatment of leukemia has been associated with a 71% incidence of engraftment and the regular occurrence of graft-versus-host disease in approximately 50% of the recipients. Twenty per cent of patients successfully engrafted died with graft-versus-host disease and concomitant viral and fungal infections.[52,53] Of 52 patients transplanted with bone marrow from HL-A identical siblings, 5 are in long-term remission from disease. One patient, from Seattle, Washington, has remained in remission from acute lymphocytic leukemia for more than 750 days.[54] The longest remission after marrow transplantation for acute myelogenous leukemia is in excess of 21 months.[55]

One of the major questions answered in these series of marrow transplants to patients with leukemia has related to the effect of random donor blood transfusion support to patients prior to attempts at marrow transplantation. It had generally been felt that transfusions, particularly transfusions of blood products with donor histocompatibility antigens, would significantly jeopardize future marrow transplants. Several animal studies have indicated that transfusions would diminish the incidence and/or duration of bone marrow engraftment.[56–59] In general, leukemic patients heavily transfused with random donor blood products engrafted at the same rate as did patients who received infrequent transfusions.

The level of immunosuppression required for successful engraftment in man has been further examined in leukemia transplant studies wherein several regimens have been employed, including total body gamma irradiation (TBI), cyclophosphamide, antilymphocyte serum (ALS), and combinations of the preceding as well as a four-drug combination, including cyclophosphamide, cytosine arabinoside, 6-thioguanine and BCNU.[60] All of these immunosuppressive regimens were found to be equally effective in producing engraftment; however, cyclophosphamide, used singly, was often associated with an incomplete level of engraftment, as detected by a mixture of donor and host markers during the post-transplant period.[51] Antilymphocyte serum, as a single agent for immunosuppression, was found to provide no antitumor activity but did offer the advantage of protecting the patient from graft-versus-host disease when transplanted with histoincompatible bone marrow.[61,62]

Table 3 summarizes published experience with 27 patients who were transplanted with HL-A identical bone marrow for refractory aplastic anemia. As noted, several regimens for pretransplant immunosuppression have been utilized. The majority have received post-transplant chemotherapy in an effort to modify graft-versus-host disease if it were to occur. The most commonly used agent was methotrexate.[73] Cyclophosphamide was used as the primary immunosuppressant in 15 patients, 11 of whom were successfully engrafted. Eight of 9 patients transplanted in Seattle were successfully engrafted using a cyclophosphamide regimen modified from Santos.[67,68] Graft-versus-host disease has occurred in approximately 26% of these patients, despite the use of methotrexate in doses recommended to modify or abolish this disease. More recently, TBI (1000 rads, midline tissue dose) has been used for immunosuppression without any greater success.[71] In fact, the incidence of graft failure and the post-transplant complication rate has been significantly higher after TBI as compared to cyclophosphamide preparation. Whether the failure of 2 patients to engraft after TBI is indicative of a microcirculatory failure within the marrow space cannot be determined; however, it is interesting to speculate that patients receiving cyclophosphamide in immunosuppressive doses may have their microenvironment altered in such a way that transplanted hemopoietic stem cells can be received, nourished, and engrafted. Whether a defect

Table 3
HL-A Identical Bone Marrow Transplantation for Refractory Aplastic Anemia

Pretransplant Immuno-suppression	Post-transplant Immuno-suppression	No. Patients	No. Takes*	No. Failures	No. GVH	No. Fatal GVH	Duration Engraftment (Days)	Survival (Days)	Reference
ALG	—	5	3	2	0	0	76–90+	30–231+	62–64
CYT	—	2	1	0	0	0	3–10	3–10	65,66
CYT	MTX	10	9	0	2	2	27–498+	0–498+	67–69
CYT	CYT	1	1	0	1	1	32	32	50
CYT+ALG	—	2	0	0	0	0	—	10	65,70
TBL	MTX	6	4	2	2	2	14–180+	10–180+	71
TBI+ALG	MTX	1	1	0	0	0	28	28	72
Totals	—	27	19 (70%)	4 (15%)	5 (26%)	5 (26%)	3–498+	0–498+	

ALG Antilymphocyte Globulin
CYT Cyclophosphamide
MTX Metrotrexate
TBI Total Body Irradiation
GVH Graft = versus = host disease
* Does not include patients living insufficient time to detect engraftment

in microenvironment actually exists and is responsible for clinical disease in humans cannot be presently answered, although the failure to engraft several patients with bone marrow from identical twins, and more recently the failure to engraft marrow from HL-A identical donors after TBI, may support this concept. Antilymphocyte serum alone has permitted successful engraftment of 3 patients, although the quality of engraftment has been in question. Following ALS, donor red blood cell marker antigens are easily identified in the recipients post-transplant, but complete recovery of hematopoietic function (granulocyte and platelet production) has failed to occur. An animal model for the study of ALS in marrow transplantation has been devised recently by Speck.[74] In rabbits made temporarily aplastic with benzene or ^{32}P, he has demonstrated temporary engraftment of histoincompatible bone marrow after treatment with ALS. Unique features of these engraftments have been the development of "split" grafts wherein recipient animals have engraftment of donor cells in bone marrow with normal B-cell function. However, T-cell function remains host type and there is no graft-versus-host reaction. Using a primate model, Merritt, et al have also demonstrated "split" grafts in animals prepared with TBI and ALS.[75] This type of selective hematopoietic engraftment without associated graft-versus-host disease may, in fact, be very important for safe hematologic reconstitution of patients with isolated defects in red-blood cell, leukocyte, or platelet precursors. Additional animal experiments will have to be performed to elucidate critical mechanisms responsible for these "split" engraftments. It is essential that all human bone marrow chimeras be examined thoroughly for completeness of chimerism periodically post-transplant.

DISCUSSION

The approach to the patient with aplastic anemia requires the most sophisticated diagnostic capabilities available to the hematologist. Advances in the techniques of supportive care (transfusion, patient isolation, and treatment of infection) lengthen patient survival temporarily. The decision to use HL-A matched siblings in a program of prolonged transfusion support or for bone marrow transplantation must be made early in a patient's illness.[76] As such, a patient with aplastic anemia should have his entire family and close relatives HL-A typed so that individuals matched with the patient for HL-A antigens can be identified. In the event an HL-A identical sibling is identified, a decision must be made as to whether to use that individual for transfusion support or to withhold HL-A matched transfusion support until bone marrow transplantation is undertaken.

One of the most difficult decisions the managing physician must reach is when to attempt marrow transplantation if a suitable donor is found (Figure 2). As more experience has been gained using marrow transplantation for the permanent hematologic reconstitution of these individuals, it has been recognized that survival statistics favor early marrow transplantation. In general, patient survival after conservative medical management, using androgenic steroids (including oxymetholone) and supportive care measures such as

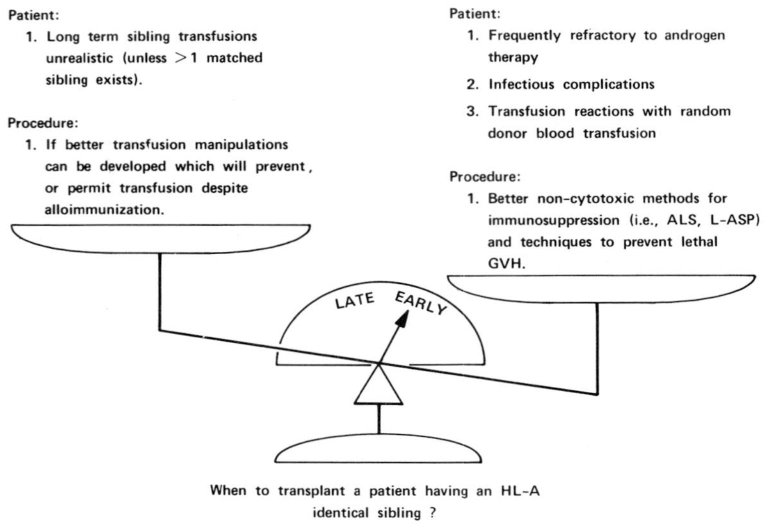

Figure 2

splenectomy, immunosuppressive drugs, transfusion, and patient isolation, have been disappointingly low (Table 1: mean = 39%). In fact, it is unclear whether these therapeutic measures have lengthened life at all in patients with profound marrow aplasia. In the largest series of patients receiving HL-A matched bone marrow, 5 of 9 have had long-term permanent hematologic reconstitution. Whether these figures will hold up as additional transplants are performed remains to be seen. Most certainly, the management of patients through a bone marrow transplant can be greatly facilitated by the availability of random donor and HL-A matched blood component transfusion support. For this reason, if for no other, a marrow transplant contemplated in a patient with an HL-A and MLC matched sibling should be performed early in his course.

For the 85% of patients for whom no suitable HL-A matched donor exists, the opportunity for a successful marrow transplant remains infrequent. Whether phenotypically HL-A matched, random bone marrow donors can be successfully utilized in such situations remains undefined. Whether protocols incorporating ALS, bone marrow fractionation for the elimination of immunocompetent cells,[77] blocking antibodies,[78] or in vitro incubation of bone marrow with selective immunologic inhibitors of B- and T-cell lymphoid populations[79] will be successful in permitting marrow transplantation between mismatched individuals, represents exciting frontiers in transplantation biology. Until these techniques are fully developed or unless better medical management can be provided for patients not having siblings suitable for marrow donation, the outlook for patients with refractory aplastic anemia is poor.

In cases where bone marrow transplantation is contemplated, it is important to minimize sensitization to random donor blood products. In general, red blood cells, freed of contaminating leukocytes together with the judicious use of single donor platelet concentrate transfusions for prophylactic treatment of thrombocytopenia will increase the period of available random donor transfusion support.

It is hoped that better techniques for the transplantation of bone marrow will soon replace the necessity for rigorous supportive care measures required to prevent complications in these patients.

REFERENCES

1. Li FP, Alter BP, Nathan DG: The mortality of acquired aplastic anemia in children. Blood 40:153–161, 1972
2. Greenberg PL, Nichols WC, Schrier SL: Granulopoiesis in acute myeloid leukemia and preleukemia. N Engl Med 284:1225–1232, 1971
3. Krantz SB, Kao V: Studies on red cell aplasia. II Report of a second patient with an antibody to erythroblast nuclei and remission after immunosuppressive therapy. Blood 34:1–13, 1969
4. Dicke KA: Personal communication, 1972
5. Shahidi NT, Diamond LK: Testosterone induced remissions in aplastic anemia of both acquired and congenital types. N Engl J Med 264:953, 1961
6. Lewis SM: Course and prognosis in aplastic anemia. Br Med J 1:1027–31, 1965
7. Vincent PC, DeGrouchy GC: Complications and treatment of acquired aplastic anemia. Br J Hematol 13:977–99, 1967
8. Allen DM, Fine MH, Necheles JF et al: Oxymetholone therapy in aplastic anemia. Blood 32:83–9, 1968
9. Hiraki K, Arimori S: Treatment and prognosis of aplastic anemia. Saishin Igaku 24:749–756, 1969
10. Nora AH, Fernbach DJ: Acquired aplastic anemia. Tex Med 65: 38, 1969
11. Killander A, Lundmark KM, Sjölin S: Idiopathic aplastic anemia in children-results of androgen treatment. Acta Pediatr Scand 58:10–4, 1969
12. McCredie KB: Oxymetholone in refractory anemia. Br J Haematol 17:265–73, 1969
13. Sanchez-Medal L, Gomez-Leal A, Duarte L et al: Anabolic steroids in the treatment of acquired aplastic anemia. Blood 34: 283–300, 1969
14. Heyn RM, Ertel IJ, Tubergen DG: Course of aplastic anemia in children treated with supportive care. JAMA 208:1372–8, 1969
15. Keiser G: Erworbene Panmyelopathien. Schweiz Med Woohenschr 100:1938, 1970
16. Corneo G, Cortellaro M, Maiolo AT: Aplastic anemia: some clinical and laboratory aspects and an evaluation of the androgen-glucocorticoid treatment. Acta Haematol 46:50–9, 1971
17. Davis S Rubin AD: Treatment and prognosis in aplastic anemia. Lancet 1:871–873, 1972
18. Aksoy M, Dincol K, Erdem S et al: Details of blood changes in thirty-two patients with pancytopenia associated with long-term exposure to benzene. Br J Ind Med 29:56–64, 1972
19. Giralt M, Torres A, Raichs A: Treatment of acquired aplastic anemia with androgens–42 cases. Rev Clin Esp 124:353–60, 1972
20. Speck B: Personal communication, 1972
21. Penland WZ, Perry S: Portable laminar-air-flow isolator. Lancet 1:174–176, 1970
22. Levine AS, Graw RG Jr, Young RC: Management of infections in patients with

leukemia and lymphoma: current concepts and experimental approaches. Semin Hematol 9:141–179, 1972
23. Huggins CE, Russell PS, Winn HJ, etal: Frozen blood in transplant patients: Hepatitis and HL-A isosensitization. Transplant Proc 5:809–812, 1973
24. Grumet EC, Yankee RA: Long-term platelet support of patients with aplastic anemia: effect of splenectomy and steroid Therapy. Ann Inten Med 73: 1–7, 1970
25. Van Der Weyden M, Firkin BG: The management of aplastic anemia in adults. Br J Haematol 22:1–7, 1972
26. Yankee RA, Grumet FC, Rogentine GN Jr: Platelet transfusion. The selection of compatible platelet donors for refractory patients by lymphocyte HLA typing. N Engl J Med 281:1208–1212, 1969
27. Graw RG Jr, Herzig GP, Perry S, et al: Normal granulocyte transfusion therapy-treatment of septicemia due to gram-negative bacteria. N Engl J Med 287:367–371, 1972
28. Bortin MM: Compendium of reported human bone marrow transplants. Transplantation 9:571–587 1970
29. Robins MM, Noyes WD: Aplastic anemia treated with bone marrow transfusion from identical twin. N Engl J Med 265:974–979, 1961
30. Fernbach DJ, Trentin JJ: Isologous bone marrow transplantation in identical twin with aplastic anemia, Proceedings of the Eighth International Congress of Haematology. Vol. 1. Tokyo, Pan Pacific Press, 1962, pp. 150–154
31. Kurnick NB: Discussion.[30]
32. Melvin KEW, Davidson JNG: Aplastic anemia treated by transplantation of isologous bone marrow. N Z Med J 63:93–95, 1964
33. Mills SD, Kyle RA, Hallenbeck GA et al: Bone marrow transplant in an identical twin. JAMA 188:1037, 1964
34. Pegg DE, Fleming WD, Compston N: A case of aplastic anemia treated by isologous bone marrow infusion. Postgrad Med J 40:213–216, 1964
35. Thomas ED, Phillips JH, Finch CA: Recovery from marrow failure following isogeneic marrow infusion. JAMA 188:1041-1043, 1964
36. Chaplin H: Personal communication.[39]
37. Israels MCG: Personal communication.[39]
38. McKenna PJ, Tocantins LM: Personal communication.[39]
39. Pillow RP, Epstein RB, Buckner CD et al: Treatment of bone marrow failure by isogeneic marrow infusions. N Engl J Med 275:94–97, 1966
40. Thomas ED, Rudolph RH, Fefer A et al: Isogeneic marrow grafting in man. Exp Hematol 21: 16–17, 1971
41. Harvey LE, Firkin BG: Repeated isogenic transplants in bone marrow failure. Med J Aust 2:538–540, 1968
42. Knospe WH, Crosby WH: Aplastic anemia: a disorder of the bone marrow sinusoidal microcirculation rather than stem cell failure? Lancet 1:20–2, 1971
43. Knospe WH, Blom J, Goldstein HB et ad: Delayed bone marrow aplasia in rats protected against lethal irradiation by allogeneic marrow transplantation. Radiat Res 47:199–212, 1971
44. Trentin JJ: Determination of Bone Marrow Stem Cell Differentiation by stromal Hemopoietic Inductive Microenvironments (HIM). Am J Pathol 65:621–628, 1971
45. Terasaki PI, Singal DP: Human histocompatibility antigens of leukocytes. Ann Rev Med 20:175–188, 1969
46. Bach FH.: Transplantation: pairing of donor and recipient. Science 168:1170–1179, 1970

47. Thomas ED, Storb R: Technique for human marrow grafting. Blood 36:507–515, 1970
48. Thomas ED, Buckner CD, Rudolph RH, et al.: Allogeneic marrow grafting for hematologic malignancy using HL-A matched donor recipient sibling pairs. Blood 38:267–287, 1971
49. Santos GW, Burke PJ, Sensenbrenner LL et al: Marrow transplantation and graft-versus-host-disease in acute monocytic leukemia. Exp Hematol 18:20–22, 1969
50. Santos GW, Sensenbrenner LL, Burke PJ et al: The use of cyclophosphamide for clinical marrow transplantation. Transplant Proc 4:559, 1972
51. Graw RG Jr, Yankee RA, Rogentine GN et al: Bone marrow transplantation from HL-A matched donors to patients with acute leukemia-toxicity and Anti-leukemic effect. Transplantation 14:79–90, 1972
52. Graw RG Jr, Herzig GP, Rogentine GN et al: Graft versus host reactions complication HL-A matched bone marrow transplantation. Lancet 2:1053, 1970
53. Krueger GRF, Berard CW, Elias PM et al: Morphology of graft-versus-host reaction in HL-A matched bone marrow transplantation and its differential diagnosis. Am J Pathol 63: 179–202, 1971
54. Thomas ED: Personal communication
55. Bleyer WA, Graw RG Jr, Halterman RH, et al: Bone marrow transplantation in acute leukemia: graft-versus-host reaction and immunoincompetence. Transplant Proc (In press)
56. Da Costa J, Ameil JL, Mathé G: Immunization against transplanted allogeneic hematopoietic cells by previous transfusions. Vox Sang 9:420–30, 1964
57. Van Putten LM, Van Bekkum DW, De Vries MJ et al: The effect of preceding blood transfusions on the fate of homologous bone marrow grafts in lethally irradiated monkeys. Blood 30:749–757, 1967
58. Storb R, Epstein RB, Rudolph RH et al: The effect of prior transfusions on marrow grafts between histocompatible canine siblings. Immunol 105: 627–633, 1970
59. Storb R, Rudolph RH, Graham JC et al: The influence of transfusions from unrelated donors upon marrow grafts between histocompatible canine siblings. J Immunol 107:409–413, 1971
60. Graw RG Jr, Yankee RA, Leventhal BG et al: Bone marrow transplantation in acute leukemia employing cyclophosphamide. Exp Hemato 22:118–125, 1972
61. Amiel JL, Schwarzenberg L, Mathé : Bone marrow grafts and histocompatibility. Transplant Proc 3:1072–1077, 1971
62. Mathé G, Amiel JL, Schwarzenberg L et al: Bone marrow graft in man after conditioning by antilymphocyte serum. Transplant Proc 3:325–332, 1971
63. Mathé G, Amiel JL, Schwarzenberg L et al: Bone marrow graft in man after conditioning by antilymphocyte serum. Br Med J 2:131–136, 1970
64. Rogentine GN, Merritt CB, Rosenberg SA et al: Allogeneic bone marrow transplantation in aplastic anemia. A case Report. Exp Hematol 21:21, 1971
65. Meuwissen HJ, Rodey G, McArthur J et al: Bone marrow transplantation-therapeutic usefulness and complications. Am J Med 51:513–532, 1971
66. Hilgartner MW, Lanzkowsky P, Nachman RL, et al: Bone marrow transplantation for aplastic anemia following hepatitis, Proceedings of the American Pediatric Society, Atlantic City, New Jersey, April, 1970, p. 82
67. Buckner CD, Clift RA, Fefer A et al: Aplastic anemia treated by marrow transplantation. Transplant Proc 5:913–916, 1973
68. Buckner CD: Personal communication, 1972

69. Bortin MM, Saltzstein EC, Waisbren BA et al: Bone marrow transplantation for aplastic anemia. Transplantation 12:573–575, 1971
70. Speck B, Dooren LJ, DeKonig D et al: Conical experience with bone marrow transplantation: failure and success. Transplant Proc 3:409–413, 1971
71. Buckner CD: Personal communication, 1972
72. Rogentine GN: Personal communication, 1972
73. Storb R, Epstein RB, Graham TC et al: Methotrexate regimens for control of graft-versus-host disease in dogs with allogeneic marrow grafts. Transplantations 9:240–246, 1970
74. Speck B, Kissling M: Successful bone marrow grafts in experimental aplastic anemia using antilymphocyte serum for conditioning. Eur Rev Etud Clin Biol 16:1047–1051, 1971
75. Merritt CB, Darrow CC II, Vaal L et al: Bone marrow transplantation in rhesus monkeys following irradiation, Transplantation 14:9–20, 1972
76. Graw RG Jr, Yankee RA: Principles of hematologic supportive care. Med Clin North Am 57:441–461, 1973
77. Dicke KA, Van Hooft JIM, Van Bekkum DW: The selective elimination of immunologically competent cells from bone marrow and lymphatic cell mixtures II. Mouse spleen cell fractionation on a discontinuous albumin gradient. Transplantation 6: 562–570, 1968
78. Buckley RH, Amos DB, Kremer WB et al: Incompatible bone marrow transplantation: use of immunologic enhancement. N Engl 285:1035–1042, 1971
79. Richie ER, Gallagher MJ, Trentin JJ: Prevention of graft-versus-host disease (GVHD) by Fab fragments derived from ALG. Transplant Proc 5:873–876, 1973

Frank H. Gardner

30
Use of Androgens in the Treatment of Bone Marrow Suppression

Androgens have been used during the past 15 years in pharmacologic doses to stimulate erythropoiesis.[1,2] Aside from replacement therapy in known organ deficiencies, current clinical benefits are associated with dosage schedules suggesting that possibly only a small portion of the testosterone administrated may be active at the stem cell site.[3] Previous reports have indicated that erythropoiesis can be induced in normal adult male and female subjects if a massive androgen schedule is used for 1 to 3 months.[4,5] With the associated effects of fluid retention and depletion of plasma volume during testosterone treatment, there is an awareness that the peripheral blood measurements may have false interpretations as to the ultimate hormonal effect.[6]

During the past decade, increased serum and urinary values of erythropoietin (ESF) after androgen administration have been used as evidence for the mechanism involved to stimulate the committed erythroid stem cell.[7,8] Indeed, with all of the testosterone esters used currently, ESF levels will become elevated with prolonged administration. A plasma ESF response is associated with all severe anemias, other than those associated with severe renal disease.[9] Elevated ESF per se does not assure stimulation of erythropoiesis, for high levels are observed in severe aplastic anemia. Levels of ESF may be increased by androgen without giving a marrow erythroid response.[10] However, some patients with aplasia may respond to androgens, and whether the additional increment of ESF from hormonal therapy is necessary to stimulate the erythroid cell is not resolved at this time. Human bone marrow culture will respond to testosterone, as evidenced by the erythropoiesis measured by radioiron incorporation.[11] A greater ^{59}Fe incorporation response is obtained if ESF is added to the culture, but the erythroid response is quite satisfactory without ESF. From such in vitro measurements one may imply that the erythroid

Aided in part by a grant from The John A. Hartford Foundation and by grant AM 11188-05-06 from the National Institutes of Health.

precursor is stimulated by the androgen, and maturation is facilitated by the presence of ESF.[12]

During the past few years, the initial observation that 5β-H steroid metabolites could stimulate porphyrin synthesis in chick embryo hepatocyte has stimulated further investigation with these agents in erythropoiesis.[13,14] Rodents will respond in the exhypoxic system to stimuli from a variety of 5β-H metabolites, as measured by increased radioiron incorporation.[15,16] These short-time measurements of heme synthesis are not associated with increased ESF levels.[16] Such observations suggest that these hormonal agents are available for direct stimulation of the bone marrow without intermediary utilization of ESF. These metabolites will also stimulate erythropoiesis in human bone marrow culture.[17] From this bulk of information evidence has begun to accumulate for direct stem cell response to hormonal agents in human bone marrow as well as rodent study systems. The agents evaluated in the past have been used primarily for erythroid response. At the present time, we do not have evidence or measurements that maturation in granulocyte and megakaryocyte stem cells can respond similarly in the marrow compartment. The direct effect of these steroid metabolites should lead to a further search to determine if such specificity is available for granulocytes and platelets.

GENERAL OBSERVATION OF HEMATOPOIESES BY ANDROGENS ON MARROW FUNCTION

In the treatment of hypoplastic bone marrow, therapy with androgens initially is associated with an increase in red cell mass. Only with prolonged treatment may we expect to see improvement in the severe thrombocytopenia (Figure 1).[18] In some instances, therapy may be needed for 6 to 18 months to see such a response. The granulocyte increment is more rapid and may more closely parallel recovery of erythropoiesis. One may postulate that the massive stimulus, by androgens, of the primary stem cell compartment into a committed erythroid division has an associated contribution to myeloblasts and megakaryocytes. The rapid response of the erythroid compartment would suggest that the primary stem cell is called upon for more rapid proliferation. If the stimulus continues to assure adequate erythropoiesis and some degree of recovery, a possible feedback may divert stem cell maturation toward the other primary bone marrow committed compartments.

The androgen response observed in extramedullary hematopoiesis with myelofibrosis is of special interest. More frequently one may observe a leukocytic response of varying magnitude with a variety of androgens (Figure 2).[19] The elevated white count would appear to be correlated with the time interval of specific androgen therapy. Hence, when androgen therapy is discontinued, the leukocyte elevation returns to pretreatment levels.[18] There is no adequate explanation as to why the myeloid precursor outside of the marrow compartment has such a response when only minimal leukocytosis is observed in normal subjects receiving androgens. A minimal or moderate thrombocytosis is also noted in the androgen response of myelofibrosis, but is not comparable to the high levels of leukocytes.[19,20] Such data are helpful to indicate that a

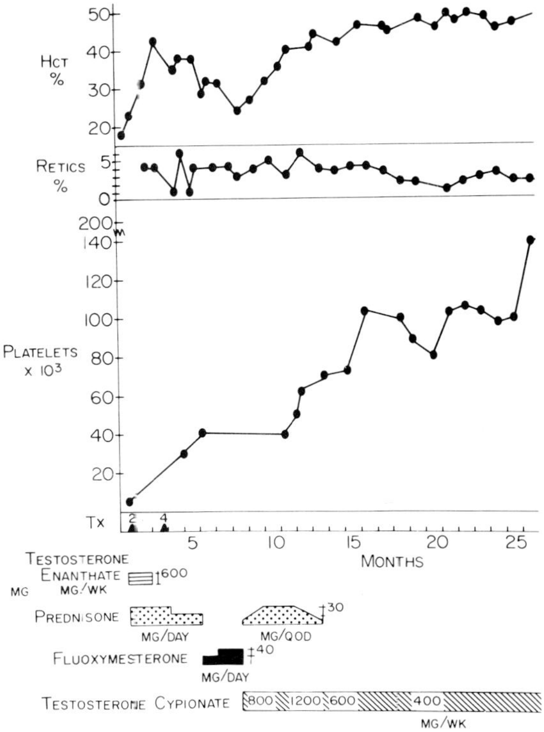

Fig. 1. 37-year-old male with drug-induced aplastic anemia. Patient had an initial rapid elevation of hematocrit with testosterone enanthate therapy. This response was not sustained with fluoxymesterone as a maintenance drug, and he recovered only after testosterone cyprionate. Prednisone was prescribed initially because of a ^{51}Cr RBC T½ life-span of 17 days. Note the slow increments in platelet counts over the initial 15 months' therapy. Most hypoplastic anemias have marked delay in recovery of platelet levels.

hormonal mechanism is available to mobilize leukocytes in this disorder. With leukocytosis, there is a marked uricemia which may also be related to the androgen response.

In vitro testing of monocytes from adult volunteers who had received 4-chlorotestosterone demonstrated an increased ingestion of colloidal carbon as compared to a placebo-treated control group.[21] This enhanced function of monocytes may be useful to improve monocytic function and protect a patient from bacterial infection when neutrophil reserves are inadequate.[22] Animal models have helped to confirm such data. Hence, mice infected with *N asteroids* had a prolonged survival if treated with 4-chlorotestosterone acetate. This same androgen ester doubled the survival time of mice infected with *staphylococcus aureus*.[23] In part, the animal response may be related to improved function of the reticuloendothelial (RE) system. In rabbits treated with testosterone, 4-chlorotestosterone acetate, and nandrolone phenylpropionate, par-

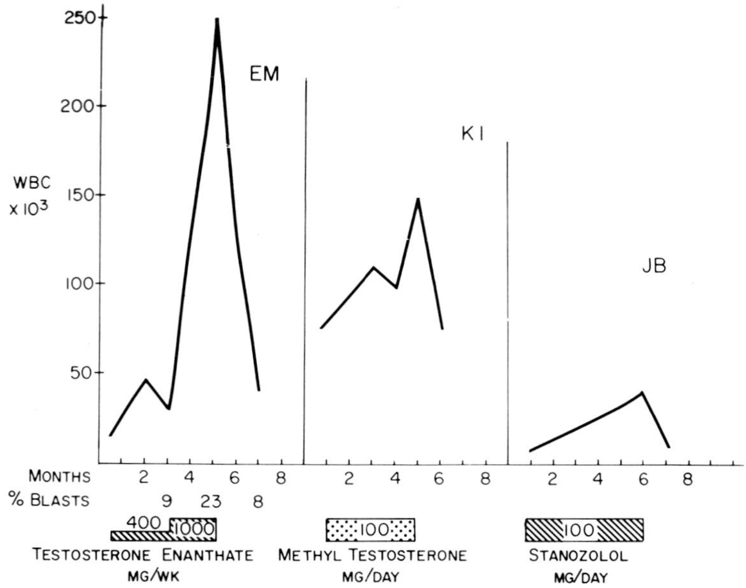

Fig. 2. Androgen leukemoid response in myelofibrosis and myeloid metaplasia. Three different patients receiving three different androgen preparations had marked leukocytosis only during the time the hormone was prescribed. Note the rapid return to pretreatment levels in these patients when testosterone was discountinued. Patient EM had the highest leukocyte count, and a large number of myeloblasts disappeared when treatment was stopped. Despite this marked leukocytosis, transfusions were required, and there was no evidence of induced erythropoiesis.

ticulate material was cleared more rapidly than in control animals.[24] Cortisone prolonged particle clearance in this model, as one might expect.

The protective effect of different types of androgens in mice receiving irradiation has been studied by Horn.[25] As we may appreciate, from the variety of androgens noted, he observed different protective responses to the various androgens used (fluoxymesterone, testosterone propionate, nandrolone phenylpropionate, and dehydroisoandrosterone). These observations emphasize the need to define methods to measure the relationship of androgen structure to stem cell response.

Many patients with depressed marrow function may have one or all precursors diminished. In the elderly patient, the marrow cytologic examination may indicate hypo- to hyperplasia with a suggestion of increased myeloid forms. In essence, the physician may not be able to diagnose a preleukemic state but he may well suspect its presence. We need to recognize that there always will be a moderate risk in our efforts to stimulate the bone marrow. Hence, we are becoming more suspicious that androgens in these disorders may well have a stimulating effect on the abnormal stem cell.[26,27] In one sense, clinical trials with androgens may be provocative, bringing forth frank leukemia from a smoldering latent phase (Figure 3). In all instances, until better parameters are available, this risk must be accepted. Indeed, as one looks over case reports of refractory anemia in elderly patients, there are numerous

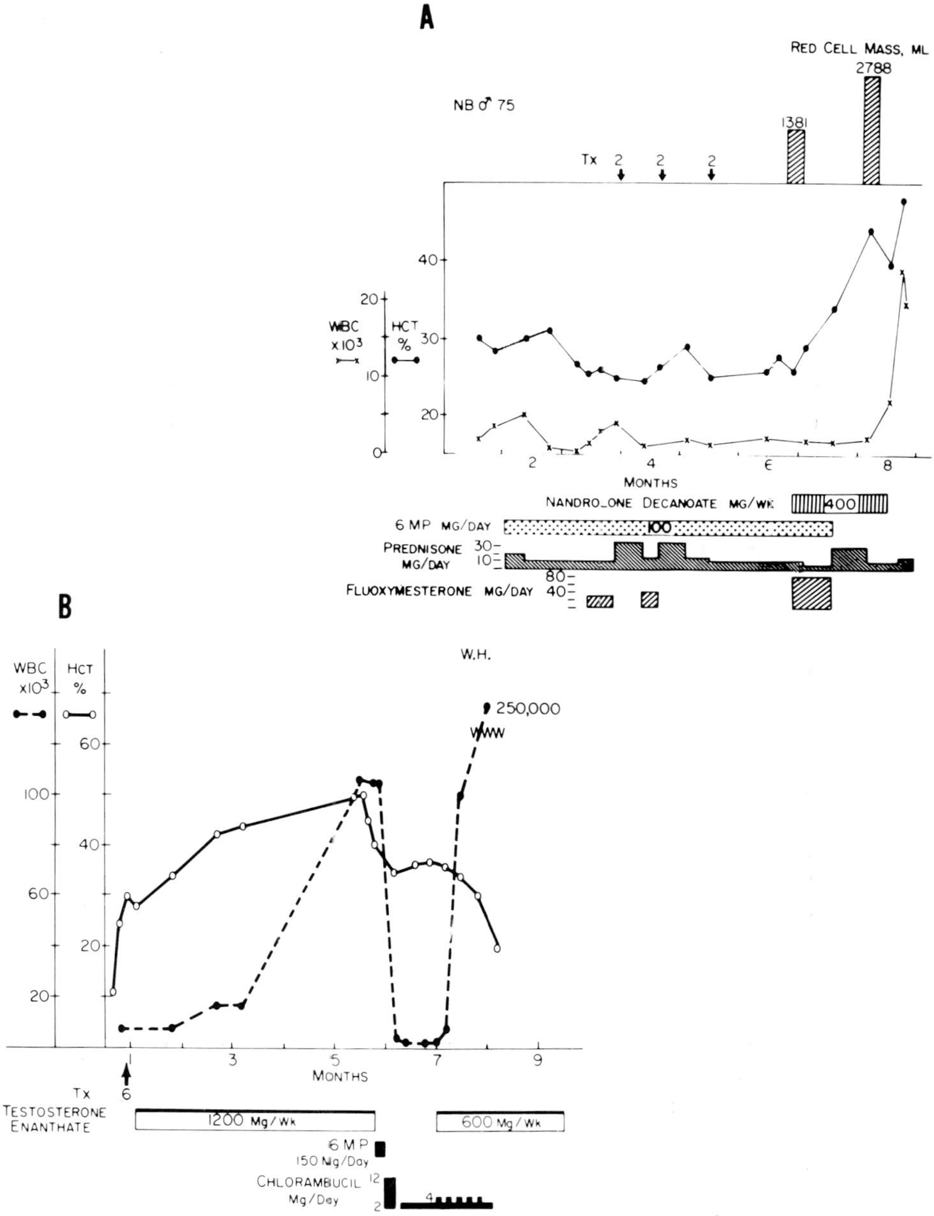

Fig. 3. Leukemia induction with androgen. A-NB, a 74-year-old male. Onset of anemia with carcinoma of nasopharynx. Peripheral leukopenia with monocytosis associated with intense myeloid hyperplasia of bone marrow. The morphology was considered to be preleukemic, and he was treated with moderate doses of 6-mercaptopurin (6-MP) and prednisone. No erythroid response obtained with small doses of fluoxymesterone, but a marked increase in red cell mass was observed with large doses of nandrolone decanoate. The patient shortly thereafter had an explosive elevation of myelomonocytic "blast" cells in peripheral blood. (Data kindly provided by Dr. Scott Murphy.) B-WH, a 72-year-old female. Onset of severe anemia with predominantly monocytoid cells in a peripheral blood smear. Had excellent response of anemia to androgens during 5 months intensive therapy. On return to clinic at fifth month, the patient had a marked leukocytosis (110,000 mm³), with predominant "blast" cells interpreted as lymphosarcoma leukemia. Chemotherapy caused a rapid reduction of white count, and when androgen treatment reinstituted leukocytosis and anemia recurred.

references to the use of androgens in treatment programs. Many of these patients suddenly develop acute leukemia.[28] While there may be an initial gratifying erythroid response to testosterone, we do not have adequate evidence to suggest that such treatment will decrease morbidity or provide better therapy for the patient with acute leukemia. One rare disorder of elderly females must be mentioned, namely, hypochromic anemia with hypoferremia associated with increased iron stores in the marrow and normoblastic hyperplasia.[29] These patients have had excellent responses to androgens and maintained a normal red cell mass with prolonged androgen therapy.

With these general comments, specific disorders should be mentioned.

BONE MARROW FAILURE

Aplastic Anemia

If we exclude risks of the preleukemic state in the elderly patients with pancytopenia, we can expect, in the adult, that about 50% of the patients with bone marrow aplasia will respond to androgen therapy.[30] At the present time, the recovery rate may favor drug-induced aplasia, but more recent data with pesticides are less suggestive.[31] From the clinical history and bone marrow examination, the physician usually has a poor prediction of response to androgens, for a single random sampling of bone marrow is not sufficient. How-

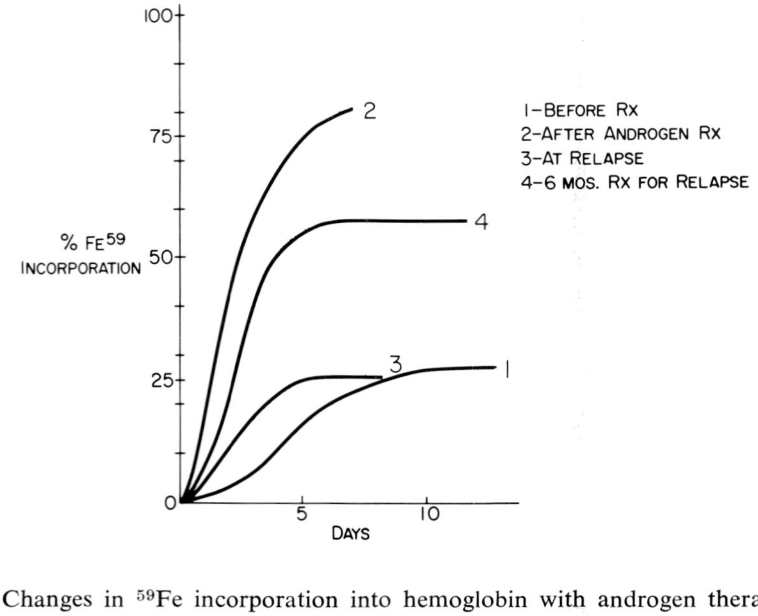

Fig. 4. Changes in ^{59}Fe incorporation into hemoglobin with androgen therapy in a patient with aplastic anemia. The pretreatment (curve 1) improved dramatically after 9 months of therapy with methyltestosterone (curve 2). When therapy was discontinued, radioiron incorporation declined to the initial pretreatment range within 6 months (curve 3). Thereafter, when therapy (northandrolone) was restarted (curve 4), the incorporation pattern returned to the normal pattern. (Redrawn from graphs provided by Dr. Y. Najean[35].)

ever, if one observes only stroma, plasma cells, and lymphocytes with a severe pancytopenia, prognosis is grave. This has been emphasized by the review of aplasia in children.[32,33] To have any hope of response to androgens, some stem cell lineage must remain. We have been impressed that radioiron incorporation into hemoglobin has helped to assay potential recovery (Figure 4). If patients have evidence of 20% or greater incorporation of radioiron into the small circulating hemoglobin mass, one may be optimistic for eventual recovery.[34] When initiated, androgen therapy should be maintained for 9 to 18 months.[35] Only in recent years have we become aware that there is no real specific androgen structure that will guarantee recovery. Hence, a patient may not respond to one agent but may have an excellent response to another androgen.[18] Probably many of our past failures have been related to the limited number of testosterone esters that have been tried. From current animal data in our laboratory, we have been especially impressed with the marked erythroid response associated with the use of nandrolone decanoate.[36,37] Patients should have a 3-month trial with a testosterone preparation, and, if there is no response, as manifested by decreased transfusions or a reticulocytosis, another androgen should be substituted (Figure 5). Unfortunately, other measurements, such as ESF or erythrocyte fetal hemoglobin, have not been useful in predicting

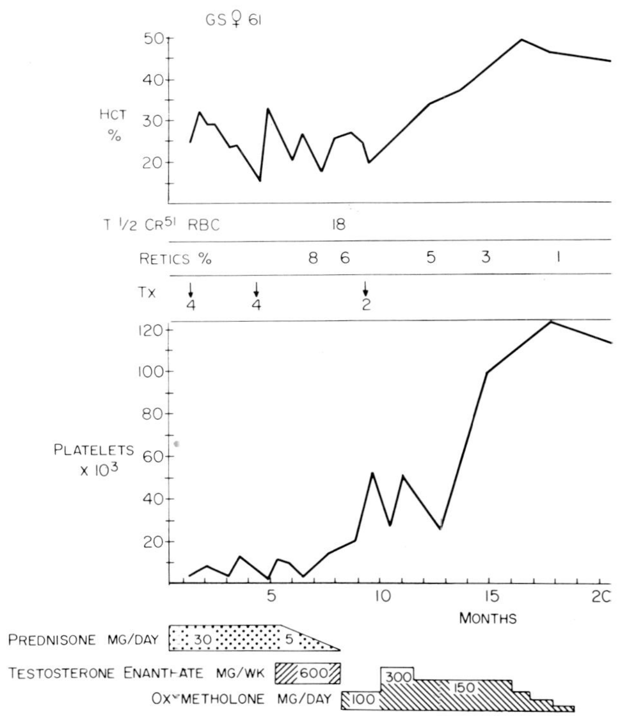

Fig. 5. GS, a 61-year-old female with drug-induced aplastic anemia. There was no response to testosterone enanthate during 3 months of therapy. After oxymetholone, hematocrit rose dramatically while the rise in platelet count was slower. Note also the altered hormone responses outlined in Figure 7.

response.[33] The clinician must recognize that even an initial favorable response to testosterone does not mean prolonged remission. One may expect to see relapses many months or years after androgen therapy has been discontinued.[18,38] As a general rule, in the treatment of aplasia androgens have been continued in our clinic until the patient has recovered from thrombocytopenia.

Our laboratory experience has not indicated that concurrent adrenal corticoids are helpful. Indeed, with large doses of prednisone in the range of 60 to 80 mg daily, one may well expect a delayed response to androgens and altered catabolic effects on the stem cell to hinder proliferation. There has been no convincing evidence that corticoids have helped to control bleeding associated with amegakaryocytic thrombocytopenia. If there is documented evidence of hemolysis by red cell survival measurements, thrombocytopenia by lysis, or increased RE sequestration, then small daily doses of prednisone (30 mg) along with androgen may be useful. We need to recognize that possible induction of pustular acne from the combination therapy may pose a serious threat of infection to these patients.

Myelofibrosis and Myeloid Metaplasia

As indicated with hypoplastic anemia, a fibrotic marrow necessarily does not indicate that adequate stem cells are unavailable for an androgen response. A physiologic measurement to demonstrate a nidus of hematopoiesis has been quite predictive.[19] Utilizing the uptake and release of iron from the bone marrow (sacrum) and spleen by isotopic surface scanning of a pulse dose of radioiron, the clinician may define those patients who can respond to androgen stimulation. Much of the past data, again, have been limited to the evaluation of a single androgen preparation. However, as noted above, with hypoplastic anemia the physiologic evidence that some functional marrow or hematopoietic tissue is available, as well as the demonstration of ^{59}Fe incorporation into hemoglobin, can suggest to the physician that the patient may respond to androgens (Figure 6).[19] As noted earlier, these patients may have quite marked leukocytosis and moderate thrombocytosis from androgen therapy.[19,39] Indeed, granulocytes and platelets may respond, while the hematocrit may not necessarily improve (Figure 2).

With a hematologic response one can expect to observe increasing splenomegaly and hyperuricemia. Androgens have been of value in our laboratory in that a more adequate hemogram is obtained which can be used as a guide for chlorambucil or busulfan in shrinking the spleen and decreasing hyperuricemia as well as hypermetabolic symptons. Again, as with the hypoplastic anemias no specific hormone always can be used successfully. A similar pattern of trial-and-error should be followed at 3-month intervals if there is no initial hematopoietic response (Figure 7). At the present time, there is incomplete data on isotope bone scans aside from ^{59}Fe studies. However, with the increasing use of technetium sulfur colloid skeletal scanning, there has been some suggestion that the prolonged use of androgens in patients with myelofibrosis may reactivate hematopoietic areas of marrow.[40] These scanning observations may, in part, explain the ability for treated patients with myelofibrosis to maintain relative normal blood values after androgens have been discontinued.[12,19,39]

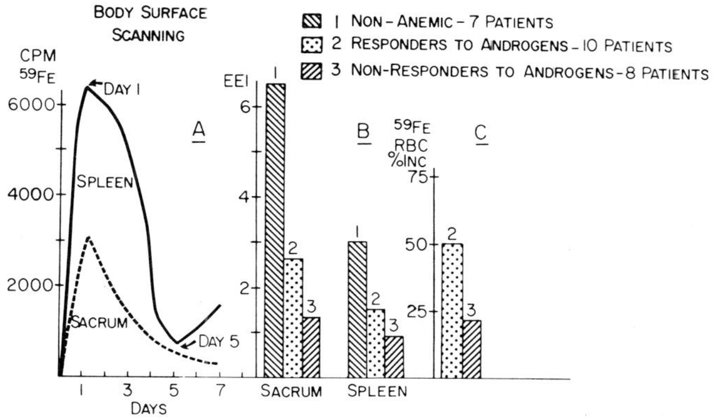

Fig. 6. Evaluation of bone marrow activity in myelofibrosis with myeloid metaplasia. By body surface scanning, the ratio of radioactivity on day 1 is compared with day 5. **Chart A.** From such data, an effective erythropoietic index (EEI) can be calculated. From the data plotted in Chart A, the EEI for the sacrum would be:

$$\text{sacrum EEI} = \frac{\text{CPM day 1 (6300)}}{\text{CPM day 5 (900)}} = 7.0$$

Similarly, the ratio for the spleen EEI is 6.0. In **Chart B,** averages of 7 patients with myelofibrosis and no anemia are plotted to compare with anemic patients with myelofibrosis studied before treatment. The nonresponders to androgen treatment are compared with those that had a good hematocrit elevation with androgen treatment, the responders. One may observe that there is a marked difference in the EEI for the two groups receiving androgens, and such a measurement can predict the response to testosterone therapy. Similarly, patients responding to therapy (**Chart C**) had a better incorporation of ^{59}Fe into hemoglobin. (Redrawn from Gardner, et al.[19])

MARROW INFILTRATION

Chronic Lymphocytic Leukemia (CLL)

It is difficult to define when the lymphocytic replacement begins to compromise the erythropoietic capacity of the marrow. The careful study of Wasi and Block[41] demonstrated that normal hemoglobin levels persist despite an 85% to 90% lymphocytic infiltration. However, as infiltration continues, with leukocyte counts above 150,000 mm^3, one may expect the onset of anemia not associated with immune hemolysis. In most instances, therapy with androgens alone have been only partially successful.[42,43] However, in combination with prednisone and an alkylating agent, androgens would appear to initiate hemoglobin synthesis, both of the "early" peak pattern as well as the regular incorporation in circulating hemoglobin (Figure 8).[44] Once again these responses would appear to be nonspecific but useful to expand residual erythroid-committed stem cells. The improved radioactive iron incorporation noted by Barrett, Cline, and Berlin[44] is the most convincing data to demonstrate the expanded erythroid compartment (note the comparison in graphs A and B, Figure 8). Patients receiving chronic testosterone therapy over prolonged intervals (years) do appear to have a higher absolute granulocyte count which is useful to combat infection.[42,45] No data have been presented to demonstrate

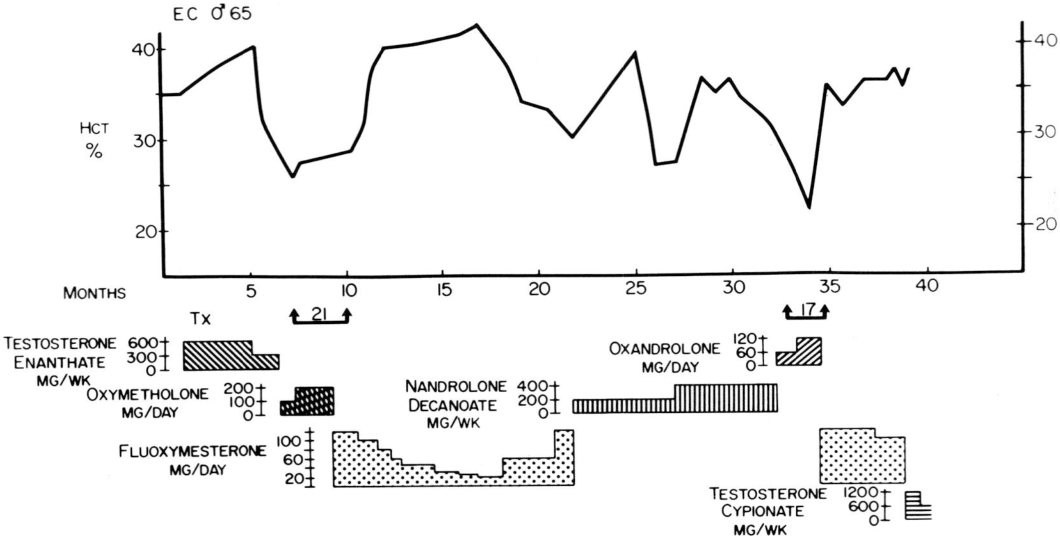

Fig. 7. A 65-year-old male with myelofibrosis and agnogenic myeloid metaplasia with an excellent effective erythropoietic index (EEI) of 4, suggesting a response to androgens. Although the patient had an initial response to testosterone enanthate, the presence of fluid retention caused his therapy to be changed to oxymetholone. During the next 3 months, he had no hematologic response and required frequent transfusions. There was a rapid and sustained elevation of hematocrit with fluoxymesterone. The hematocrit began to decline with a lower dose of the androgen; an increase in the dose of fluoxymesterone to the high initial dosage (120 mg per day) did not prevent the onset of anemia.

The hematocrit did rise with weekly injections of nandrolone decanoate, but again it declined after 4 months. A larger weekly dose of 400 mg was able to elevate the hematocrit for the next 3 months; thereafter there was a decline despite the high dosage of nandrolone. Multiple transfusions were required when the androgen was changed to oral oxandrolone for 10 weeks. The patient again responded to large doses of oral fluoxymesterone. Alterations in his liver enzymes had necessitated the change to a parenteral preparation, testosterone cyprionate, and the hematocrit has been maintained in the 36%–38% range. The ineffective response of one androgen preparation should be evaluated at 3-month intervals, for some patients may respond to another testosterone ester.

improvement after testosterone therapy in the low IgM protein values observed in CLL.[46] However, observations of higher granulocyte counts may be one of the most important facets of androgen therapy to protect the patient from infection, and represents the major value of such therapy in CLL.[2,47,48]

Multiple Myeloma

In many respects marrow infiltration with plasma cells can be compared to the myelophthisic anemia of CLL. In most instances, complications with bone lesion or renal compromise will alert the physician to the disease before there is total marrow replacement. While our laboratory experience has indicated a good response to the anemia of myelomatosis,[2,49] no careful protocol

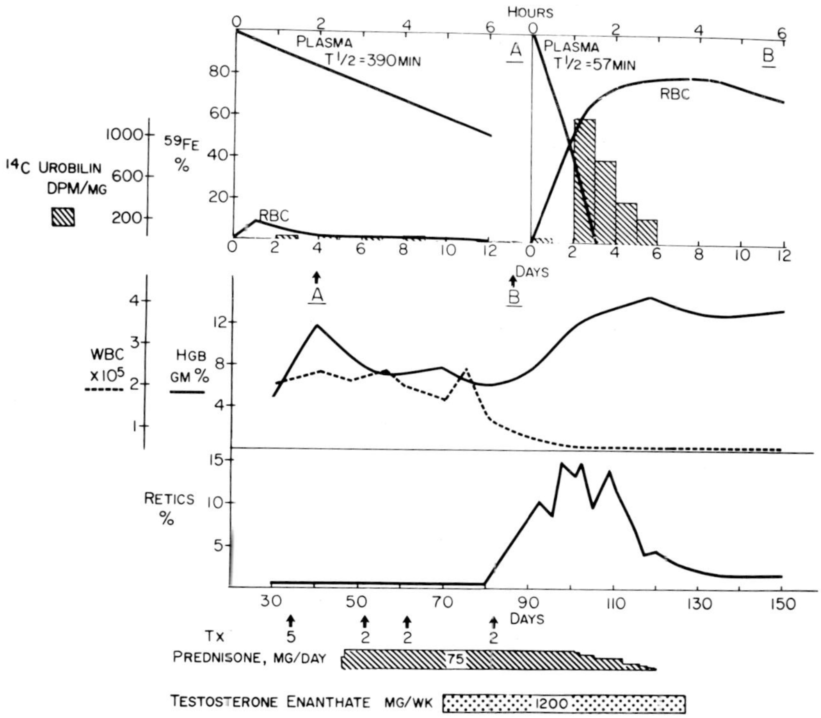

Fig. 8. AH, a 57-year-old male with chronic lymphocytic leukemia. In the initial phase (**Chart A**), the ^{59}Fe clearance is prolonged, ^{59}Fe incorporation is almost nil, and there is little "early peak" of ^{14}C urobilin incorporation. No evidence of reticulocytosis or a reduction of leukocytosis was observed until intensive androgen therapy was started on day 70. Thereafter, there was a marked increase in bone marrow activity associated with relatively normal ^{59}Fe RBC incorporation (**Chart B**). The early peak of ^{14}C urobilin excretion was greater than normal, which may imply marked proliferation of the erythroid stem cell compartment by the androgen. (Redrawn from Barrett, et al[44] and data kindly provided by Dr. N. Berlin.)

study has been done to demonstrate lessened morbidity with this program. Androgen-induced erythroid hyperplasia may well confuse the interpretation of plasma cell infiltration, if morphologic evaluation is used to judge response to specific alkylating agents.

Prophylactic Protection from Marrow Suppression

Without doubt one of the major areas of interest to the physician is the possible use of androgens to protect bone marrow from the toxic aplasia associated with chemotherapy or irradiation. Casual references have been made to such a protective effect, but no adequate series is available for conviction.

Irradiation

Early in the use of androgens, comment was made that the prophylactic use of androgens prior to irradiation could be useful to prevent severe neutropenia associated with the large abdominal portals used in irradiation in lymphosarcoma.[2] Similar observations were defined in the response with ^{32}P in the treatment of multiple myeloma.[49] However, neutrophil and platelet protection was minimal, and the major benefit was control of anemia. This response also has been emphasized most recently by Evans and Elias who used testosterone to treat a large series of patients with lung cancer.[50] In this group with matched controls, patients receiving nandrolone phenylpropionate throughout irradiation had higher hemoglobin levels at the end of the treatment program with 4500 rads than the controls. In a study of irradiated mice, Gallagher, Warnecks, and Zimmer[51] noted that irradiated recipients who received spleen suspension plus testosterone enanthate had a more rapid recovery of radioiron incorporation than did control animals. Such data implied a more rapid proliferation of infused stem cells. Fragmentary reports indicate that the committed erythroid cell can respond and be protected by androgen therapy during irradiation. Unfortunately, the data are inadequate for the recovery of granulocytes and platelets during irradiation.

Chemotherapy protection with androgens is equally sparse, but clinical studies of Brodsky and Kahn[52] have been encouraging. Ten patients with carcinoma treated with 5-fluorouracil or cyclophosphamide had a comparative response of the white count during a course of therapy followed by prophylactic use of testosterone enanthate (600 mg weekly) for 6 to 7 weeks before the same chemotherapy program was started. The marked neutropenia improved during the second trial period (Figure 9). Similar data were observed in lymphoma and myeloma patients who received melphalan. A group of female patients with genital cancer was treated with nandrolone decanoate every 3 weeks to control neutropenia while they received cyclophosphamide. However, this program was not protective, and 12 of the 13 patients had to discontinue therapy. When the androgen program was reinstituted at 10-day intervals, only 2 of the 9 patients had neutropenia, and the onset was slower and the recovery more rapid.[53] These data further emphasized the need to evaluate different hormone preparations and dosage schedules in coordinated clinical trials. In contrast to these favorable results, Kennedy and Newton were not able to show such granulocyte protection in a group of patients receiving hydroxyurea.[54] In part, the timing or preparation of the patient with an induction interval of testosterone treatment prior to the onset of chemotherapy may explain the different observations. Nevertheless, nonspecific responses to increased leukocytes with improvement in phagocytic function[21] imply that this aspect of therapy does warrant evaluation.

The suppressed bone marrow, because hemorrhage from amegakaryocytic or nonfunctional megakaryocytic thrombocytopenia is feared often is treated with prednisone along with androgens. Unless there is hemolysis or lytic thrombocytopenia, it is unlikely that many of the corticoid preparations will be useful.[55] There is an impressive collection of animal and clinical studies to emphasize the inhibition of marrow proliferation from moderate-to-high doses of corticoids. Regeneration of marrow after intense irradiation in the rat is impaired so that fatty marrow persists if cortisone is given during the recovery phase.[56] Similarly, red cell regeneration with drug hemolysis in the rabbit is blunted with triamcinalone therapy.[57] Altered bone marrow function is demonstrated more clearly in patients with idiopathic thrombocytopenic purpura (ITP). In this instance, thrombocytosis may develop initially with prednisone,

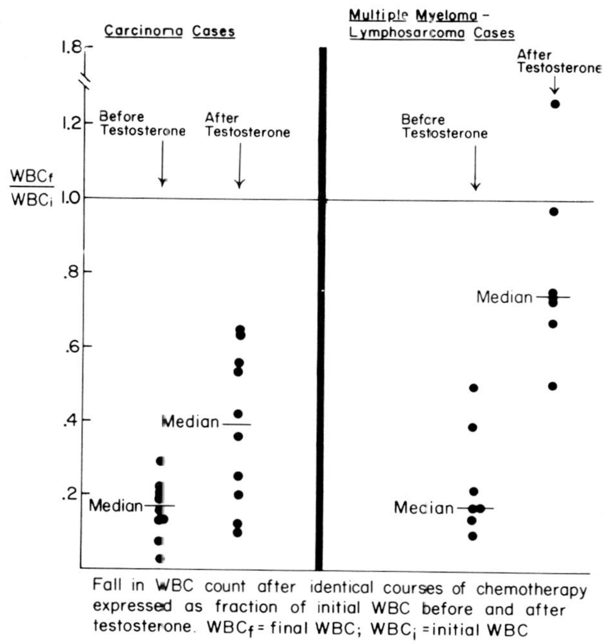

Fig. 9. Comparison of WBC after identical courses of chemotherapy in the same patient with different types of tumors. WBC_f is the final count when chemotherapy is completed, compared with the initial WBC, WBC_i, prior to onset of therapy. This ratio, WBC_f/WBC_i, has been compared during 2 courses of identical chemotherapy, except that the course during testosterone enanthate therapy (600 mg weekly) had 6 to 8 weeks of pretreatment with androgen before chemotherapy was started. The higher ratio indicates that the WBC was better maintained after chemotherapy. (Figure kindly supplied by Dr. I Brodsky and reproduced by permission from the publisher.[52])

but if the same high initial dose is continued severe thrombocytopenia will recur.[58] This finding has been noted in adults and children and is associated with impaired maturation of megakaryocytes. In adults receiving massive doses of prednisone (500 mg daily), the total leukocyte and granulocyte count begin to decline to low levels.[59] Immune mechanisms are altered even in normal subjects, with decreased synthesis of IgG; the blastogenic response of lymphocytes to phytohemagglutin is diminished.[46] One may appreciate, from such a brief commentary, that many beneficial effects of androgen could be masked or even obliterated if moderate-to-large doses of corticoids are used concurrently.

SUMMARY

During the past 15 years, data have been collected to demonstrate that androgens can be used to treat various types of anemia and to induce an increased red cell mass (erythrocythemia) in normal subjects. While the mechanism has been attributed to a stem cell response from increased plasma levels of erythropoietin, current information would suggest that some androgen metabolites may initiate direct replication of the erythroid committed stem cell. This stem cell compartment has responded quickly; the anemia improved but platelet and leukocyte levels rose slowly. Indeed, prolonged therapy over many months is required before recovery from thrombocytopenia is observed.

Currently, with depressed bone marrow function we have no criteria by which a response to testosterone therapy can be predicted. In most instances, an interval of 3 months is required. Probably as an estimate in adults, about half of the patients with bone marrow hypoplasia and pancytopenia will have an erythroid response to testosterone therapy. The use of isotope to assess radioiron incorporation has been helpful to predict an erythroid response in patients with bone marrow hypoplasia as well as myeloid metaplasia with myelofibrosis. Comparative cooperative trials of different hormone preparations as well as drug schedules are needed to determine how various types of hypoplasia should be treated. The patient with depressed hematopoiesis associated with marrow infiltration has responded more uniformly to androgen therapy, especially anemias associated with chronic lymphocytic leukemia and multiple myeloma. In all instances of comparison, women appear to have a more rapid erythroid response than men do to currently available testosterone preparations.

Different laboratory groups have observed favorable erythroid responses to a variety of parenteral and oral androgen preparations. At the present time, there are no data to document adequately the superior efficacy or safety of one preparation over another. Individual patients have demonstrated that they can have an erythropoietic response to one androgen preparation after another had been unsuccessful. Other patients may become refractory to a specific androgen despite continued therapy; anemia may recur after an initial erythroid response. Despite such a recurrence, another testosterone ester may again stimulate erythropoiesis. These preliminary observations with pharmacologic doses of androgens would suggest that the steroid metabolite reacting with the stem cell may be altered or conjugated differently to prevent recognition, stimulation, or interaction with the erythroid committed cell. Until there is a better understanding of the metabolism of testosterone and its relationship to the effector cell, the clinician should evaluate several androgen preparations in patients with depressed bone marrow function. Cooperative clinical trials will be needed to obtain information on response rates and dosage schedules.

REFERENCES

1. Kennedy BJ, Gilbertsen AS: Increased erythropoiesis induced by androgenic hormone therapy. N Engl J Med 256:719, 1957
2. Gardner FH, Pringle JC Jr: Androgens and erythropoiesis I. Preliminary clinical observations. Arch Intern Med 107:846, 1961
3. Jepson JH: Agents influencing the production and action of erythropoietin in man. JR Coll Physicians Lond 2:381, 1968
4. Nathan DG, Piomelli S, Cummings JF et al: The effect of androgens on body composition and erythropoiesis in octogenarian males. Ann NY Acad Sci 110: 965, 1963

5. Gardner FH, Nathan DG, Piomelli S et al: The erythrocythaemic effects of androgen. Br J Haematol 14:611, 1968
6. Besa EC, Gorshein D, Gardner FH: Blood volume changes in normal and various anemic states in man following androgens. Ann Intern Med 76:869, 1972
7. Jepson JH: Mechanism of action of androgens on erythropoiesis, Proceedings of Symposium on Use of Androgens in Hypoplastic Anemia. Edited by T Necheles. (In press).
8. Alexanian R: Erythropoietin and erythropoiesis in anemic man following androgens. Blood 33:564, 1969
9. Fried W, Kilbridge T: Effect of testosterone and of cobalt on erythropoietin production by anephic rats. J Lab Clin Med 74:623, 1969
10. Shahidi NT: Aplastic anemia in childhood and the results of androgen therapy, Proceedings of Symposium on Use of Androgens in Hypoplastic Anemia. Edited by T Necheles. (In press).
11. Reisner EH Jr: Tissue cultures of bone marrow II. Effect of steroid hormones on hematopoiesis in vitro. Blood 27:460, 1966
12. Gardner FH, Pringle JC Jr: Androgens and erythropoiesis II. Treatment of myeloid metaplasia. N Engl J Med 264:103, 1961
13. Granick S, Kappas A: Steroid induction of porphyrin synthesis in liver cell culture I. Structural basis and possible physiological role in the control of heme formation. J Biol Chem 242:4587, 1967
14. Levere RD, Kappas A, Granick S: Stimulation of hemoglobin synthesis in chick blastoderms by certain 5β-androstane and 5β-pregnane steroids. Proc Natl Acad Sci USA 58:985, 1967
15. Gorshein D, Gardner FH: Erythropoietic activity of steroid metabolites in mice. Proc Natl Acad Sci USA 65:564, 1970
16. Gordon AS, Zanjani ED, Levere RD et al: Stimulation of mammalian erythropoiesis by 5β-H steroid metabolites. Proc Natl Acad Sci USA 65:919, 1970
17. Gorshein D, Reisner EH Jr, Gardner FH: Tissue culture on bone marrow V. The effect of cyclic AMP and 5β-H steroids on heme synthesis. (In press).
18. Gardner FH: Erythropoietic activity of different androgens, Proceedings of Symposium on Use of Androgens in Hypoplastic Anemia. Edited by T Necheles. (In press)
19. Gardner FH, Nathan DG: Androgens and erythropoiesis III. Further evaluation of testosterone treatment of myelofibrosis. N Engl J Med 274:420, 1966
20. Silver RT, Jenkins DE Jr, Engle RL Jr: Use of testosterone and busulfan in the treatment of myelofibrosis with myeloid metaplasia. Blood 23:341, 1964
21. Magliulo E, Giraldi M, Cattaneo E, et al: Effects of 4-chlorotestosterone acetate on the phagocytic activity of human monocytes. Results of a double-blind trial. Clin Exp Immunol 10:469, 1972
22. Baehner RL, Johnston RB Jr: Monocyte function in children with neutropenia and chronic infections. Blood 40:31, 1972
23. Ghione M: Ant-infective action of an anabolic steroid. Proc Soc Exp Biol Med 97:773, 1958
24. Umehara S, Ito H, Takahashi M et al: Influences of various hormones and the autonomic nervous system on the RES activity in rabbits, Reticuloendothelial System Proceedings of the Fourth International Symposium on RES, May 1964. Tokyo. Japanese Society for Promotion of Science, p 425
25. Horn Y: Leucopoietic properties of four different androgenic hormones in irradiated rats. Scand J Haematol 8:470, 1971
26. Gardner FH: The use of testosterone in anemia. Mod Treat 1:634, 1964
27. Gordon Smith EC, Lewis SM: Treatment of aplastic anaemia and allied dis-

orders with oxymetholone, Proceedings of a Symposium on Steroids in Modern Medicine. Edited by VH James, L Martini. Amsterdam, Excerpta Medica, 1972, p 8

28. Delamore IW, Geary CG: Aplastic anaemia, acute myeloblastic leukaemia, and oxymetholone. Br Med J 2:743, 1971
29. Haurani FI, Green D: Primary defective iron reutilization. Am J Med 42:151, 1967
30. Nejean Y, Dresch C, Schaison G, et al: Etude de l'effet de l'androgenotherapie au cours des insuffisances medullaires. Presse Med 74:2537, 1966
31. Sanchez-Medal L: The hemopoietic action of androstanes, Progress in Hematology. Edited by EB Brown, CV Moore. New York, Grune and Stratton, 1971, p 111
32. Heyn RM, Ertel IJ, Tubergen DG: Course of acquired aplastic anemia in children treated with supportive care. JAMA 208:1372, 1969
33. Li FP, Alter BP, Nathan DG: The mortality of acquired aplastic anemia in children. Blood 40:153, 1972
34. Bernard J, Najean Y: Evolution and prognosis of the idopathic pancytopenias. Ser Haematol 5:1, 1965
35. Najean Y, Schaison G, Dresch C et al: Evolution tardive des pancytopenies chroniques traitées avec succes par les androgenes. Nouv Rev Fr Hematol 9:23, 1969
36. Gorshein D, Murphy S, Gardner FH: Comparative study on the erythropoietic function of androgens and their mode of action in mice. Clin Res 18:405, 1970
37. Daiber A, Herve L, Con I et al: Treatment of aplastic anemia with nandrolone decanoate. Blood 36:748, 1970
38. Dreyfus B, Amiel JL, Bernard J et al: Les androgenes sont-ils efficaces dans le traitement des aplasies medullaires. Presse Med 75:1809, 1967
39. Kennedy BJ: Effect of androgenic hormone in myelofibrosis JAMA 182:114, 1962
40. Nelp WB, Larson SM: Patterns in clinical bone marrow scanning. J Nucl Med 13:456, 1972
41. Wasi F, Block M: The mechanism of the development of anemia in untreated chronic lymphatic leukemia. Blood 17:597, 1961
42. Gardner FH: Treatment of lymphoproliferative disease, Cancer Chemotherapy II. The Twentysecond Hahnemann Symposium. Edited by I Brodsky, SB Kahn, JH Moyer. New York, Grune and Stratton, 1972, p 361
43. Yuknyavichus Y: Androgens in the therapy of chronic lymphadenosis. Ter Arkh 37:27, 1965
44. Barret PVD, Cline MJ, Berlin NI: The association of the urobilin "early peak" and erythropoiesis in man. J Clin Invest 45:1657, 1966
45. Stacher A, Bohnel J: Wirkung eines neuen anabolikum auf das hamopoietische system. Med Klin 22:976, 1962
46. Butler WT, Rossen RD, Hersh EM: Effect of high doses of methylprednisolone on immunity in man. J Clin Invest 51:18a, 1972
47. West WO: The treatment of bone marrow failure with massive androgen therapy. Ohio State Med J 61:347, 1965
48. Kennedy BJ: Androgenic hormone therapy in lymphatic leukemia. JAMA 190: 104, 1964
49. Gardner FH, Cohen P: The function of androgens and fluoride salts in the treatment of multiple myeloma. Trans Am Clin Climatol Assoc 77:226, 1965
50. Evans JT, Elias EG: The erythropoietic response to anabolic therapy in patients receiving radiotherapy. J Clin Pharmacol 12:101, 1972

51. Gallagher NI, Warnecke MS, Zimmer MJ: Effect of testosterone enanthate (NSC-1759) on erythropoiesis in irradiated mice given marrow transfusions. Cancer Chemother Rep (Part 1) 52:627, 1968
52. Brodsky I, Kahn SB: The effect of androgens on cancer chemotherapy, Cancer Chemotherapy. Edited by I Brodsky, SB Kahn, JH Moyer. New York, Grune and Stratton, 1967, p 275
53. Biedermann C, Obolensky W, Scoglio P, et al: Traitement anabolisant associe a un antimitotique dans le but de prevenir la chute des leucocytes sanguins. Ther Umsch 23:509, 1966
54. Kennedy BJ, Newton K: Effect of androgenic hormone combined with hydroxyurea (NSC-32065) on hematopoietic system of patients with cancer. Cancer Chemother Rep 49:21, 1965
55. Diamond LK: Hematological consequences of long-term corticosteroid treatment, Drug-Induced Disease. Edited by L Meyler and HM Peck. Amsterdam, Excerpta Medica, 1969, p 177
56. Thiersch JB, Conroy L, Stevens AR Jr et al: Adverse effect of cortisone on marrow regeneration following irradiation. J Lab Clin Med 40:174, 1952
57. Cohen P, Gardner FH: Effect of massive triamcinolone administration in blunting the erythropoietic response to phenylhydrazine hemolysis. J Lab Clin Med 65:88, 1965
58. Cohen P, Gardner FH: The thrombocytopenic effect of sustained high dosage prednisone therapy in thrombocytopenic purpura. N Engl J Med 265:611, 1961
59. Levenson SM, Watkin DM: Protein requirements in injury and certain acute and chronic diseases. Fed Proc 18:1155, 1959

Leif G. Suhrland
and Paul Hollister

31

Use of Vitamins and Corticosteroids in Drug-induced Hematologic Disorder

This volume contains chapters by an impressive group of experts with considerable clinical knowledge and investigative skills, and it provides an important means of disseminating new information while making maximal use of past clinical experience. It is true that new drugs undergo extensive clinical trials before being approved for specific treatment regimens. However, it may take several years before serious side effects are recognized and their mechanism of action elucidated, if at all. In many clinical studies in the past, inadequate proper controls have made it difficult to evaluate treatment with these drug-induced disorders. Recently, clinical studies in man have come under close scrutiny at a National, as well as local, level and may result in improved experimental designs with appropriate controls through broad-based cooperative study programs.

This chapter pertains to the role of vitamins and corticosteroids in the treatment of drug-induced hematologic disorders and will attempt to develop some guidelines concerning their rational administration and expectations. The literature is replete with clinical observations in these areas, but the inadequacy of proper controls together with anecdotal experiences, precludes drawing firm conclusions. In addition to these shortcomings, results in animal experiments frequently have been extrapolated to man or so closely interwoven into the fabric of the reports that the origin of the threads have become obscured in their application to human disease. However, in an effort to provide a useful overview of this topic with its enormous literature, we have been selective rather than comprehensive and have been concerned primarily with the effects on formed elements of blood.

This presentation will review current information organized under the following topics: (a) possible mechanisms of drug-induced hematologic disorders; (b) hematopoietic vitamins and their role in therapy of these disorders; (c) role of corticosteroids in hematopoiesis; (d) role of corticosteroids in the treatment of drug-induced hematologic disorders.

Although there are many ways of categorizing drug-induced hematologic

Table 1
Classification by Mechanism of Action

1. Direct toxicity—exposure dose-related
2. Idiosyncratic process—not dose-related
3. Creating or involving metabolic abnormalities
4. Involving an immunologic response
5. Unknown

disorders, for the purposes of this report, a general classification by possible mechanisms of action is shown in Table 1.

The role of vitamins in hematopoiesis has been relatively well defined during the past two decades, but their precise interrelationships still are not well understood.[1–3] Folic acid, B_{12} and B_6 are necessary for normal hematopoiesis, and drug-induced or conditioned deficiencies of these vitamins are well documented.[4–5] Drug-induced folic acid abnormalities are more frequent and may produce anemia, leukopenia, thrombocytopenia, or a combination of these. A number of drugs have been implicated in producing peripheral blood abnormalities, and these are shown in Table 2.

In alcohol-induced toxicity, hematologic abnormalities may be due to (a) direct toxic effect of alcohol, (b) development of folate deficiency, (c) combination of these. In such conditions, cessation of alcohol and a normal diet usually are sufficient to return blood counts to normal. Pharmacologic doses of folic acid are seldom required. Even when a sideroblastic anemia is present, suggesting an abnormality in B_6 metabolism, cessation of alcohol ingestion and a normal diet frequently is all that is necessary. Pyridoxol phosphate has been found to be effective when pyridoxine failed, but only when alcohol consumption was continued.[17]

Antituberculous drugs associated with a low serum folate and megaloblastic proliferation in bone marrow include: INH, pyrazinamide, and cycloserine. If the drug is discontinued or folic acid is given orally, these abnormalities disappear. The anticonvulsants and oral contraceptives may interfere with intestinal absorption of folate, but the precise mechanisms are uncertain.[18,19] However, by providing an adequate folate intake in the diet or by added folic acid, the hematoxic effects of these drugs may be avoided.

Pharmacologic doses of other vitamins, including B_{12} and B_6 have not been shown to be of therapeutic benefit in these drug-induced disorders. However, one should be aware that folate deficiency may occur with certain drugs and usually can be prevented by an adequate dietary intake of folic acid.

Table 2
Drugs Associated with
Folic Acid Deficiency

1. Alcohol–ethanol[7–10]
2. Antituberculous Drugs[11]
3. Anticonvulsants[12–15]
4. Oral Contraceptives[16]

In an attempt to provide a rational basis for the use of corticosteroids in drug-induced blood dyscrasias, we will review the pharmacologic effects of corticosteroids on cellular elements of blood and the immune systems.

One of the striking effects is upon the peripheral leukocyte count. Normally, in man, leukocytosis regularly occurs after the administration of corticosteroids and persists until the drug is discontinued.[20,21] There are two phases of this type of leukocytosis. The first develops immediately, reaches a peak in 2 to 4 days, then declines. This is characterized by rapid onset with mature leukocytes and is due to reduced migration of leukocytes from the vasculature and mobilization of the marginal granulocyte pool. A second but sustained leukocytosis develops, with a gradual rise to a peak after 5 to 10 days of treatment. This leukocytosis may be 2 to 4 times higher than the basal leukocyte count.

The mechanism of this second rise in peripheral leukocyte count is not clear. Alterations in the kinetics of all leukocyte pools have been described: marrow pool, marginal pool, circulating pool, and tissue pool of leukocytes.[22,23] Evidence for increased leukopoiesis is based primarily upon animal studies. It was found that a marked leukocytosis occurs in mice after the injection of serum from subjects receiving corticosteroids during the second rise in leukocyte count but not during the initial rise or in the controls. This suggests a humoral myeloid stimulant or leukopoietin factor but has not been supported in man. Furthermore, studies on in vitro human bone marrow cultures failed to show any direct leukopoietic effect from corticosteroids.[24] Using radioactive white cells, it has been shown that the marginal leukocyte pool, which accounts for 50% of the peripheral vascular leukocytes, is mobilized and becomes part of the countable circulating leukocytes. Finally, there is decreased utilization of leukocytes secondary to impaired migration from the vascular space. This has been established firmly by determining the leukocyte content of inflammatory exudates, in the presence and absence of corticosteroids, through a skin window technique.[25] In addition to the inhibition of leukocyte migration from the vascular space, corticosteroids also interfere with lysosomal release (degranulation) and phagocytosis. For example: in man, erythrophagocytosis is markedly inhibited by either oral or parenteral corticosteroids.[26] Eosinophils and basophils are also decreased in peripheral blood by corticosteroids but the mechanism is not known. There is some suggestion that the eosinopenia may be due to inhibition of the release of eosinophils from marrow.[27,28]

Corticosteroids have selective inhibitory effects upon the lymphoid and immune systems.[29] Compared to other species, man is a relatively steroid-resistant species. However, the lymphoid system is comprised of a heterogeneous population of lymphoid cells with variable corticosteroid sensitivity. Conversion of cell-mediated positive tuberculin to a negative skin reaction has been observed within 2 weeks after corticosteroid administration. Although inhibition by corticosteroids have been shown to inhibit humoral antibody production in a number of steroid-sensitive animals, these data are lacking for man.

Corticosteroids do not increase platelet production nor do they increase the life-span of platelets in normal man.[30] They do increase capillary resistance to rupture in man. This is evidenced by an arrest of petechiae formation in the presence of thrombocytopenia after corticosteroid therapy and occurs without a rise in platelet count.[31] Capillary resistance has been studied before and after corticosteroids, with a negative pressure apparatus, in patients with rheumatoid arthritis, systemic lupus erythematosis, ankylosing spondylitis, and idiopathic thrombocytopenia purpura. Resistance to the formation of petechiae, generally doubled within 48 hours of therapy, exceeding normal resistance in nonthrombocytopenic subjects and a return to at least normal resistance in thrombocytopenic subjects.

Corticosteroids have not been demonstrated to have any effect upon erythropoiesis in man, nor have there been studies in man evaluating the effects of corticosteroids on erythropoietin production. They do not induce a reticulocytosis and, in the absence of immune hemolytic anemia, do not affect RBC survival.[30] Observations on in vitro human bone marrow cultures fail to demonstrate stimulation of erythropoiesis by corticosteroids.[24]

This review of the pharmacologic effects of corticosteroids on cellular elements of blood and the immune system will provide some basis for the discussion of the role of these compounds in the treatment of drug-induced hematologic disorders. Corticosteroids have been administered for a variety of drug-induced disorders involving erythrocytes but have limited value in these conditions. In immune hemolytic disease secondary to such drugs as α-methyldopa or penicillin, discontinuing the drug usually suffices. If a severe hemolytic state exists, corticosteroids might be useful temporarily to slow the rate of red cell destruction, perhaps by inhibiting erythrophagocytosis. In G-6-PD deficiency, corticosteroids have no role in treatment, but in drug-induced aplastic anemia their role is more controversial and less certain. Some reports suggest that corticosteroids should be given a trial, alone or in combination with androgens.[32] However, there is no convincing evidence that corticosteroids hasten the recovery of bone marrow from its hypoplastic state. In leukopenic states and in agranulocytosis, corticosteroids are potentially dangerous and should be used only with considerable caution. Although in some leukopenic conditions the peripheral leukocyte count might be increased, other effects of corticosteroids on leukocytes would seem to create a hazardous biologic state. On the other hand, the role of corticosteroids in the treatment of drug-induced thrombocytopenia is quite different and may be very beneficial to the patient. If the degree of thrombocytopenia is such that spontaneous bleeding occurs or has a high expectancy of occurring, then corticosteroids may control serious or life-threatening bleeding. This takes place usually without any increase in platelet count or enhanced platelet function and is presumably due to the effect of corticosteroids on the permeability of vessel walls.

SUMMARY

Vitamins in the treatment of drug-induced hematologic disorders have a limited use. In alcohol, with or without folate deficiency, withdrawal plus an adequate dietary source is usually sufficient. In more profound deficiencies, pharmacologic doses of folic acid hasten recovery. Vitamins B_{12} and B_6 have no proven value in drug-induced hematologic disorders.

The role of corticosteroids in drug-induced hematologic disorders remains uncertain. However, the following guidelines for their use are based upon a review of their pharmacologic effects on the hematopoietic system and clinical observations on the treatment of drug-induced hematologic disorders.

1. The underlying disease must receive appropriate attention.
2. Corticosteroids may be useful to control bleeding in severe thrombocytopenia.
3. Corticosteroids may be useful in short-term management of severe hemolytic states.

REFERENCES

1. Beck WS: Vitamin B_{12} deficiency, Hematology. New York, McGraw-Hill, 1972
2. Harris HW, Kellermeyer RW: The Red Cell Production Metabolism, Destruction, Normal and Abnormal. Cambridge, Harvard, 1970
3. Herbert V: Folic acid. Ann Rev Med 16:359, 1965
4. Reynolds EH, Milner G, Matthews DM et al: Anticonvulsant therapy megaloblastic haemopoiesis and folic acid metabolism. Q J Med 35:521, 1966
5. Thedering F: Pernicious anemia and its variants. Vitam Hormon 26:539, 1968
6. Williams JO, Mengel CE, Sullivan LW et al: Megaloblastic anemia associated with chronic ingestion of an analgesic. N Engl J Med 280:312, 1969
7. Sullivan LW, Herbert V: Suppression of hematopoiesis by ethanol. J Clin Invest 43:2048, 1964
8. Lindenbaum J, Hargrove RL: Thrombocytopenia in alcoholics. Ann Intern Med 68:526, 1968
9. Cowan Dale H, Hines John D: Thrombocytopenia of severe alcoholism. Ann Intern Med 74:37, 1971
10. Lindenbaum J, Lieber CS: Hematologic effects of alcohol in man in the absence of nutritional deficiency. N Engl J Med 281:333, 1969
11. Klipstein FA, Berlinger FG, Reed LJ: Folate deficiency associated with drug therapy for tuberculosis. Blood 29:697, 1967
12. Ryan GMS, Forshaw JWB: Megaloblastic anemia due to phenytoin sodium. Br Med J 2:242, 1955
13. Klipstein FA: Subnormal serum folate and macrocytosis associated with anticonvulsant drug therapy. Blood 23:68, 1964
14. Druskin MS, Wallen MH, Bonagura L: Anticonvulsant-associated megaloblastic anemia. N Engl J Med 267:483, 1962
15. Pearson D: Megaloblastic anemia due to glutethimide. Lancet 1:110, 1965
16. Shojania AM, Hornady G, Barnes PH: Oral contraceptives and serum folate level. Lancet 1:1376, 1968
17. Hines John D, Cowan Dale H: Pathogenesis of alcohol-induced sideroblastic bone-marrow abnormalities. N Engl J Med 283:445, 1970
18. Reynolds EH, Hallpike JF, Phillips BM et al: Reversible absorptive defects in anticonvulsant megaloblastic anemia. J Clin Pathol 18:593, 1965
19. Streiff RR: Malabsorption of polyglutamic folic acid secondary to oral contraceptives. Clin Res 17:345, 1969
20. John TJ: Leukocytosis during steroid therapy. Am J Dis Child 111:68, 1966
21. Strausz I, Kekes E, Acnes S: Mechanism of prednisone-induced leucocytosis in man. Acta Haematol 33:40, 1965
22. Cartwright GE, Athens JW, Wintrobe MM: The kinetics of granulopoiesis in normal man. Blood 24:780, 1964

23. Boggs DR: The kinetics of neutrophilic leukocytes in Health and in disease. Sem Hematol 4:359, 1967
24. Reisner Jr EH: Tissue culture of bone marrow. II. Effect of steroid hormones on hematopoiesis in Vitro. Blood 27:460, 1966
25. Boggs DR, Athens JW, Cartwright GE et al: The effect of adrenal glucocorticosteroids upon the cellular composition of inflammatory exudates. Am J Pathol 44:763, 1964
26. Greendyke RM, Bradley EM, Swisher SN: Studies on the effects of administration of ACTH and adrenal corticosteroids on erythrophagocytosis. J Clin Invest 44:746, 1965
27. Hudson G: The marrow reserve of eosinophils. Effect of cortical hormones on the foreign protein response. Br J Haematol 10:122, 1964
28. Cade CF: Histamine, eosinophils and basophils in the blood. J Physiol (Lond) 136, 1957
29. Claman H: Corticosteroids and lymphoid cells. N Engl J Med 8:388, 1972
30. Videbaek A: Glucocorticoids in hematology. Acta Med Scand Suppl: 500:35, 1969
31. Robson HN, Duthie JJR: Capillary resistance and adrenocortical activity. Br Med J:971, 1950
32. Shahidi NT, Diamond LK: Testosterone induced remission in aplastic anemia of both acquired and congenital type. N Engl J Med 264:953, 1961

Index

a
4 b
5 c
6 d
7 e
8 f
9 g
0 h
1 i
8 2 j